AF851060

TOXICOLOGY ANNUAL VOLUME 2

TOXICOLOGY ANNUAL VOLUME 2

CHARLES L. WINEK, Editor

Chief Toxicologist, Allegheny County Coroner's Office; Professor of Toxicology, Duquesne University School of Pharmacy; Adjuvant Professor of Toxicology, University of Pittsburgh School of Medicine; Adjuvant Professor of Education, Duquesne University School of Education, Pittsburgh, Pennsylvania.

SYDNEY P. SHANOR, Associate Editor

Professor of Pharmacology-Toxicology, Duquesne University School of Pharmacy, Pittsburgh, Pennsylvania.

MARCEL DEKKER, INC. New York and Basel

The Library of Congress has cataloged this serial as follows:

Toxicology annual 1974-
New York, M. Dekker.
v. 24 cm.

Key title: Toxicology annual, ISSN 0361-3410

1. Toxicology--Periodicals

RA1190.T7 615.9'005 76-641009

ISBN: 0-8247-6594-X

These papers originally appeared in Clinical Toxicology, Volume 10, Numbers 1 and 2, edited by Richard T. Rappolt, Sr.

MARCEL DEKKER, INC.
270 Madison Avenue, New York, New York 10016

Current printing (last digit):
10 9 8 7 6 5 4 3 2 1

PRINTED IN THE UNITED STATES OF AMERICA

TO THE MEMORY OF
DR. JOSEPH PULLEKINES

CONTRIBUTORS

DAVID J. BRUSICK, Ph.D. Director, Department of Genetics, Litton Bionetics, Inc., Kensington, Maryland

JAMES J. BURGUN, Ph.D. Duquesne University School of Pharmacy, Department of Pharmacology and Toxicology, Pittsburgh, Pennsylvania

WALTER J. DECKER, Ph.D., F.A.A.C.T. U.S. Army Medical Laboratory, Brooke Army Medical Center, Fort Sam Houston, Texas*

GORDON O. GUERRANT, Ph.D. Proficiency Testing Branch, Licensure and Proficiency Testing Division, Center for Disease Control, Public Health Service, U.S. Department of Health, Education, and Welfare, Atlanta, Georgia

CHARLES T. HALL, Ph.D. Proficiency Testing Branch, Licensure and Proficiency Testing Division, Center for Disease Control, Public Health Service, U.S. Department of Health, Education, and Welfare, Atlanta, Georgia

KEITH B. HAMMOND, M.S., F.I.M.L.S. Pediatric Microchemistry Laboratories, University of Colorado Medical Center, Denver, Colorado

LAWRENCE CHARLES KIER, Ph.D. Kier Laboratories, Inc., Denver, Colorado

BARBARA R. MANNO, Ph.D. Associate Professor, Department of Pharmacology and Therapeutics, Louisiana State University Medical Center, School of Medicine in Shreveport, Shreveport, Louisiana

---

*Present address: Department of Pharmacology, and Toxicology, University of Texas Medical Branch, Galveston, Texas

JOSEPH E. MANNO, Ph. D. Associate Professor and Chief, Section of Toxicology, Department of Pharmacology and Therapeutics, Louisiana State University Medical Center, School of Medicine in Shreveport, Shreveport, Louisiana

ANTHONY S. MANOGUERRA, Pharm. D. Assistant Professor, College of Pharmacy, University of Minnesota, and Supervisor, Poison Control Center, Department of Emergency Medicine, Hennepin County Medical Center, Minneapolis, Minnesota

FREDERICK W. OEHME, D. V. M., Ph. D. Professor of Toxicology, Medicine and Physiology, Comparative Toxicology Laboratory, Kansas State University, Manhattan, Kansas

DONALD L. OPDYKE, Ph. D. Research Institute for Fragrance Materials, Inc., Englewood Cliffs, New Jersey

PATRICIA A. F. PRANITIS, B.A. Connecticut State Department of Health, Toxicology Laboratory, Hartford, Connecticut

ANDREW L. REEVES, Ph. D. School of Medicine, Wayne State University, Detroit, Michigan

MELVIN DWANE REUBER, M. D. Columbia, Maryland

ABRAHAM STOLMAN, Ph. D. Connecticut State Department of Health, Toxicology Laboratory, Hartford, Connecticut and University of Connecticut, School of Medicine, Farmington, Connecticut

LAWRENCE C. WEAVER, Ph. D. Professor and Dean, College of Pharmacy, University of Minnesota, Minneapolis, Minnesota

JEAN K. WESTON, M. D. Department of Clinical Engineering, George Washington University School of Medicine, Washington, D. C.

KATHLEEN WESTON, M. D. Purcellville, Virginia

CHARLES L. WINEK, Ph. D. Duquesne University School of Pharmacy, Department of Pharmacology and Toxicology, Pittsburgh, Pennsylvania

FOREWORD

This is a continuing and successful series of Toxicology Annuals containing informative articles dealing with various aspects of the overall field of toxicology. The contributing authors are all experts in their respective fields, and each has prepared an article that represents years of academic achievement, practical experience, and in several instances, original research.

The editor, Dr. Charles L. Winek, and the associate editor, Dr. Sydney P. Shanor, have demonstrated keen editorial ability in compiling this fine book. There is scarcely an important or major area of toxicology that has not been considered in putting this volume together. Moreover, Drs. Winek and Shanor have fashioned a book which is remarkably uniform in quality and clarity.

The editors, collectively, have more than three decades of extensive, active experience in academic, industrial, and forensic toxicology, and both have lectured and written extensively on numerous toxicology subjects. Their long experience as academicians has given them an additional advantage in preparing this volume, namely, the ability to organize and present materials with precision and lucidity.

This and each future addition to this new series should become an integral part of every toxicologist's library, no matter what field of subspecialization he or she is engaged in. Forensic scientists, coroners and medical examiners, anatomic and clinical pathologists, industrial scientists, police and crime laboratories, pharmacologists, and medical clinicians involved in drug treatment programs will find this book equally rewarding and enlightening.

CYRIL H. WECHT, M.D., J.D.

PREFACE

Toxicology Annual Volume 2, prepared in manuscript form in 1975, represents the second in a continuing series of books devoted to the entire field of toxicology. As this volume goes to press, the 1976 (Volume 3) and 1977 (Volume 4) _Annuals_ are being prepared. Volume 3 is already completed with regard to contributors and topics. It is the hope and intention of the editor to have the _Annuals_ appear in the latter part of the indicated titular year.

Because _Toxicology Annual 1974_, the first book of the series, was promoted by the publisher as a 1975-1976 book, some confusion existed in ordering the _Annual_. By numbering rather than dating the volumes, we trust this will be remedied.

A new feature of Volume 2 is a section of Free Communications. Original papers not previously published, containing data on safety or hazards of chemicals, will be included.

As with the first _Annual_, I thank all of the contributors who have spent their valuable time in preparing chapters. I thank Helen Roderick, my excellent secretary for her many efforts in getting this volume to the publisher. I thank the folks at Marcel Dekker for the fine cooperation in the preparation of Volume 2.

Charles L. Winek

CONTENTS

TOXICOLOGY ANNUAL VOLUME 2

Veterinary Toxicology: The Epidemiology of Poisonings in Domestic Animals

FREDERICK W. OEHME, D.V.M., Ph.D.

Professor of Toxicology, Medicine and Physiology
Comparative Toxicology Laboratory
Kansas State University
Manhattan, Kansas

Epidemiology is defined as the science of the prevalence of a disease or diseases in a community. In human medicine this refers essentially to contagious or infectious diseases and their spread throughout a population. In veterinary medicine, infectious diseases are only a portion of the disease problem. Disorders produced by chemicals (poisonings) and improper management are at least equally important; and since animals are almost entirely dependent upon humans for providing the essentials of proper nutrition, housing, and their total environment, animal diseases produced by chemicals have relatively more importance in veterinary medicine than in human medicine.

Not only is the relative incidence of diseases more variable in domestic animals, but pets and livestock are different beasts from humans. Their anatomic differences are obvious. Coupled with differences in structure are physiologic differences in organ size and function, and in capacity and limitations of tissue activity. Differences are also found when the biochemistry of individual tissues and animals are examined. Enzyme capabilities in the digestive tracts, metabolism and biotransformation systems in the liver, and transport and other enzymatic processes throughout the body differ markedly from species to species and between domestic animals and humans. Indeed, the occurrence of these variations is the basis for the entire group of comparative sciences [1-5].

Of equal or more disease-producing significance than anatomic, physiologic and biochemical differences are the effects of domestication and the resulting characteristics that our animal population have developed through years of close affiliation with humans. Domestic animals have essentially become creatures of habit and have maintained the specific feeding, grazing, watering, and daily routine habits that humans have imposed. Irregularities in diets and routine produced by mismanagement leave the animals with little alternative. Due to their complete domestication, animals have become entirely dependent upon humans for their total care and well-being. They thus have become subject to the whims of human beings, their attempts to become efficient or "cut-corners," and also to stupidity and errors. The domestic animal is forced to feed and be housed where the human wills. Feed, water, and therapeutic or prophylactic application of chemicals make animals susceptible to errors in dosages, feed ingredients, faulty applications of chemicals, and general mismanagement, with the potential for toxicity always present.

With such a wide variety of potential sources of errors due to animals' complete lack of independence and total acceptance of their environment, it is common to find chemical poisonings occurring under wide circumstances. The epidemiologic pattern of animal poisonings is closely related to man's ability to properly manage his pets and livestock. The following are examples of some of the common animal poisonings and reflect the variety and importance of this area to the veterinary practitioner.

DRUGS AND HOUSEHOLD PRODUCTS

Errors in the choice of a therapeutic compound, in its route or mechanism of application, and in its dosage are common lapses of judgment that result in poisoning. The faulty selection of a worming preparation, the administration of a new chemical by an other-than-recommended route of administration, and the overdosage of an anesthetic are dangerous and frequently fatal errors. The mistaking of propylene glycol for mineral oil and the administration of 1 gallon of the wrong material to horses has resulted in a characteristic toxic reaction [6]. Not only are such errors subject to frank poisoning, but adverse reactions and the multitude of possible acute and chronic variations may also occur.

Household chemicals are a popular source for human poisonings. This is also becoming common in veterinary medicine due to the increased number and diversity of chemicals found and used in the home. Aspirin, vitamin and mineral pills, birth control tablets, marijuana and drugs of abuse, disinfectants, and germicides are only a few of such hazardous materials [6, 7]. Because types of household pets vary from birds through rodents to dogs and cats, a wide variation in toxic response is possible. Hence, owners used to exposing their previous pets to the usual household chemicals may find toxicities developing upon the introduction of a new species of household animal. The phenolic disinfectants are one group of commercial compound for which this species variation is potentially of importance.

Figure 1 illustrates the normal phenolic components of urine from four different animals. The wide variation in phenol metabolites is obvious and reflects the variability in ability to detoxify phenolic materials. Figure 2 is the plasma disappearance of radioactive phenol in cats, dogs, pigs, and goats following the intravenous administration of identical single doses. The pig and goat demonstrate the ability to rapidly detoxify and eliminate phenol from the blood. This represents not only liver metabolism, but also excretion, primarily via the kidneys. The dog is intermediate in its rate of plasma clearance, while the cat has a relatively slow capability of removing the toxic phenol from the plasma. As long as the plasma level of the toxic chemical remains high, toxicity is a potential problem. It would further be expected that pigs and goats have little potential for phenol poisoning, dogs would have an average potential for toxicity, and cats would be presented with a greater hazard from exposure to phenolic materials [8-10].

If dogs and cats are exposed to similar doses of phenolic compounds and their survival time measured, cats respond with greater toxicity than dogs. Dogs are more capable of excreting the toxic phenolic material than cats [9-11]. Thus, the capacity of dogs to metabolize and excrete the phenolic compounds is apparently related to that species ability to withstand doses lethal to cats. Although this species difference has been experimentally demonstrated for a wide variety of household chemicals (aspirin, cleaning fluids, petroleum products, insecticides, disinfectants), the phenolic dosages used to document this effect were greatly in excess of the household exposure to which pets are subjected under usual conditions of household use.

Nevertheless, were it not for our faulty judgment in applying such compounds directly to and around our domestic animals, toxicities due to errors in selection of the chemical, application route, dosage, or species difference ("I think I'll bathe my cat with this new shampoo; it worked so well on my dogs last year!"), the incidence of poisoning due to drugs and household products would be greatly reduced.

PESTICIDES

This group of chemicals includes insecticides, rodenticides, herbicides, and fungicides; the latter two have the least potential for toxicity. The newer herbicides and fungicides are in general relatively safe, and only the use of some of the older, more toxic chemicals or exposure to

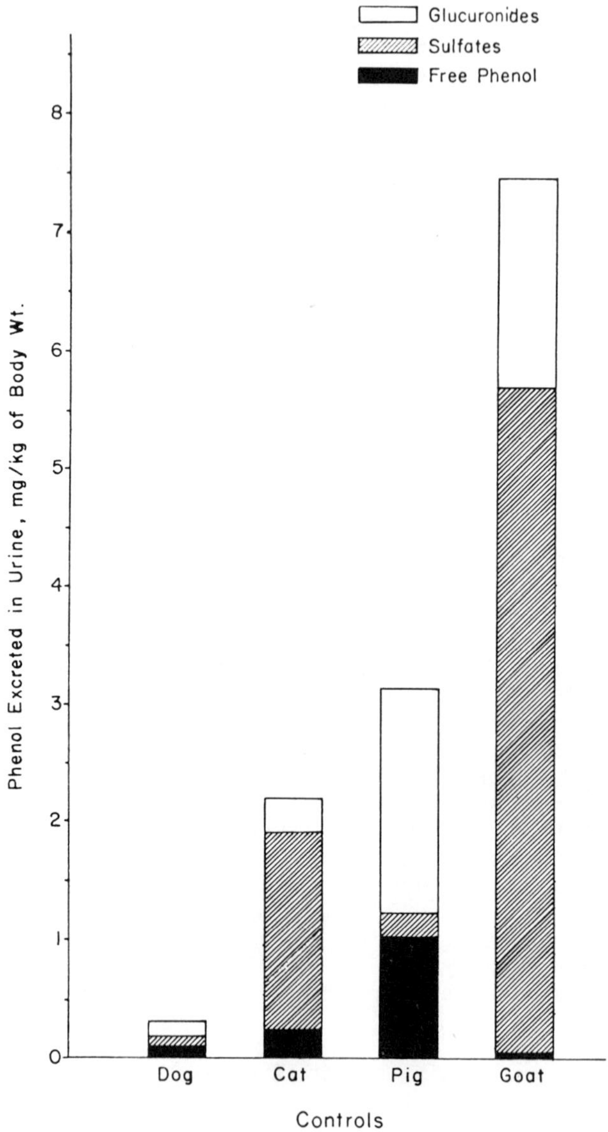

FIG. 1. Phenolic components of urine from four different species of control animals [8].

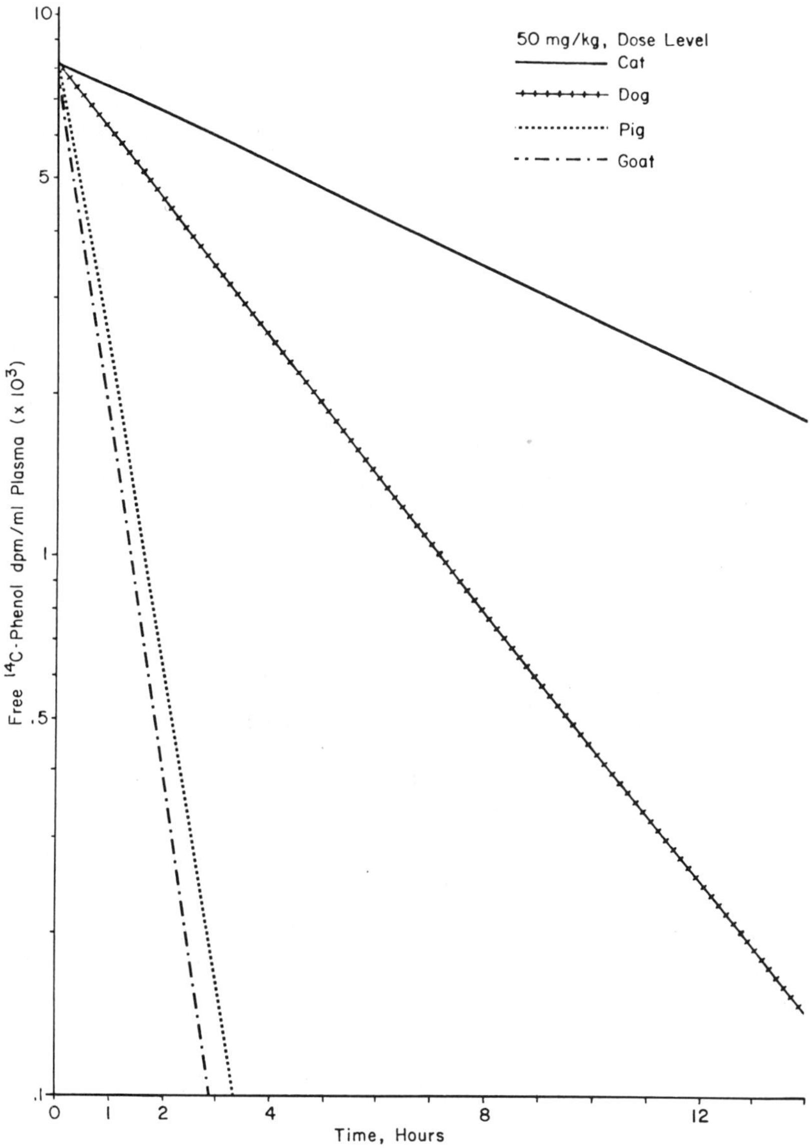

FIG. 2. Plasma disappearance of identical iv doses of [^{14}C]phenol in four animal species [8].

organic solvents used to carry the chemicals in their application are likely to produce poisoning.

However, rodenticides are an important group of chemicals causing animal poisonings. Strychinine is probably the most common cause of poisonings in dogs and is frequently used to "cleanse" the neighborhood of undesirable dogs [5, 7, 12-14]. The fact that strychnine can be purchased under the guise of rodent bait greatly increases the hazard of poisoning. Other compounds used for rodent control are at least equally toxic, but the limited distribution of such materials as 1080 (sodium monofluoracetate), ANTU (alpha-naphthyl thiourea), phosphorus, metaldehyde, and red squill makes incidence of their toxicity much less than that of strychnine. Warfarin is a readily available compound used to control rats and mice, but toxicity is limited by the necessity for repeated dosages to be ingested before poisoning usually occurs.

The insecticides are a much more complicated and diverse group of foreign compounds [13, 14, 16]. As causes of animal poisonings, the chlorinated hydrocarbons and the organophosphorus and carbamate materials are hazardous. Fortunately, effective treatments are available for the organophosphorus and carbamate compounds; the chlorinated hydrocarbons are less effectively treated. The widespread use of insecticides around large and small animals result in considerable hazard to these species. Poisoning usually occurs from accidental exposure via spray drift or due to the intentional application of the insecticide to control livestock or pet insects. In the latter instance, toxicity may result from improper dilution of the concentrated material or too frequent application of acceptable amounts. Both problems are diminished by users properly reading the labels of the respective products and abiding closely by the specified recommendations.

While direct toxicity to the exposed animals is a foremost concern, many of the pesticides are capable of accumulating in feed or food supplies following their application to the environment. Hence, the widescale use of insecticides to animals on pasture may result in hay or feedstuffs growing on neighboring fields developing residues of these foreign chemicals. Likewise, if proper precautions in marketing the exposed cattle are not followed, the meat and by-products from such animals may contain high residues of the applied chemicals. Such matters are of vital interest to governmental regulatory agencies and provide a significant concern in their efforts to protect not only animal, but also human health [17].

The government's concern with the accumulation of foreign compounds in not only foods, but also the general environment, has resulted in the consideration of restrictions on the use of many of the pesticides currently in use. Foremost in such action was the recent banning of DDT from routine usage in the United States. This has been followed by other chlorinated hydrocarbons being examined as a preliminary for similar restrictions. Many of the rodenticides (strychnine, 1080, ANTU, warfarin), and some of the heavy metal materials used as herbicides and fungicides, are being re-evaluated by regulatory agencies because of their hazard and adverse environmental impact. Whether they will indeed be banned from use or only restrictions placed on their application remains to be seen.

HEAVY METAL TOXICANTS

Heavy metals are a common factor in producing animal poisonings because of their wide distribution and use as agricultural chemicals, components of greases and oils used on farm machinery, portions of waste materials found in garbage disposed on animal pastures, their presence in paints, and as feed additives, and the ever-present possibility of them being present as environmental pollution. In addition to their abundance, these compounds have the added hazard of being persistent in nature; hence their application to environmental areas and surfaces results in their presence for many years. Such problems have been demonstrated by attempts of livestockmen to dispose of arsenic, lead, and mercury-containing materials by burning or dumping on open ground. The introduction of livestock to such areas in later years has resulted in severe animal losses.

Lead

Among the variety of heavy metal chemicals potentially toxic to animals, lead is one of the most frequent causes of poisoning [6, 7, 13, 14]. It is the most common toxicant in cattle and is available through the ingestion of paint, lead solder or battery terminals, building materials, and various lead-containing sprays. The poisoning is usually acute and neurologic in effect. Blindness, incoordination, and severe convulsive siezures are observed in affected animals. As cattle become older, the lead toxicity is usually expressed as a chronic syndrome with the convulsive pattern less pronounced. Although acute cases are treated successfully with chelating agents (calcium EDTA), the identification of a lead source for the clinical outbreak is a valuable diagnostic aid for the puzzled veterinarian. Adult cattle with lead poisoning respond well to removal from the source, good nutrition, and nursing care.

This toxicity also occurs in dogs and zoo animals and appears to parallel the occurrence of environmental pollution, especially that found in heavily polluted air situations [18]. The clinical signs in dogs are more chronic than that observed in cattle and frequently are first noticed as a mild gastrointestinal disturbance. This then progresses to sporadic convulsions easily confused with epilepsy. After several weeks, affected dogs may have several convulsive seizures daily. Of interest is the marked red blood cell changes associated with this canine toxicity. Anemia, basophilic stippling, and associated change in physiologic function are seen in some 90+% of dogs affected with lead toxicity [18]. In zoo animals, the toxicity is often unobserved until unexplained deaths occur. Postmortem examination and chemical analysis of tissues has incriminated lead in many of these circumstances.

The widespread occurrence of lead has resulted in studies investigating the behavioral effects of this heavy metal. Recent studies have demonstrated that sheep chronically exposed to low levels of lead do exhibit behavioral and neurologic alterations [19]. This observation adds further substance to similar conclusions drawn in humans and supports the wide interest in eliminating or reducing lead as an environmental contaminant that is hazardous for all varieties of animal life. The use of domestic and laboratory animals as models for studies of lead toxicity has also been proposed [20]. Certain species have been found to be excellent models if variations due to differences in physiology and biochemistry are recognized.

Arsenic

Arsenic is a less frequent intoxication, but very dramatic when observed. It results from the topical application or oral absorption of arsenic-containing insecticides or orchard sprays, as well as consumption of ant and roach baits. Severe gastrointestinal irritation results in all affected animals, with a bloody diarrhea common. Deaths are acute. Treatment in the early stages with BAL (2 mg/lb) every 4 hr and the application of digestive tract protectants is useful. An organic form of arsenic, arsenilic acid, is used as a feed additive for swine. Toxicity results if feed levels greater than 250 ppm are fed for several weeks [13]; incoordination with posterior ataxis leading to paresis is seen. Interestingly, appetite and alertness of the affected animals is normal. Removal of the swine from the feed source largely results in progressive recovery.

Copper

The addition of copper to feed rations and supplements has also contributed to poisonings in sheep and swine. Because of the intentional inclusion of copper, but the omission of molybdenum in livestock rations, the resulting biologic imbalance produces a characteristic toxicity [21, 22]. While the ingestion of copper (and even the sporadic worming with copper sulfate in sheep) leads to chronic accumulation of copper in the system, the signs of poisoning are acute and lead to death 36-72 hr after onset. Icterus and hemoglobinuria may be observed, but usually the animals are "just found dead."

The necropsy examination is characteristic of a hemolytic crisis—generalized icterus, dark metallic-colored kidneys, swollen friable liver, and a bladder with brown-black urine [23]. The blood is watery and often fails to clot normally. Treatment is to correct the copper-molybdenum dietary ratio by spraying 100 mg ammonium molybdate and 1 gm sodium sulfate/head/day on the feed, adding 1 lb sodium molybdate to every 200 lb of salt, or applying 4 oz of molybdenum superphosphate/acre to the pastures.

Mercury

Fortunately, mercury poisoning due to fungicide-treated seed fed swine is now uncommon. Occasionally, however, old mercury-treated seed may be included in animal feeds and can then produce toxicity. Mercury is a potent nephrotoxin and produces nephrosis and eventually uremia [14]. At necropsy the firm, shrunken kidneys are obvious. Although the Reinsch test may be used for laboratory confirmation of the presence of mercury in the feed [13], treatment is not of benefit due to the degree of damage present when a diagnosis is usually made.

Fluoride

An occasional, but when observed, destructive intoxication is that produced by the chronic ingestion of fluoride salts. Most frequently this results from industrial effluents deposited on pastures and consumed with the forage. The condition is chronic and characteristically produces bone, teeth, and hoof abnormalities [24]. Calves may be born with teeth or bone lesions if the mothers were exposed to fluorides during pregnancy. Severe cases of fluorosis will also exhibit a chronic diarrhea difficult to differentiate from other intestinal afflictions. No effective treatment is available, but the addition of aluminum to the diet will reduce the absorption of fluoride from the digestive tract.

FERTILIZERS

The problem of synthetic materials, such as nitrates and ammonia, and also naturally occurring organic material, such as manure, contributing to animal poisonings may seem remote. Unfortunately, synthetic and natural fertilizers are an important cause of livestock toxicoses. The most obvious situation results from the excessive use of nitrate-containing fertilizers on crops and the accumulation of high nitrate levels in the harvested product. These nitrate concentrations in animal feeds can produce acute or chronic nitrate intoxication and widespread economic loss. Even the application of manure to fields can result in high levels of nitrates developing in plants growing in such areas. Not only do cash crops accumulate toxic levels of nitrate, but certain weeds, such as pigweed (Amaranthus retroflexus), are capable of building up high levels of nitrate in their organic matrix when grown on soils containing concentrations of nitrates or nitrate-releasing organic matter [6, 13, 14, 25].

An instance of a vacant feedlot that had grown a lush crop of weeds and was used to provide green pasture for cattle illustrates this problem. Within a few hours after a large group of feeder cattle were turned into the weed-covered feedlot, the owner found 17 cattle dead and numerous others in various stages of toxicity. Even though the cattle were promptly removed from the lot, approximately one-third of the animals died from nitrate poisoning. Analysis of the weeds growing in the area revealed concentrations of nitrate as high as 4.5%.

A complicating situation is the relationship between adverse growing conditions and the accumulation of nitrates in plant materials. Although levels of nitrate may be moderate in the soils supporting grain crops (particularly corn or sorghum) or a variety of weeds, under the influence of a drought or the application of plant hormone herbicides, these commonly grown plants may accumulate excessively high and toxic concentrations of nitrate [25, 26]. The widescale losses in the middle 1950s due to livestock consuming drought-affected corn and sorghum was largely due to nitrate toxicity. The application of 2,4-D to weeds frequently permits these plants to develop transient toxic concentrations of nitrate; if consumed during this temporary phase, nitrate poisoning may result [25].

NATURAL TOXINS

Toxicoses due to plants and animals are not usual in humans, but livestock and pet poisonings due to a variety of poisonous plants or toxic venoms are a significant part of veterinary toxicology [3, 6, 7, 25-30]. The basic factor underlying most plant poisoning problems is mismanagement. Livestock are frequently allowed to graze wide areas of natural range land. When weather conditions are bad, pastures may provide less forage than expected and limited plant material for animal consumption and overgrazing frequently results. Under conditions of repeated overgrazing, naturally occurring desirable pasture grasses die out and weeds, many of them poisonous, take over the range. While such weeds are normally unpalatable, hungry livestock may be forced to consume them and thereby become poisoned. Although most owners recognize overgrazing and the resulting hunger that results in their animals, mismanagement aggravates the loss of native pasture grasses and speeds the introduction and multiplication of poisonous plants. When owners do not provide supplemental feeding for animals on such poor pasture land, the livestock are forced to consume the noxious weeds.

Poisonous Plants

A variety of poisonous plants are available to livestock and household pets and present hazards to their health. The cyanide-producing forages are the most common cause of animal sicknesses due to plants. Usually the sorghums (Johnson grass, sudan grass, milo) are responsible for losses. In addition, arrowgrass (Triglochin spp.), elderberry (Sambucus spp.), wild cherry (Prunus spp.), and the pits of several common fruits (apple, peach, apricot) contain compounds with the potential of releasing cyanide upon ingestion. Toxicities usually result from ignorance on the part of owners who feed such plant materials to their animals or who throw fence-row clippings into pastures to utilize the material for forage. Adverse weather conditions and wilting frequently increase the toxic potential.

Halogeton (Halogeton glomeratus) and black greasewood (Sarcobatus vermiculatus) are two plants that contain high levels of oxalic acid in their plant matrix. Although these plants are only commonly found in the ranges of western states, the oxalic acid is an extremely potent toxin and upon ingestion combines with serum calcium or magnesium. The clinical situation resulting from the sudden drop in the blood level of calcium and magnesium causes large-scale acute deaths. The loss of thousands of sheep annually in the Rocky Mountain area is directly due to the ingestion of one or both of these poisonous plants [31]. Only recently a loss of several thousand sheep in one herd resulted in the erroneous claim that the release of experimental nerve gas had caused their death. Upon detailed examination it was found that owner-error had resulted in the sheep consuming the oxalate-containing plants and the large-scale deaths. Since the calcium and magnesium oxalate salts formed are excreted in the urine and become crystalized in the kidney tubules, causing an inability to pass urine, animals that survive the acute syndrome commonly develop renal failure.

Locoweeds (Astragalus spp. and Oxytropis spp.) are other common and characteristic causes of livestock losses in the western states. The plants are not usually consumed by livestock but under adverse growing conditions and inadequate natural forage, cattle, sheep, and horses may be forced to consume them. Once livestock taste the plants they may develop a liking for their flavor and will then preferentially consume them, even if other feed is supplied. Although horses and ruminants may consume locoweeds, horses are much more sensitive to the toxic principle's effect. Hence, as in one incident when cattle and horses were grazing the same pasture, horses developed locoweed poisoning well before cattle showed even the earliest signs of intoxication [32]. The clinical syndrome is one of weight loss and mental derangement. Animals become easily aggravated and undergo bizarre temperament changes. Deaths frequently result from self-inflicted injuries due to running through fences, falling down wells, or drowning in ponds or streams. The toxin has an affinity for the nervous system and characteristic microscopic lesions are detected in the neurons of the brain [32-34].

Selenium is a chemical found in certain types of rock and hence specific types of soils [22]. Plants growing on such soils may accumulate levels of selenium in their plant structure varying from only a few parts per million to several 10,000 ppm. While any plant growing on soils containing selenium may build up low levels of this chemical, specific plants, such as poison vetch (*Astragalus* spp.) and woodyaster (*Xylorrhiza* spp.), have the ability to selectively take up and accumulate massive amounts of selenium. Some of these plants (golden-weed, *Oonopsis* spp., and princesplume, *Stanleya* spp., for example) will only grow on soils high in selenium; hence they are called "indicator plants," since they indicate the fact that selenium is present in the soils on which they are growing. Toxicity due to selenium will produce various clinical signs, depending upon the concentration of the chemical in the consumed plants. Low levels of selenium may result in weight loss, deformed hooves and hair loss, and birth of deformed young. Larger amounts of selenium cause liver damage. A nervous syndrome, similar to that seen with locoism, commonly develops if large amounts of selenium are ingested.

Several other poisonous plants produce such rapid death that owners may report only that the animals were found dead. Waterhemlock (*Cicuta* spp.) grows in wet areas and contains the highest toxin concentrations in chambers just above the roots. Animals become exposed by crushing the plant in the stream in which it is growing and then consuming the toxin-containing water, or they may actually consume one or more mouthfuls of the plant material. The toxin is so severe that violent muscle spasms may knock the animal off its feet and cause death within minutes. Cattle poisoned by waterhemlock have been found with walnutsize pieces of the plant still in their mouths.

Common oleander (*Nerium oleander*) is not only responsible for sudden animal losses but has also resulted in several human fatalities. Only a small amount of the plant material or toxin-containing sap is required to produce poisoning. Cases have developed from individuals consuming meats cooked using oleander branches as spits. The toxin affects cardiac function and produces a rapid death in all species of animals.

Cocklebur (*Xanthium* spp.) is a weed capable of infesting almost any barren ground. It appears in the early spring as one of the first forms of green vegetation. Since the plant is so common, it is fortunate that its most potent state is during the early growth period, but unfortunately this is just when other green vegetation is limited. Cattle and hogs may be browsing pastures when early spring rains produce cocklebur sprouting. The resulting sprouts contain high concentrations of hydroquinone, a potent liver toxin capable of producing massive liver necrosis and death within a few hours. The mature cocklebur plant is not palatable to livestock, but the burrs containing the seeds may sprout in the fall following a warm rain. Hence, poisoning may not only occur in the spring, but also in the fall when sprouting cockleburs again provide lush forage for grazing animals.

The Japanese yew (Taxus cuspidata) is an ornamental plant that recently has been shown to produce acute poisonings in animals consuming clippings. The plant is frequently installed around fences and animals may become exposed to clippings or may browse the plant directly through the fence. The toxic principle has not yet been fully defined, but horses and ruminants have been found dead by amazed owners following access to this plant [35]. Even though oleander and yew are attractive plants to beautify landscapes around homes and other structures, their toxicity provide great hazards not only for pets and livestock, but also for children accustomed to placing foreign objects in their mouths.

Perhaps the most subtle and potentially damaging hazard from plants is that which results from pregnant animals consuming weeds containing one or more teratogenic principles. Numerous instances of such effects have been reported and many have been confirmed under experimental circumstances [36-38]. The types of defects recorded vary from skeletal to soft-tissue alterations and in many cases multiple anomalies are documented. The study of such occurrences is a vast field for future research.

Fungal Toxins

Some of the lower members of the plant family, the fungi, are capable of producing a variety of toxins. This particular group of poisons, mycotoxins, has become a focal point for scientific investigation during the past decade [39]. The aflatoxins are a group of mold poisons produced by specific strains of the fungi Aspergillus flavus and Pencillium spp. [39]. As with all fungi, a source of nourishment and proper amounts of moisture and heat must be present to support growth. Under suitable conditions, these fungi, and others capable of producing toxins, will grow and in their growth processes will produce their toxins [40]. Hence, the toxins are products of fungal growth; the mere presence of the fungus does not necessarily indicate that its particular toxin is also present. Conversely, the toxin can be present and viable fungi may no longer exist in the sample. Mold toxins commonly develop in stored grains and on certain feedstuffs subjected to unusual weathering or storage conditions. Although moldy feed is usually grossly identifiable, the spoiled feed may be mixed into a ration or otherwise offered for livestock consumption through ignorance or by intention. Animals will usually reject extremely spoiled feed, but well-diluted feeds or rations offered hungry cattle may result in acceptance and toxicity.

Most fungal toxins affect the liver and produce lesions varying from frank necrosis to biochemical interference with enzymes or blood-clotting mechanisms. Digestive tract disturbances, photosensitization, poor feed utilization, abortions, and reproductive failures have been also associated with mycotoxin consumption [41]. Although cancer has never been associated with clinical instances of mycotoxicoses, the experimental production of tumors by aflatoxins in some laboratory animals has resulted in concern over the concentrations of this toxin in grains destined for human consumption. Only a few of the toxins of potential fungal origin have presently been identified [42]. There is no doubt that this interesting area will continue to attract the attention of toxicologists, chemists, and animal scientists for some time to come.

Toxins of Animal Origin

A wide variety of animal-origin toxins are found throughout the world [43, 44]. However, because of limited accessibility and usual close confinement, only a few toxins produced by animals are hazardous to domestic animals and therefore of concern to the veterinarian. These intoxications are due to toxins produced by ticks, toads, and snakes.

FEED ADDITIVES

The use of chemicals added to livestock rations for the purpose of increasing feed efficiency and reducing disease is a characteristic unique to animal production [45]. Although this practice has greatly benefited the livestock economy, the practice is not without danger. Whenever foreign compounds are added to feeds, the possibility of error and resulting animal or human hazard increases. While the presence of chemical residues in human foods and their potential contribution to adverse effects in humans is of most concern to public health officials, animals directly consuming feeds containing feed additives are also likely to become grossly toxic. This may be due to improper mixing of the ration, incomplete following of feeding recommendations, faulty husbandry, or mismanagement. In these instances, acute poisonings result from livestock consuming feeds to which they are unaccustomed or because the feed contains unusually high levels of one or more toxic materials [13]. Two such common poisonings are those produced by excessive or improper feeding of urea or salt.

The factors frequently associated with the development of urea poisoning in cattle are due to: only roughage being fed before urea was offered; no previous urea being fed; switching to high urea ration suddenly; "bully cattle" getting all the feed; cattle being unusually hungry and overeating; feeding instructions not followed carefully; accidentally feeding the wrong mixture; and improper or incomplete feed mixing processes. Urea is a protein supplement fed ruminant animals to provide an economical source of protein to the consuming individuals. The production of ammonia from the urea by the ruminal microorganisms is normally followed by incorporation of the ammonia into bacterial protein; this protein is digested in the intestinal tract of the ruminant and serves as a source of nutrient protein. Under conditions of mismanagement the production of ammonia becomes excessive and the rumen micororganisms are unable to utilize the ammonia in its entirety. Ammonia poisoning then results, with the onset of clinical signs within minutes and death frequently following in 1-2 hr.

Salt is a necessary dietary ingredient, but in excess or in the absence of sufficient fresh water it may become toxic. Toxicity occurs most commonly in swine, but also occasionally in cattle, due to a variety of management factors, leading to the accumulation of sodium ion in the central nervous system and other body tissues. If the owner then discovers that water was unavailable to the animals for a period of time, and then provides unlimited access to water, the osmotic pressure produced by the sodium results in increased central nervous system pressure due to edema and an acute neurologic and convulsive syndrome. While the condition in cattle is somewhat more chronic and digestive signs are more prominent, the underlying cause of salt poisoning is human error resulting in poor animal husbandry practices.

PETROLEUM PRODUCTS

A variety of oils, greases, benzenes, hydrocarbons, and other petroleum products are used on and around domestic animals. Some are employed directly on machinery to which livestock have access; several are utilized as solvents for sprays and materials applied to animals; others are formulated for application to buildings, and animals lick or otherwise contact the applied product; or animals may directly consume the petroleum products by gaining access to storage areas housing opened containers of these materials. In certain areas of the United States, oil wells and oil storage tanks provide the potential for cattle consuming the crude petroleum product. Proper care and precautions are frequently not taken to assure that animals are protected from exposure. Incomplete fencings of crude oil holdings or storage areas may permit inquisitive cattle to satisfy their curiosity. Ignorance of the potential toxicity of these products leads owners to utilize various petroleums directly on livestock as therapeutic aids.

Petroleum products produce a characteristic sequence of clinical signs. If applied to the skin, irritation and thickening commonly results. Photosensitization is frequent, especially in white-haired or light-skinned individuals. If consumed by mouth, the petroleum material produces digestive disturbances, may be inhaled with resulting pneumonia, and after several days can produce liver, kidney, and bone marrow dysfunction. Pregnant animals may abort and a poor-doing individual, continually losing weight and eventually dying, is a usual outcome. Poisoning due to petroleum products is a complicated and varied intoxication. Its occurrence could largely be prevented by owner education and by assuring that proper precautions are taken to prevent animal access to these materials.

POLLUTANTS

The occurrence of air, water, industrial, and other pollutions are just as much animal hazards as they are for humans. A good correlation may be observed between animal and human toxicity problems caused by chemicals polluting the environment. The animal epidemiology is frequently identical to that observed for humans [17].

Air pollution usually results from industrial fumes being released to the atmosphere, and animals in the vicinity are exposed to sulfur and nitrogen oxides, heavy metals such as zinc and lead, hydrocarbons, and various forms of particulate matter. Since most industrial plants are located in suburban and rural areas, livestock grazing surrounding pastures are increasingly likely to assume body burdens of these chemicals or to exhibit biologic responses to their inhalation. Since lead from automobile fumes accumulates in the heavier portions of the air and in particulate matter, dogs are more likely to exhibit signs of lead poisoning than are the adult humans living in the same environment.

Water pollution is a special problem for rural areas utilizing streams and wells as municipal water sources. This is in contrast to large cities that utilize upland reservoirs many miles distant from the consuming population. The sewage discharge of upstream communities and industrial complexes and agricultural enterprises (feedlots, fertilization) may result in a variety of toxic materials being present in the water used by a downstream stockman or community for drinking purposes. The same waters may enter wells supplying other farmsteads or communities.

Recent interest in nitrate concentrations in water supplies have resulted in speculation as to the potential hazard of the continuous ingestion of low-level nitrate waters [46, 47]. Water supplies in Kansas have widely varying nitrate concentrations. In one survey, a significant percentage (28.5%) had levels in excess of 50 ppm, and

19% had nitrate levels in excess of 70 ppm [48]. While the influence of nitrates on animal and human health has only partially been defined, there is little doubt that the other foreign chemicals present in water supplies due to industrial and agricultural pollution are indeed capable of producing significant toxicity.

Other pollutants can produce toxicities under circumstances that are frequently unique to the situation. Carbon monoxide is a special problem during winter weather in animals confined in tightly sealed quarters. Tractors or improperly vented heating equipment utilized within such facilities may produce lethal concentrations of this gas. Antifreeze (ethylene glycol) is a special problem for dogs and cats because of its sweet taste [49, 50]. Consumption of this material when owners discharge radiators in garages or on the ground results in toxicity due directly to the glycol or to its metabolism to oxalate, which produces renal failure through the formation of calcium oxalate crystals. As with most pollution problems, prevention is a matter of education and regulation, and prophylactic efforts are immeasurably more rewarding than the treatment of poisoned individuals.

CONCLUSIONS

The variety of foreign chemicals capable of producing animal poisonings is almost infinite. As long as such potentially toxic materials exist and are utilized by livestockmen and animal owners, hazards for animals, human and domestic alike, will be a prominent concern of the health community and of toxicologists particularly. Persons responsible for animal care must be aware of the hazards associated with the use of these foreign chemicals. They must be instructed and encouraged to use good judgment in the application of these compounds on and around our animal population. Forceful and continuing education is required to assure that safe and sensible use of toxic materials is practiced. Only if the persons handling and applying these chemicals recognize their responsibility can their use be made relatively safe, not only to the users, but also to their neighbors and to the animals in their care. User error or ignorance is the underlying cause for most animal poisonings, and effective education together with the requirement for good common sense is the prime method of reversing the increasing incidence of animal toxicities.

SUMMARY

Animals are constantly exposed to a wide variety of foreign chemicals, many of which are potentially toxic and some of which result in the clinical poisonings. Pesticides are applied on or around animals for the control of insects and rodents. These chemicals may be placed in areas without regard for accessibility to household pets and domestic livestock. Insecticides, herbicides, and fungicides are routinely and haphazardly applied to animal and environmental surfaces alike with apparent disregard for differences in absorptive capability. Fortunately, newer herbicides and fungicides are relatively nonhazardous. Drugs are considered to have therapeutic effects, but the lay and professional person's disregard for species differences and variations in recommended dosages can result in poisonings. Adverse reactions may be misnomers for errors in judgment. Failure to provide satisfactory storage facilities for animal feeds and the improper preservation and handling of feedstuffs allow the growth and development of a variety of mycotoxins. Ignorance on the part of animal owners and livestockmen can result in a number of unusual and sometimes fatal clinical syndromes. The dependence of domestic animals and livestock upon their owners for the total environment makes these animals extremely susceptible to environmental pollutants. Exposure to noxious gases, irritating and hazardous industrial materials and wastes, water contaminants, and casually discarded compounds of our own use can and frequently do result in animal illnesses and death. Persons responsible for animals may be unaware of the potential hazard or lack good judgment in the use of these chemicals. Forceful and continuing education for the safe and sensible use of all foreign compounds on and around domestic animals and livestock is needed. Persons handling and applying these materials must recognize their responsibility, not only to themselves but also to their neighbors and the animals in their care.

REFERENCES

[1] S. B. De. C. Baker, J. Tripod, and J. Jacob (eds.), The problem of species differences and statistics in toxicology, Proc. Eur. Soc. Study Drug Toxicity, Vol. XI, Excerpta Medica Foundation, Amsterdam, 1970.

[2] F. W. Oehme, Species differences: The basis for and importance of comparative toxicology, Clin. Toxicol., 3, 5 (1970).

[3] F. W. Oehme (ed.), Symposium on veterinary toxicology, Clin. Toxicol., 5, 141 (1972).

[4] F. W. Oehme (ed.), Symposium on comparative toxicology: The relationship between animals and humans, Clin. Toxicol., 7, 139 (1974).

[5] F. W. Oehme, Comparative toxicology is where it's at. . ., Clin. Toxicol., 7, 139 (1974).

[6] F. W. Oehme, Practical clinical toxicology, Proc. Ann. Conf. Vet., Kansas State University, Manhattan, 1972.

[7] F. W. Oehme, Clinical toxicology, in Scientific Presentations and Seminar Synopses of the 39th Annual Meeting, AAHA, Las Vegas, Nev., 1972.

[8] F. W. Oehme, Comparative study of the biotransformation and excretion of phenol, Dissertation, University of Missouri, Columbia, 1969.

[9] F. W. Oehme, Comparative toxicity of o-phenylphenol and an o-phenylphenol-containing disinfectant, Toxicol. Appl. Pharmacol., 19, 412 (1971).

[10] F. W. Oehme, New information on the toxicity of phenolic compounds in small animals, Gaines Newer Knowledge About Dogs, 21, 8 (1971).

[11] F. W. Oehme and T. H. F. Smith, The metabolism and urinary excretion of 0-phenylphenol in dogs and cats, Toxicol. Appl. Pharmacol., 22, 292 (1972).

[12] A. L. Aronson, "Chemical Poisonings in Small Animal Practice," in Symposium on Emergencies in Veterinary Medicine (S. I. Bistner, ed.), Vet. Clin. N. Am., 2, 379 (1972).

[13] W. B. Buck, G. D. Osweiler, and G. A. Van Gelder, Clinical and Diagnostic Veterinary Toxicology, Kendall/Hunt Publishing Co., Dubuque, Ia., 1973.

[14] E. G. C. Clarke and J. L. Clarke, Garner's Veterinary Toxicology, 3rd ed., Williams and Wilkins, Baltimore, 1967.

[15] F. W. Oehme (ed.), "Physical and Chemical Disorders," in Current Veterinary Therapy V. Small Animal Practice (R. W. Kirk, ed.), Saunders, Philadelphia, Pa., 1974, pp. 115-177.

[16] R. D. Radeleff, Veterinary Toxicology, 2nd ed., Lea and Febiger, Philadelphia, Pa., 1970.

[17] M. W. Miller and G. G. Berg (eds.), Chemical Fallout, Charles C Thomas, Springfield, Ill., 1969.

[18] B. C. Zook, Lead intoxication in urban dogs, Clin. Toxicol., 6, 377 (1973).

[19] G. A. Van Gelder, T. Carson, R. M. Smith, and W. B. Buck, Behavioral toxicological assessment of the neurologic effect of lead in sheep, Clin. Toxicol., 6, 405 (1973).

[20] N. N. Scharding and F. W. Oehme, The use of animal models for comparative studies of lead poisoning, Clin. Toxicol., 6, 419 (1973).

[21] W. B. Buck and R. C. Ewan, Toxicology and adverse effects of mineral imbalance, Clin. Toxicol., 6, 459 (1973).

[22] E. J. Underwood, Trace Elements in Human and Animal Nutrition, 3rd ed., Academic, New York, 1971.

[23] F. W. Oehme, Copper toxicity in ruminant animals, Southwestern Vet., 19, 295 (1966).

[24] J. L. Shupe, A. E. Olson, and R. P. Sharma, Fluoride toxicity in domestic and wild animals, Clin. Toxicol., 5, 195 (1972).

[25] J. M. Kingsbury, Poisonous Plants of the United States and Canada, Prentice-Hall, Englewood Cliffs, N. J., 1964.
[26] L. C. Hulbert and F. W. Oehme, Plants Poisonous to Livestock, 3rd ed., Kansas State University Printing Service, Manhattan, Ks., 1968.
[27] R. A. Evers and R. P. Link, Poisonous Plants of the Midwest and Their Effects on Livestock, Special Publication 24, College of Agriculture, University of Illinois, Urbana, Ill., 1972.
[28] I. E. Liener (ed), Toxic Constituents of Plant Foodstuffs, Academic, New York, 1969.
[29] E. M. Schmutz, B. N. Freeman, and R. E. Reed, Livestock-poisoning Plants of Arizona, University of Arizona Press, Tucson, Az., 1968.
[30] O. E. Sperry, J. W. Dollahite, G. O. Hoffman, and B. J. Camp, Texas Plants Poisonous to Livestock, Texas A & M University, Texas Agricultural Experiment Station, College Station, Tx., 1968.
[31] L. F. James, Oxalate toxicosis, Clin. Toxicol., 5, 231 (1972).
[32] F. W. Oehme, W. E. Bailie, and L. C. Hulbert, Astragalus mollissimus (locoweed) toxicosis of horses in western Kansas, J. Am. Vet. Med. Assoc., 152, 271 (1968).
[33] L. F. James, Syndromes of locoweed poisoning in livestock, Clin. Toxicol., 5, 567 (1972).
[34] K. R. Van Kampen and L. F. James, Sequential development of the lesions in locoweed poisoning, Clin. Toxicol., 5, 575 (1972).
[35] J. E. Lowe, H. F. Hintz, H. F. Schryver, and J. M. Kingsbury, Taxus cuspidata (Japanese yew) poisoning in horses, Cornell Vet., 60, 36 (1970).
[36] W. Binns, R. F. Keller, and L. D. Balls, Congenital deformities in lambs, calves, and goats resulting from maternal ingestion of Veratrum californicum: Hare lip, cleft palate, ataxia, and hypoplasia of metacarpal and metatarsal bones, Clin. Toxicol., 5, 245 (1972).
[37] R. F. Keller, Known and suspected teratogenic hazards in range plants, Clin. Toxicol., 5, 529 (1972).
[38] H. W. Leipold, F. W. Oehme, and J. E. Cook, Congenital arthrogryposis associated with ingestion of jimsonweed by pregnant sows, Am. J. Vet. Med. Assoc., 162, 1059 (1973).
[39] L. A. Goldblatt (ed.), Aflatoxin, Academic, New York, 1969.
[40] T. C. Campbell, H. L. Gurtoo, R. S. Portman, and M. U. K. Mgbodile, Influence of environmental factors on mycotoxin toxicity as evidenced by studies with aflatoxin, Clin. Toxicol., 5, 517 (1972).
[41] L. A. Goldblatt, Implications of mycotoxins, Clin. Toxicol., 5, 453 (1972).

[42] L. Stoloff, Analytical methods for mycotoxins, Clin. Toxicol., 5, 465 (1972).
[43] J. H. Brown, Toxicology and Pharmacology of Venoms from Poisonous Snakes, Charles C Thomas, Springfield, Ill., 1973.
[44] S. A. Minton (ed.), Symposium on snake venoms and evenomation, Clin. Toxicol., 3, 343 (1970).
[45] National Academy of Sciences, "Use of Drugs In Animal Feeds," Publication 1679, National Academy of Sciences—National Research Council, Washington, D.C., 1969.
[46] J. R. Olson, F. W. Oehme, and D. L. Carnahan, Relationship of nitrate levels in water and livestock feeds to herd health problems on 25 Kansas farms, Vet. Med./Small Animals Clinician, 67, 257 (1972).
[47] W. E. Ridder and F. W. Oehme, Nitrates as an environmental, animal, and human hazard, Clin. Toxicol., 7, 145 (1974).
[48] W. E. Ridder, F. W. Oehme, and D. C. Kelley, Nitrates in Kansas groundwaters as related to animal and human health, Toxicology, 2, 397 (1974).
[49] J. L. Sanyer, F. W. Oehme, and M. D. McGavin, Systematic treatment of ethylene glycol toxicosis in dogs, Am. J. Vet. Res., 34, 527 (1973).
[50] L. Penumarthy and F. W. Oehme, Treatment of ethylene glycol toxicosis in cats, Am. J. Vet. Res., 36, 209 (1975).

Laboratory Support of Drug Abuse Control Programs: An Overview*

WALTER J. DECKER, Ph.D., F.A.A.C.T.

U.S. Army Medical Laboratory
Brooke Army Medical Center
Fort Sam Houston, Texas†

INTRODUCTION

Programs designed to control drug abuse and to rehabilitate drug abusers are highly dependent upon laboratory support. Even though a given drug abuse control program may have excellent educational, communication, counselling, and treatment personnel and facilities, it is certain to run into difficulties unless specimens are subjected to chemical analyses. Few law enforcement officials would be willing to certify that a capsule, tablet, powder, liquid, or plant found on the person or premises of a suspect is an illicit drug without laboratory confirmation. Likewise, few clinicians would state that a patient undergoing rehabilitation is not using illicit drugs unless the patient's urine is found to be free of such drugs by laboratory testing. Exceptions exist, of course. Some law enforcement agents are sufficiently skilled in the morphologic identification of botanicals to state with certainty that a suspect material is marijuana, peyote, etc. A clinician faced with a patient abusing a drug for which there is currently no definitive test, or which is excreted in quantities below the sensitivity limit of the appropriate test, has a problem not solvable by the laboratory. However, most currently abused drugs, certainly in "street" form and usually in biologic materials, are amenable to laboratory identification.

---

*The opinions or assertions contained herein are the private views of the author and are not to be construed as official or as reflecting the views of the U.S. Army Medical Department, the Department of the Army, or the Department of Defense. The mentioning of trade names or manufacturers does not constitute endorsement by or approval of the U.S. Government.

†Present address: Department of Pharmacology and Toxicology, University of Texas Medical Branch, Galveston, Texas 77550.

METHODOLOGY OF URINE DRUG ANALYSIS: A HISTORICAL PERSPECTIVE

The ability to determine the presence of drugs of abuse in urine specimens is of quite recent origin. Prior to the advent of chromatographic methods in the early 1950s, difficulty of separation of mixtures of drugs and lack of sensitivity posed numerous problems. Typically [1], the urine specimen was steam distilled twice to yield an acidic and a basic fraction containing volatile compounds. The acid distillate would contain such compounds as hydrocyanic acid, chloroform, methanol, ethanol, nitrobenzene, free iodine, iodoform, phenol, chloral hydrate, formaldehyde, carbon disulfide, acetone, turpentine, phosphorus, cresols, and carbon tetrachloride. The basic distillate would contain volatile amines, ammonia, aniline, and volatile alkaloids such as nicotine and coniine. The residue in the distilling flask was than acidified and extracted four times with ethanol under reflux conditions. These extracts were combined, filtered, and evaporated to a syrupy consistency, acidified with sulfuric acid, and refrigerated to separate lipoid material. After filtration, the filtrate was extracted several times with ether to remove acid drugs, to include acetanilid, acetophenetidin, antipyrine, aminopyrine, barbiturates, salicylates, sulfa drugs, caffeine, theobromine, and theophylline. The remaining aqueous solution was made alkaline with magnesium oxide and extracted several times with chloroform to remove alkaline compounds such as strychnine, brucine, nicotine, cocaine, procaine, quinine, atropine, codeine, and morphine. The three fractions, volatile, acidic, and basic, were assayed largely by "spot tests" of varying sensitivity and specificity. The cumbersome extraction procedure described took the better part of a day to perform, and the assays up to several days to complete. Many compounds ranging from considerable to slight volatility, such as amphetamines, could not be recovered at the low levels normally found in urine. The spot tests used on the extract to detect morphine; i.e., Marquis', Mecke's, and Froehde's reagents were quite sensitive. They are able to produce their characteristic colors with 20 μg of morphine; but when a mixture of drugs is present, their selectivities are poor.

In the late 1940s, the technique of solvent extraction, long used by pharmacologists to determine oil:water partition coefficients of drugs, was applied in toxicology [2]. By this method, acidic and basic drugs could be selectively extracted from urine by adjusting the pH. Acidic drugs were concentrated in the immiscible organic solvent by making the urine acid, and basic drugs were likewise concentrated by making the urine alkaline. Amphoteric drugs, such as morphine, were extracted by adjusting the pH to the isoelectric point of the drug. In this manner, some separation of drugs in urine was attained.

The next technique adapted for further separation of drugs was paper chromatography [3]. This did indeed improve separation; individual drugs showed up as discrete spots on the paper, but the time for analysis was very long. Using the method of descending chromatography (downward solvent flow; capillary action aided by gravity), development required at least an overnight period. Ascending chromatography (upward solvent flow; capillary action hindered by gravity) took about twice as long to accomplish. The paper was slow to dry; the use of heat was deleterious to the somewhat volatile compounds. Paper electrophoresis was a faster method, but drying was again a problem [4].

Column adsorption chromatography was used to separate and purify alkaloids and barbiturates in the late 1940s [5], but the collection of fractions was quite cumbersome. Application of the adsorbent (silica gel) in a thin layer on a sheet of glass gave rise to the technique of thin-layer chromatography (TLC). This technique, first described in 1949, was adapted to forensic toxicology in the late 1950s [6]. It is much faster and more convenient than paper chromatography; development time is usually less than an hour, and air drying is accomplished in a few minutes.

Although the use of ion exchange resins in toxicology was described in 1952 [7], its application to detection of drugs of abuse in the urine did not become widespread until the middle 1960s [8]. In this technique, a piece of ion exchange paper is soaked in the diluted urine, extracting all the commonly abused drugs. The paper is dried and sent to the laboratory for elution and analysis, obviating shipment of urine specimens and decreasing the amount of solvent required.

The development of gas chromatography (GC) in 1952 [9] signalled a powerful technique for the separation and identification of drugs. The first applications appeared in the literature in the late 1950s but were confined to the analyses of volatiles such as ethanol. During the 1960s, however, almost all drugs were found to be amenable to GC analysis [10]. This technique provides the best separation of drugs of abuse and the most rapid means of analysis to date; in emergency situations, a preliminary report can be given in approximately 30 min [11].

A system for coupling gas chromatography and mass spectrometry was developed in 1959 [12]. However, most toxicologic applications did not appear until the early 1970s [13]. GC-MS analysis is the ultimate in specificity of all techniques currently available to detect drugs of abuse in biologic material. Certainty of identification approaches 100%.

Thus, the development of techniques to solve the most difficult problem of analytical toxicology, that is, separation of drugs in biologic material, has taken place essentially only during the past 20 years.

There are several other methods in current use which have varying degrees of sensitivity and specificity. These include colorimetry, ultraviolet spectrophotometry, fluorometry, and immunoassays. They can be very valuable in pinpointing drugs of abuse in urine. Colorimetric methods for a number of drugs were developed during the 1930s [14].

These and later such tests were developed primarily for the quantitation of specific drugs.

Similarly, the assays employing ultraviolet spectrophotometry were designed to quantitate specific drugs or chemical classes of drugs such as barbiturates [15] and diphenylhydantoin [16]. Fluorometry as a technique to detect drugs of abuse was developed during the 1940s [17] but was expanded markedly during the heroin "epidemic" of the late 1960s and early 1970s [18]. Its specificity in the detection of morphine in the urine is very high.

The latest methodology to be applied to screening urines for drug abuse is that of immunoassay. Four individual techniques have been developed: free radical assay technique (FRAT), hemagglutination inhibition (HI), enzyme-multiplied inhibition assay (EMIT), and radioimmunoassay (RIA). FRAT is quite useful in detecting morphine in urine but suffers a great disadvantage in that it requires a very expensive, dedicated instrument, an electron spin resonance spectrometer. The other three systems, EMIT, HI, and RIA are currently in quite common use, particularly EMIT and RIA. A summary of the advantages and disadvantages of the three has recently been published [19].

ENZYME MULTIPLIED IMMUNOASSAY TECHNIQUE (EMIT)

Advantages	Disadvantages
1. Rapid results, convenient for screening purposes.	1. Some false positive results owing to native lysozyme activity in urine.
2. Results obtained objectively.	2. pH may be critical in aged samples.
3. Quantitative evaluation in the range 0.5 to about 5 $\mu g/ml$.	3. Less sensitive than other immunoassay methods.
4. Detects total morphine (free + glucuronide conjugate).	4. Technique requires instrumentation.
5. Assays for opiates, barbiturates, amphetamines, methadone, and cocaine are available.	5. High price of reagents.
6. Minimal technical skills required.	

HEMAGGLUTINATION-INHIBITION (HI)

Advantages	Disadvantages
1. Low price of reagents, no equipment, simple technique.	1. Time required to complete the complete the analysis.
2. Sensitivity of the assay easily adjusted.	2. Subjective reading or interpretation of results.
3. Detects total morphine (free + glucuronide conjugate).	3. Urine sediment may cause difficulties in interpreting the results.
4. Sensitivity.	4. Quality control on available reagents variable.

RADIOIMMUNOASSAY (RIA)

Advantages	Disadvantages
1. Quantitative data for morphine in the range 1 to 60 ng/ml.	1. Time required to complete the analysis.
2. Results obtained objectively.	2. Technical skills required for handling radioactive materials.
3. Detects total morphine (free + glucuronide conjugate).	3. High price of reagents.
4. Sensitivity.	4. Requires expensive instrumentation.

Recently, there has been a great demand by smaller medical facilities to have available simple, inexpensive, and rapid procedures for identifying drug misuse, in other words, spot tests [20, 21]. Analytical toxicology has come full circle.

GENERAL CONSIDERATIONS

Obtaining a proper specimen—proper both qualitatively and quantitatively—is of extreme importance. When blood is the specimen of choice, this problem is minimal. The clinician drawing the blood can, with relative sureness, identify the subject with the specimen. Similarly, he can usually obtain sufficient specimen for the test or tests to be performed. If urine is required, certain difficulties can arise. Unless the urine is obtained by catheter—medical and legal considerations make this unfeasible in most situations—it becomes vastly more of a problem to identify the subject with the specimen. Minimal micturition at the time the specimen is demanded or the deliberate discarding of part of the specimen by the subject will reduce the quantity available to the analyst. Substitution or adulteration of the subject's urine by tap water, apple juice, the famous Florida fortifier of athletes, or last, but not least, other peoples' urine have been employed to evade detection of drug abuse. Several solutions have been offered to prevent such frauds. The most obvious is direct observation of micturition [22], a procedure often objected to as invasion of privacy, and certainly posing a difficulty when the individual is subject to the "bashful kidney" syndrome. Measurement of urine specific gravity has been proposed as an alternative, but there is no assurance that a determined subject will not substitute a "clean" urine or devise (rather easily) an "artificial" urine in the "normal range" of specific gravity. A second alternative is microscopic examination of the specimen for casts, typical crystals, etc., but neither does this exclude a substituted or adulterated urine.

In regard to another aspect of urine specimen quality, it has been shown that drug degradation or adsorption can occur between collection and analysis. A number of drugs can be decomposed by light (particularly in the ultraviolet range) and by heat. The latter becomes particularly significant if specimens are transported long distances, spending long hours on shipping docks and in hot warehouses. Drugs are, after all, carbon sources; microorganisms will consume them as well as any organic material in urine. Boric acid, one gram per specimen bottle, has been used to prevent loss of drugs by microbiotic metabolism. Certain constituents of urine, notably in the sediment formed upon standing, can strongly adsorb drugs. Thorough mixing of liquid phase and sediment just prior to taking an aliquot for analysis can prevent falsely low results. Several plastics used for specimen containers and cap liners can adsorb drugs; these materials must be avoided. Polyethylene seems to be inert in this respect and is the material of choice [23].

Thin layer chromatography is probably the most widely used drug screening technique at the present time. It is inexpensive, relatively rapid, and encompasses a broad scope of drugs of abuse. As a result of its scope, it is also prone to yielding false positives, usually resulting from metabolic products, over-the-counter medications, and lawfully prescribed drugs. Therefore, it is virtually mandatory to confirm, by an independent technique, any positive result obtained [24]. Some analysts use another solvent system or spot tests for this purpose. These are relatively reliable methods when budgetary considerations preclude instrumental analyses, but confirmation by gas chromatography and/or ultraviolet spectrophotometry is much more certain. Indeed, it is very easy to mask a portion of the thin layer plate before spraying with visualizing reagents; if a positive spot appears, an unsprayed corresponding portion of the plate can be scraped off, eluted, and subjected to instrumental testing [25]. Screening performed by free radical immunoassay, radioimmunoassay, hemagglutination inhibition, or fluorometry is no less subject to the requirement for confirmation.

Confirmed positive results from highly reliable laboratories can, under certain circumstances, wrongly indicate drug abuse. Such results must be interpreted in light of the medical history of the individuals involved. A case in point is the identification of both codeine and morphine in a subject's urine. Codeine is biotransformed into morphine by O-dealkylation to a limited degree but not vice versa [26]. If the subject in question was legally prescribed codeine, both of these opium alkaloids can be found in his urine. A very high codeine:morphine ratio would indicate legal use of codeine, whereas a low codeine: morphine ratio is a sure indication of abuse of heroin or morphine. The possibility of a false positive result due to methodologic problems is always present.

On the other hand, drug abusers are not always detected by these reliable laboratories, by virtue of the considerations mentioned previously. Other reasons include collection of specimen too long after the last "fix"; here, the amount of drug in the specimen may be below the analytical method's detection limit. Also, even the most highly respected laboratories have occasional lapses of quality control; if they did not, they would not need quality control monitors. Indeed, quality control is the key to adequate laboratory support of drug abuse control programs.

QUALITY CONTROL

To paraphrase a venerable quotation, the price of good laboratory results is eternal vigilance. The means by which a laboratory strives to produce reliable results is embodied in the concept of quality control or quality assurance. Quality control is not merely a noble aspiration of laboratory scientists; it is demanded by law in many parts of the world. In the United States, federal, state, and municipal agencies have statutory requirements for quality control extending even to the "dipstick" laboratories of private physicians. The Clinical Laboratories Improvement Act of 1967, Code of Federal Regulations Title 42, Chapter 1, Subchapter F, Part 74 provides a model for such regulation; the toxicology laboratory is specifically delineated in Subpart B of the Act. The Center for Disease Control of the U.S. Public Health Service is the monitoring agency for the Act. An introductory memorandum supplied to laboratories applying for licensure by this agency succinctly sets down requirements for quality control; pertinent sections are quoted here.

"The Clinical Laboratories Improvement Act of 1967, which required that clinical laboratories engaged in interstate commerce be licensed by the Secretary of the Department of Health, Education, and Welfare, has provided an opportunity to develop standards for laboratories throughout the country. The standards, as set forth in the Act and regulations, have been developed through the cooperative effort of many professional organizations and Federal and state governmental agencies. They are designed to assure that high quality laboratory service is maintained. The Secretary will license laboratories meeting the standards.

"The essential elements in a performance evaluation program are: quality control within the laboratory; adequate facilities, equipment and records; qualified personnel; and satisfactory achievement in a proficiency testing program.

"The internal quality control program should be designed to disclose any significantly variant laboratory result which falls outside of an established satisfactory limit. The program should also include action to correct any such deviation. Internal quality control also includes proper calibration and maintenance of equipment and instruments.

"Participation in a proficiency testing program is essential to good performance evaluation. Proficiency testing is now limited to a few of the more common laboratory procedures. As experience is gained, additional tests will be included. To determine the true content or identity of a proficiency testing sample, the sample is referred to three or more (frequently ten or more) laboratories for exhaustive examination. When the identification or content has been established, the samples are distributed to the participating laboratories. The basis for determining satisfactory achievement varies among disciplines; but in general, the laboratory's results are compared with those of other laboratories which perform the specific test as a routine service. A laboratory which inserts the proficiency testing samples into its routine daily runs should find the program no burden. However, if a laboratory consistently handles proficiency testing samples with special care, participation may require a disproportionate part of the work time.

"After submitting the application for licensure, the laboratory should expect a visit from a laboratory examiner of the laboratory Licensure Section of the Center for Disease Control. Since the laboratory director's presence during the first on-site visit is highly desirable, advance arrangements will be made whenever possible. His presence will expedite the on-site visit and provide an opportunity for him to ask questions about the performance evaluation program. During the on-site visit, the laboratory examiner may wish to confirm personnel qualifications by examining employee records and transcripts. Using a checklist as a guide, the examiner will review the quality control programs, the adequacy of facilities and equipment, and the completeness of records maintained by the laboratory and of reports to physician clientele.

"Any laboratory soliciting or accepting specimens in interstate commerce after July 1, 1969 is required to hold a valid license or Letter of Exemption issued by the Secretary, Department of Health, Education, and Welfare."

The Letter of Exemption refers to a provision of the Act that, if the laboratory complies with requirements of an accrediting or licensing body that has standards equal to or more stringent than those of the Act, the laboratory can be exempted from licensure by the Center for Disease Control. Such is the case in the State of New York where the standards of quality control are given so strictly that clinical laboratories certified by the state are readily given Letters of Exemption. Similarly, those laboratories accredited by the College of American Pathologists are exempted. External quality control surveillance programs administered by the Center for Disease Control, the College of American Pathologists, and other agencies provide, on a periodic basis, specimens of serum or urine to be tested by the clinical laboratory. The specimens, usually lyophilized for stability, are either prepared by the submitting agency (the Center for Disease Control) or obtained under contract from a commercial supplier of quality control material (the College of American Pathologists). Grading of results of the survey is accomplished by the use of the results of carefully selected reference laboratories (the Center for Disease Control) or by consensus of surveyed laboratories (the College of American Pathologists). Results of the agencies' evaluation are then returned to the surveyed laboratories. Unacceptable performance on the part of a laboratory can, and often does, result in the suspension or revocation of the laboratory's license or accreditation.

These unfortunate situations can be avoided by a total commitment to a constantly applied internal quality control program; if a clinical laboratory has an effective internal program, external surveys are rarely difficult. This commitment can be brought about only with the complete and affirmative cooperation of the entire professional staff of the clinical laboratory—its director, supervisors, technologists, and technicians. The staff must learn to appreciate and practice quality control procedures at every working moment. A great deal of education and persuasion is often initially required; but after a time, an almost infective enthusiasm develops. The key to developing a positive attitude to quality control is pride of workmanship. One of the methods to stimulate this is to post quality control charts in a prominent location—a well-travelled hallway, for example. In this manner, evidence of good workmanship is displayed for all to see. Another is to establish incentive awards for quality production–a long weekend off, a small cash bonus, a certificate of achievement, a laboratory luncheon for the honoree, and so on.

Formulation of an internal quality control program does not require a sophisticated knowledge of statistics, as many neophytes believe. Indeed, statistical calculations play a rather small role in the job of a quality control manager. The most important attribute of the manager is vigilance. This person must be able to detect promptly factors, patterns, and trends which may result in a procedure going out of control; for example, a constant decrease in the values plotted on a quality control chart. The manager must then quickly follow up this lead by discussing the problem with the supervisor responsible for the procedure to find the reason for the discrepancy and to determine corrective measures. In the example at hand, the falling values might be traced to the fact that the control serum was not kept at the refrigerator temperature recommended by the manufacturer; the solution to the problem, then, would be to obtain new control serum and to keep it at the recommended temperature. It is very important that the manger follow the corrective action for a period of time to ensure its continuation.

The use of quality control serum or urine in every analytical procedure cannot be emphasized enough. Purified drug standards will not suffice. They are helpful in determining unmetabolized drug Rf's on a thin layer chromatographic plate, the retention time of an unmetabolized drug in gas chromatography, or the absorption coefficient of an unmetabolized drug for ultraviolet spectrophotometric quantitation, but they should not be used for quality control purposes. The reasons for this are several. First, the extraction efficiency is usually not the same for aqueous solutions and biologic fluids (urine and blood). Hence, control serum and urine carried through the toxicologic analytic procedure will lead to more accurate quantitation. Next, many, if not most, drugs are metabolized in the living organism to compounds behaving differently in the analytical procedure than the parent drugs. As examples, most of the morphine found in the urine of addicts is in the form of the glucuronide, and methadone has at least five chemically identified metabolites. Unfortunately, only one drug is currently offered in control urine as a metabolite—morphine glucuronide, obtained from hospitalized patients prescribed morphine for control of pain. All other commercial control material is prepared by adding unmetabolized drugs to a drug-free urine pool. It is expected that manufacturers will soon offer other "physiologic" control sera and urines. Another reason for using drugs in biologic matrices for control purposes is to test the analysts' findings in a single-blind manner. The laboratory supervisor should, on a continuing but intermittent basis, insert control materials into the analyst's workload and review the results with the analyst. Still another reason is that biologic material contains biochemical compounds that can be mistaken for drugs—spots on thin layer plates and peaks on gas chromatograms. These extraneous materials can be noted and rejected when control sera or urines are employed.

Many laboratories passively accept the values and ranges of control material specified by the manufacturer. This can be very misleading since particular analytical procedures usually vary either slightly or greatly from laboratory to laboratory. Each laboratory should calculate its own mean, standard deviation, and coefficient of variation for each procedure. Generally, ten assays of the control material performed on two different days (20 data points) should suffice.

SUMMARY

Labeling an individual a drug abuser has serious sociologic and legal implications that only laboratory testing can effectively allay. A proper specimen (both qualitatively and quantitatively) must be obtained for analysis. Positive identification of specimen with subject is of paramount importance. The problems of specimen substitution—other people's urine, tap water, apple juice—directly impinge here, as does the possibility of drug degradation by heat, light, and microbial attack and of drug adsorption by the container and urinary sediment. Confirmation of positives indicated by screening tests (thin layer chromatography and immunoassays) by gas chromatography and/or ultraviolet spectrophotometry is, in most situations, mandatory. An effective quality control program is an absolute requirement. Even under ideal circumstances, laboratory results can sometimes wrongly indicate the abuse of drugs; and conversely, drug abuse can take place without detection by the laboratory. As in any clinical situation, laboratory tests are only a part (albeit an important one) of the entire evaluation of the individual involved.

REFERENCES

[1] F. R. Davision, Handbook of Materia Medica, Toxicology, and Pharmacology, 4th ed., Mosby, St. Louis, 1949, pp. 112-118.
[2] J. W. Jailer and L. R. Goldbaum, Studies on plasma concentration and tissue distribution of sodium pentothal, J. Lab. Clin. Med., 31, 3 (1946).
[3] R. Munier and M. Machebouef, Preliminary experiments on paper microchromatography of various alkaloids with the use of liquid phases miscible with water, Bull. Soc. Chem. Biol., 32, 904 (1950).
[4] S. Kaye and L. R. Goldbaum, in Legal Medicine (R. B. H. Gradwohl, ed.), Mosby, St. Louis, 1954, pp. 677-678.
[5] A. Stolman and C. P. Stewart, Isolation and determination of morphine, codeine, and heroin from viscera and body fluids by adsorption, Analyst, 74, 544 (1949).
[6] G. Machata, Thin layer chromatography in toxicology, Mikrochim. Acta, 47, 79 (1960).

[7] L. Levi and C. G. Farmilo, Determination of narcotics by ion exchange, Can. J. Chem., 30, 793 (1952).
[8] V. P. Dole, W. K. Kim, and I. Eglitis, Detection of narcotic drugs, tranquilizers, amphetamines, and barbiturates in urine, JAMA, 198, 349 (1966).
[9] A. T. James, and A. J. P. Martin, Gas-liquid partition chromatography: the separation and estimation of volatile fatty acids from formic acid to dodecanoic acid, Biochem. J., 50, 679 (1952).
[10] B. S. Finkle, E. J. Cherry, and D. M. Taylor, A GLC-based system for the detection of poisons, drugs, and human metabolites encountered in forensic toxicology, J. Chromat. Sci., 9, 393 (1971).
[11] H. L. Thompson and W. J. Decker, Analysis of blood: a simplified gas chromatographic approach for toxicologic purposes, Am. J. Clin. Pathol., 49, 103 (1968).
[12] R. S. Gohlke, Time-of-flight mass spectrometry and gas-liquid partition chromatography, Anal. Chem., 31, 535 (1959).
[13] C. E. Costello, H. S. Hertz, T. Sakai, and K. Biemann, Routine use of a flexible gas chromatograph-mass spectrometer-computer system to identify drugs and their metabolites in body fluids of overdose victims, Clin. Chem., 20, 255 (1974).
[14] C. H. Thienes and T. J. Haley, Clinical Toxicology, 5th ed., Lea and Febiger, Philadelphia, 1972.
[15] L. R. Goldbaum, Determination of barbiturates—ultraviolet spectrophotometric method with differentiation of several barbiturates, Anal. Chem., 24, 1604 (1952).
[16] J. E. Wallace and H. E. Hamilton, Diphenylhydantoin microdetermination in serum or plasma by UV spectrophotometry, J. Pharm. Sci., 63, 1795 (1974).
[17] B. B. Brodie, S. Udenfriend, W. Dill, and G. Downing, The estimation of basic organic compounds in biological material. II. Estimation of fluorescent compounds, J. Biol. Chem., 168, 311 (1947).
[18] L. R. Goldbaum, P. Santinga, and A. M. Dominguez, A procedure for the rapid analysis of large numbers of urine samples for drugs, Clin. Toxicol., 5, 369 (1972).
[19] S. J. Mulé, M. L. Bastos, and D. Jukofsky, Evaluation of immunoassay methods for detection, in urine, of drugs subject to abuse, Clin. Chem., 20, 243 (1974).
[20] W. J. Decker and J. J. Treuting, Spot tests for rapid diagnosis of poisoning, Clin. Toxicol., 4, 89 (1971).
[21] L. R. Lewis and W. J. Decker, Evaluation of SCREENDEX, a multireagent system for detection of drug abuse and drug overdose, Clin. Toxicol., 6, 201 (1973).

[22] AMA Council on Mental Health and Committee on Alcoholism and Drug Dependence, Oral methadone maintenance techniques in the management of morphine-type dependence, JAMA, 219, 1618 (1972).

[23] D. J. Beach, Walter Reed Army Institute of Research, personal communication.

[24] R. L. Coumbis, C. C. Fulton, J. P. Calise, and C. Rodrigues, The necessity for elution and identification of drugs indicated by thin-layer chromatography, J. Chromatogr., 54, 245 (1971).

[25] W. J. Decker, Recovery of drugs from thin-layer chromatographic plates, Clin. Toxicol., 5, 371 (1972).

[26] A. Goldstein, L. Aronow, and S. M. Kaplan, Principles of Drug Action: The Basis of Pharmacology, 2nd ed., John Wiley, New York, 1974, p. 247.

Beryllium in the Environment

ANDREW L. REEVES

School of Medicine
Wayne State University
Detroit, Michigan

The name "beryllium" for element No. 4 of the periodic table is derived from the mineral beryl, a semiprecious stone with remarkable optical properties. Beryl was known since ancient times and is mentioned in the Bible and in the works of Aristotle and Pliny. Beryl is beryllium aluminum hexametasilicate; Vauquelin in 1798 was the first to prepare from it the oxide [104] and Wöhler in 1828 was the first to prepare the metal [123].

Beryllium is an indispensable material in today's technology, but it has become that only relatively lately. As recently as 50 years ago, the element was still a laboratory curiosity. However, in the 1920s it was discovered that an alloy of copper with 2-4% beryllium had superior resistance to fatigue. This alloy became a popular material in the construction of computers, switchboards, aircraft engines, and precision instruments. By 1940 beryllium had become a ubiquitous material of our civilization.

The first report in the medical literature on occupational disease in a beryllium worker appeared in 1933. Weber and Engelhardt [117] reported on pulmonary and dermal lesions in an employee of a beryllium extraction plant; beryllium was extracted from ore as the fluoride and the effects were generally ascribed to the fluoride moiety of the product. Toxicity of its own for a light metal was then not regarded as likely, and two further reports by Marradi-Fabroni [59] and Gelman [32] were also viewed with similar prejudice. Until about the beginning of World War II, beryllium was generally accepted as a biologically innocuous material.

World War II caused an upsurge in the demand for beryllium by all belligerent parties. Compounds of the metal were needed in the manufacture of radio tubes, filament coatings, vacuum electrodes, and cathode heating elements. Moreover, beryllium was destined to play a special role in the development of atomic energy.

When beryllium atoms are bombarded with alpha particles, their nuclei disintegrate and yield a profusion of neutrons. This reaction led Chadwick in 1933 to the discovery of the neutron, and a radium-beryllium source provided the neutrons for the historic experiment of Fermi that led to the discovery of uranium fission. Beryllium turned out to be one of the most efficient materials for slowing down the speed of neutrons; it is also an excellent neutron reflector. The Manhattan Project alone required more beryllium than the total world consumption until 1940.

The general public had its first opportunity to get acquainted with beryllium when light bulb manufacturers in the early 1940s started to use zinc beryllium silicate as an ingredient of the phosphors that give fluorescent tubes their glow. It was in this industry that pulmonary berylliosis was finally rediscovered and established as a new industrial disease.

The great debate on the causation of this syndrome [26, 27, 42, 116] was a fascinating but also infuriating episode of modern medical history. General acceptance of the environmental etiology required several outbreaks of cases, some involving fatalities. Not until the 1950s was berylliosis firmly established as a compensable occupational disease.

Some confusion in this situation was doubtless due to the fact that the clinical course of beryllium disease has been extremely variable. The acute form was first described by VanOrdstrand et al. [103] in Ohio. The "Ohio cases" were essentially chemical pneumonias, caused by inhalation of soluble beryllium compounds with acidic pH in relatively high dose. The acute inflammation was rarely fatal and recovery after weeks or months was the rule. It was chiefly encountered in the beryllium extraction industry, and no nonoccupational cases were described thus far.

The chronic form seemed a totally different syndrome. It was first encountered in the fluorescent lamp industry in Massachusetts by Hardy and Tabershaw in 1946 [39], and it was immediately apparent that chronic disease may result from much smaller exposures than that required for causing the acute disease. Also, insoluble compounds in this case appeared no less and perhaps more hazardous than soluble compounds. However, the pathogenicity of beryllium oxide seemed to depend on the firing temperature during its production: "high-fired" dusts (produced at about 1500°C) were definitely less toxic than "low-fired" dusts (produced at about 500°C) [85, 90]. This observation is perhaps explainable on the grounds of differences in crystal structure [16], but the biologic reasons for the varying reaction are not understood.

Clinical course of chronic berylliosis was very insidious, with gradual onset after a more or less symptomless incubation period of months or years. Histopathology of the cases was described as granulomatous inflammation of pulmonary tissue [109], resembling Boeck's sarcoid [36, 41]. Chelation therapy with aurintricarboxylic acid [47, 54, 88, 118], or with certain organophosphates [7, 50] and administration of corticosteroids [19, 37, 49, 64] was tried with more or less success. However, the disease often progressed to the point of general debilitation with lethal outcome. Alarmingly, cases were observed not only among beryllium workers, but also in the general population surrounding a beryllium plant [10, 25]. These "neighborhood cases" originated from within about a mile around the plant. Beryllium concentration of the stack emissions was measured and found in the order of magnitude of 0.1 γ/m^3 [93]. A woman who became sick with chronic berylliosis lived at a distance of 2 miles; it developed that she used to wash at home the work clothing of her husband, a worker in the plant. Evidently, she obtained her exposure during the wash.

It is easy to imagine the impact of these developments on contemporary industrial medicine and hygiene. On one hand, there were cases of a dangerous and often lethal illness, apparently caused by almost unbelievably low atmospheric concentrations of beryllium. On the other hand, incidence among exposed persons was sporadic, inconsistent, and distinctly not concentration-dependent. In the case of the woman with the laundry, for instance, the husband, who wore the contaminated clothing, did not get the disease and there were other instances where the number of neighborhood cases equalled or exceeded the number of cases within the plant. Certain factories, including some that were not exactly models of cleanliness, reported zero incidence of berylliosis among their workers. These reports were received with a certain skepticism occasionally, but unbiased inspection has sometimes sustained them. In fact, the cleanest plants apparently had the most cases. Perhaps they had better health surveillance; perhaps the sex distribution of workers was a factor. It was found that women were more susceptible to chronic berylliosis than men [20].

In addition to these problems, it was soon realized that beryllium had dermatologic effects as well [21]. Exposed persons (frequently young lads who used defunct fluorescent tubes as baseball bats, and then cut themselves with beryllium-contaminated broken glass) developed granulomatous ulcerations of the skin which did not heal readily and suggested an allergic etiology [61]. On the basis of these observations and of the epidemiologic distribution of neighborhood cases, Sterner and Eisenbud suggested in 1951 that berylliosis was an autoimmune disorder which affected only certain sensitive individuals [91]. This idea was then ahead of its time and had to remain unproven.

In any case, it seemed that there were persons with extraordinary sensitivity towards beryllium, and they had to be considered in the setting of a threshold limit value. That is why beryllium was assigned one of the lowest figures on the TLV list (2 γ/m^3) and on the air quality standard list (0.01 γ/m^3). The severity of these limits is best realized by comparison with such well-known poisons as arsenic, cyanide, or dimethyl sulfate, which have corresponding limits 200-2000 times higher. Manufacture of beryllium phosphors was all but discontinued by the early 1950s, and cases of industrial berylliosis, as well as neighborhood cases, have again become great rarities.

In spite of this, beryllium is again attracting toxicologic attention, attributable to two new applications of the metal. Both are connected with space exploration, which is indicative of their potential importance. First, beryllium oxide has become a substantial component of the ceramic formulation used in the manufacture of space vehicle reentry cones. The heat-reflecting and insulating properties of beryllium oxide are so favorable that it is regarded as an indispensable ingredient—the oxide is the "high-fired" variety, which is supposed to be much less toxic than the "low-fired" variety [85, 90]. Furthermore, evaporation of the cone during reentry is minimal and occurs at such altitude that this application does not appear to be a measurable or hazardous source of environmental beryllium.

The second potential application of beryllium in astronautics is a source of more concern. The metal turned out to be the ideal rocket fuel; in view of its low molecular weight it packs more energy per unit volume than any other solid and chemically stable material. Space propulsion technologists of various nations competing with each other in this area must resist a strong temptation in the formulation of their rocket fuel, especially for near-terrestrial use. Of course we have assurances that no such use of beryllium fuels has been or will be contemplated; the discharge of tons of beryllium anywhere near the Earth from rocket exhaust would be a scary prospect. However, who determines what is no longer "near the Earth"? Is it possible that during a period of increased competition or national emergency, the planners would be pressured to assume certain risks? This dilemma must have occurred to scientists of several nations, and it is perhaps significant that the study of beryllium toxicology in the Soviet Union has experienced a great renaissance during the last 10 years. Quality and quantity of published work in Russian has risen from near-zero to considerable heights [2-7, 45, 46, 50, 52, 64, 66-69, 105-107]. In Western Europe, beryllium analysis of food crops and tobacco recently yielded values of 0.07-0.33 γ/g [124].

Unfortunately, we have no dependable indicators of the trend of global atmospheric beryllium concentrations during the last several decades. Comparison with older measurements poses certain problems, because the methodologies have changed. Gas chromatography and atomic absorption spectrophotometry are recently introduced methods which offer greatly improved accuracy over the older methods of emission spectrography [89, 95] or fluorescence photometry [13, 53]. The amounts to be determined are of course small, and occasional reports claiming increase of atmospheric beryllium levels by a factor of two or even three deserve little confidence if based on determinations subject to error of the same magnitude. This question is at present not resolved.

Another question occasionally raised concerns the prevalence of Boeck's sarcoid, believed to be on the rise. Is that due to improved programs of detection, or are unrecognized cases of berylliosis sometimes reported as sarcoid? If so, could that be due to low-level generalized environmental contamination, affecting only the most susceptible individuals in the population? This question must also remain unanswered at present. To be sure, no documentation exists to prove that presumed cases of sarcoidosis are indeed on the increase—much less that they are attributable to environmental beryllium. Clearly, more research is urgently needed on this subject.

In any case, even if these fears turn out to be groundless, it cannot be denied that the handling, transport, and storage of the considerable quantities of beryllium in use today do involve certain risks. Threshold limit values regulate only the situation during occupational handling. But what will happen in the case of a traffic accident during transport? Or in the case of fire of a beryllium plant? Is then the potential contamination of the environment for perhaps hundreds of miles inevitable? Newly established "public emergency limits" attempt to control such a situation. Public emergency limits are meant to regulate the storage and handling of all dangerous materials in such a way that even in the case of an unforeseen accident no disastrous results should follow. For beryllium, a public emergency limit of 100 $\gamma/m^3/10$ min has been suggested—if the period of expected contamination is longer, the limit must be proportionally lower. However, extrapolation in the other direction for higher momentary burden is not permissible. With this limit, the cumulative total exposure of a population would not exceed the air quality standard of 0.01 γ/m^3 even in the unlikely event that such an accident occurred once every three months in a single area—a very pessimistic assumption. All transport, testing, storage, or other handling of beryllium has to be planned in such a way that even in the case of an accident the degree of environmental contamination will not exceed this limit. Obviously, some guesswork was involved in setting this figure, but it is better to have this figure for the planning of these activities than none.

Investigations on the experimental toxicology of beryllium were commenced soon after the discovery of industrial berylliosis and yielded surprising results. Gardner and Heslington [31] observed in 1946 bone sarcoma in rabbits after intravenous beryllium injection, and Vorwald et al. [112] in 1955 produced pulmonary carcinoma in rats after inhalation. A certain species specificity was evident from these studies: rabbits developed bone sarcoma also after inhalation [24]; monkeys developed pulmonary carcinoma after inhalation [111]; while guinea pigs showed no malignant changes either after injection or after inhalation [110].

The main question remained, of course; whether beryllium was carcinogenic in humans. Development of the tumors in the animal models did take considerable time—about a year in rats, i.e., almost half of the average life expectancy—therefore it would have been premature to base very optimistic expectations on the fact that no beryllium-connected human cancer cases were observed during the initial years. In the early reviews [92, 94] this question was left unanswered. However, 10-15 years have passed in the meantime, during which all reported human exposures were collected in a "Beryllium Case Registry" [30, 38]. This material as well as other sources of cases were epidemiologically examined by Mancuso recently [57, 58]. The conclusion from this study was that the prevalence of lung cancer among beryllium-exposed persons, when compared with a control cohort matched with respect to age, sex, income, and smoking habits, was not elevated. However, the prevalence of lung cancer did show positive correlation with the prevalence of other pulmonary disorders, including berylliosis. On the other hand, incidence of pulmonary cancer among beryllium workers was inversely related to length of employment in the plant. Therefore, the sum of evidence, at least thus far, favors the view that humans, like the guinea pig, are susceptible to berylliosis but resistant to beryllium cancer.

The significance of this parallelity of responses was not immediately recognized. In the early years, the animal of choice for beryllium research had been the rat, because in rats it was relatively easy to produce pulmonary cancer with beryllium [86, 87, 113, 114]. It could be shown that chemical specificity was a key factor in the carcinogenesis and corresponding compounds of aluminum which were precisely matched to the molarity, pH, and buffering capacity of carcinogenic beryllium compounds, were without neoplastic effect [76, 82]. Observations were also made on the enzymatic metabolism of these tumors [71, 72, 75]; on the absorption, transport, and excretion of the carcinogen [28, 70, 79, 81, 99-101]; and on the influence of age and sex on the carcinogenic response [74]. The apparently higher sensitivity of the female sex to inhaled beryllium was reproduced experimentally and attributed to a less efficient lymphatic clearance of the lungs in females [73].

The biochemical basis of beryllium toxicity was also investigated. In 1949, it was discovered that beryllium is a most powerful inhibitor of alkaline phosphatase [23, 33, 48]. Additional enzymes inhibited by beryllium include phosphoglucomutase [1], deoxythymidine kinase [56], lactate dehydrogenase [72] as well as, at higher concentrations, a large number of others [84]. Protein metabolism [45, 52, 66] as well as nucleic acid metabolism [29, 55, 120, 121] in the presence of beryllium was studied. Endocrine factors, especially adrenal imbalance, appeared to play a role [15].

In the lungs, beryllium was found in the alveolar cells. Electron microscopic [83] as well as biochemical [122] studies showed that inhaled beryllium first accumulated in the lysosomes, then became translocated to the nuclei [46, 113, 114]. Witschi [120, 121] found inhibition of replication of DNA in the nuclei in the presence of beryllium, but no binding of DNA to beryllium. Protein or RNA biosynthesis was not inhibited, and beryllium apparently became attached to an unidentified cellular component [96]. High concentrations of beryllium also had hemolytic activity, causing precipitation of hemosiderin in the lung capillaries [67-69].

These studies have yielded some very interesting results, but it cannot be said that they have fully elucidated the fundamental biochemical reaction responsible for the development of berylliosis or of beryllium cancer. Rather, it appears now that this fundamental reaction must be sought not in the realm of enzymology or nucleic acid metabolism, but in the realm of immunology.

Guinea pigs are noted not only for apparent resistance to beryllium cancer, but also for the capability of developing cutaneous hypersensitivity to beryllium [2-4, 11, 12, 14, 97, 105-107]. Similar hypersensitivity was already known to exist in humans and was employed by Curtis [17, 18] for the diagnosis of berylliosis [34, 63, 115]. The Curtis test has not received general acceptance because of fear that it might reactivate dormant cases; also, it gave false negative results in some instances [125]. In humans, the reaction was described as granulomatous hypersensitivity [35, 40], with beryllium functioning as the hapten [98, 108]. Some kind of a beryllium-protein combination [8, 51] seemed to be the complete antigen, perhaps a complex of cutaneous alkaline phosphatase [9]. Other immunologic tests besides skin reactivity were explored as diagnostic tools for the recognition of chronic berylliosis. They included lymphocyte transformation [22, 34, 43, 62, 102] and macrophage migration inhibition [40, 44, 60, 65, 119]. The relation between these features and pulmonary berylliosis is just beginning to emerge. It was recently observed that inhalation of beryllium sulfate can suppress an already established cutaneous hypersensitivity in guinea pigs, and if the hypersensitivity is reinforced through periodic booster shots, then the animals develop an alleviated response to beryllium inhalation in the lungs [77-80]. Apparently, some kind of immunization to pulmonary berylliosis is possible, at least in the guinea pig. Whether the principle also works in humans is not known at present.

However, the suggestion of Sterner and Eisenbud that berylliosis was an autoimmune disorder is clearly reinforced by these experiments. This explains the inconsistent observations in population groups; the bizarre dose-response relations; the apparent disadvantage of the cleanest plants where cutaneous contact with beryllium was not the rule; and also the therapeutic results with corticosteroids which have a general immunosuppressive effect.

Possibly, the situation also contains clues to the puzzling resistance of guinea pigs to beryllium cancers. It should be noted that species that are prone to develop cancer from beryllium, specifically rats, do not develop cutaneous hypersensitivity to beryllium. This question clearly needs additional research. A dangerous environmental pollutant might thus become the key of understanding of autoimmune disorders and their relationship to cancer resistance.

REFERENCES

[1] W. N. Aldridge and M. Thomas, Biochem. J., 98, 100 (1966).
[2] O. G. Alekseeva, Gig. Tr. Prof. Zabol., 9, 20 (1966).
[3] O. G. Alekseeva, Gig. Tr. Prof. Zabol., 11, 29 (1967).
[4] O. G. Alekseeva, A. P. Volkova, and N. V. Svinkina, Farmakol. Toksikol., 29, 353 (1966).
[5] O. G. Arkhipova and N. K. Demokidova, Farmakol. Toksikol., 30, 352 (1967).
[6] O. G. Arkhipova, P. P. Dvizhkov, T. A. Kochetkova, and A. S. Ivanova, Gig. Sanit., 33, 26 (1968).
[7] O. G. Arkhipova, T. Y. Medved, M. V. Rudomino, and M. I. Kabachnik, Gig. Tr. Prof. Zabol., 11, 19 (1967).
[8] S. Belman, J. Am. Chem. Soc., 85, 2154 (1963).
[9] S. Belman, J. Occup. Med., 11, 175 (1969).
[10] C. Chesner, Ann. Int. Med., 32, 1028 (1950).
[11] G. Chiappino, G. Barbiano di Belgiojoso, and A. M. Cirla, Boll. Ist. Sieroter. Milan, 47, 669 (1968).
[12] G. Chiappino, A. M. Cirla, and E. C. Vigliani, Arch. Pathol., 87, 131 (1969).
[13] J. Cholak and D. B. Hubbard, Anal. Chem., 20, 73 (1948).
[14] A. M. Cirla, G. Barbiano di Belgiojoso, and G. Chiappino, Boll. Ist. Sieroter. Milan, 47, 663 (1968).
[15] J. J. Clary and H. E. Stokinger, J. Occup. Med., 15, 255 (1973).
[16] G. C. Crossmon and W. C. Vandemark, Arch. Indust. Hyg. Occup. Med., 9, 481 (1954).
[17] G. H. Curtis, Arch. Dermatol. Syphilol., 64, 470 (1951).
[18] G. H. Curtis, Arch. Indust. Health, 19, 150 (1959).
[19] J. M. DeNardi, Arch. Indust. Hyg. Occup. Med., 3, 543 (1951).
[20] J. M. DeNardi, Arch. Indust. Health, 19, 110 (1959).
[21] J. M. DeNardi, H. S. VanOrdstrand, and M. G. Carmody, Ohio State Med. J., 45, 567 (1949).
[22] S. D. Deodhar, B. Barna, and H. S. VanOrdstrand, Chest, 63, 309 (1973).
[23] K. P. DuBois, K. W. Cochran, and M. Mazur, Science, 110, 420 (1949).
[24] F. R. Dutra, R. J. Largent, and J. L. Roth, Arch. Pathol., 51, 473 (1951).

[25] M. Eisenbud, R. C. Wanta, C. Dustan, L. T. Steadman, W. B. Harris, and B. S. Wolfe, J. Indust. Hyg. Toxicol., 31, 282 (1949).
[26] Editorial, Product Engineering, 20/9, 155 (1949).
[27] Editorial, Lancet, 260, 1357 (1951).
[28] I. Feldman, J. R. Havill, and W. F. Neuman, Arch. Biochem. Biophys., 46, 443 (1953).
[29] B. Festy, J. B. LePecq, C. Paoletti, and R. Truhaut, Ann. Biol. Clin., 23, 37 (1965).
[30] D. G. Freiman and H. L. Hardy, Human Pathol., 1, 25 (1970).
[31] L. U. Gardner and H. F. Heslington, Federation Proc., 5, 221 (1946).
[32] I. Gelman, J. Indust. Hyg., 18, 371 (1936).
[33] R. S. Grier, D. B. Hood, and M. B. Hoagland, J. Biol. Chem., 180, 289 (1949).
[34] C. Groetenbriel, W. F. VanGanse, and J. Oleffe, Acta Tuberc. Pneumol. Belg., 61, 363 (1970).
[35] J. M. Hanifin, W. L. Epstein, and M. J. Cline, Invest. Dermatol., 55, 284 (1970).
[36] H. L. Hardy, Am. Rev. Tuberc., 74, 885 (1956).
[37] H. L. Hardy, F. C. Bartter, and A. E. Jaffin, Arch. Indust. Hyg. Occup. Med., 3, 579 (1951).
[38] H. L. Hardy, E. W. Rabe, and S. Lorch, J. Occup. Med., 9, 271 (1967).
[39] H. L. Hardy and I. R. Tabershaw, J. Indust. Hyg., 28, 197 (1946).
[40] W. R. Henderson, K. Fukuyama, W. L. Epstein, and L. E. Spitler, J. Invest. Dermatol., 58, 5 (1972).
[41] H. L. Higgins, Conn. State Med. J., 11, 330 (1947).
[42] F. Hyslop, E. D. Palmes, W. C. Alford, A. R. Monaco, and L. T. Fairhall, The Toxicology of Beryllium, U.S. Natl. Inst. Health, Bethesda, 1943.
[43] J. M. Jones and H. E. Amos, Intern. Arch. Allergy & Appl. Immunol., 46, 161 (1974).
[44] J. M. Jones and H. E. Amos, Intern. Arch. Allergy & Appl. Immunol., 48, 22 (1975).
[45] S. F. Kharlamova, Gig. Tr. Prof. Zabol., 12, 58 (1968).
[46] S. F. Kharlamova and I. N. Potapova, Farmakol. Toksikol., 31, 357 (1968).
[47] M. E. King, A. M. Shefner, and R. Ehrlich, Ind. Med. Surg., 33, 566 (1964).
[48] F. W. Klemperer, J. M. Miller, and C. J. Hill, J. Biol. Chem., 180, 281 (1949).
[49] E. M. Kline, S. R. Inkley, and W. H. Prischard, Arch. Indust. Hyg. Occup. Med., 3, 549 (1951).
[50] T. A. Kochetkova and O. G. Arkhipova, Arkh. Pathol., 31, 52 (1969).

[51] N. D. Krivanek and A. L. Reeves, J. Am. Indust. Hyg. Assoc., 33, 45 (1972).
[52] N. G. Kurysheva, Gig. Tr. Prof. Zabol., 13, 51 (1969).
[53] H. A. Laitinen and P. Kivalo, Anal. Chem., 24, 1467 (1952).
[54] A. Lindenbaum, M. R. White, and J. Schubert, Arch. Biochem. Biophys., 52, 110 (1954).
[55] M. Z. Luke, L. Hamilton, and T. Hollocher, Biochem. Biophys. Res. Commun., 62, 497 (1975).
[56] K. D. Mainigi and E. Bresnick, Biochem. Pharmacol., 18, 2003 (1969).
[57] T. F. Mancuso, Environ. Res., 3, 251 (1970).
[58] T. F. Mancuso and A. A. El-Attar, J. Occup. Med., 11, 422 (1969).
[59] S. Marradi-Fabroni, Med. Lavoro, 26, 297 (1935).
[60] J. J. Marx and R. Burrell, J. Immunol., 111, 590 (1973).
[61] C. P. McCord, Ind. Med. Surg., 20, 336 (1951).
[62] R. L. Naeye, Chest, 63, 306 (1973).
[63] H. K. Niemöller, Intern. Arch. Gewerbepathol. Gewerbehyg., 19, 27 (1962).
[64] A. A. Orlova and V. V. Ozerova, Gig. Tr. Prof. Zabol., 10, 17 (1966).
[65] M. J. Palazzolo and A. L. Reeves, Soc. Toxicol. Ann. Mtg. Abstr., 14, 11 (1975).
[66] J. V. Pavlova, S. F. Kharlamova, and N. G. Kurysheva, Gig. Tr. Prof. Zabol., 14, 56 (1970).
[67] I. N. Potapova, Arkh. Pathol., 29, 61 (1967).
[68] I. N. Potapova, Gig. Tr. Prof. Zabol., 14, 57 (1970).
[69] I. N. Potapova and M. S. Tolgskaya, Arkh. Pathol., 31, 69 (1969).
[70] A. L. Reeves, Arch. Environ. Health, 11, 209 (1965).
[71] A. L. Reeves, Proc. Am. Assoc. Cancer Res., 7, 227 (1966).
[72] A. L. Reeves, Cancer Res., 27, 1895 (1967).
[73] A. L. Reeves, Intern. Arch. Gewerbepathol. Gewerbehyg., 24, 226 (1968).
[74] A. L. Reeves, Am. Indust. Hyg. Assoc. J., 30, 110 (1969).
[75] A. L. Reeves, E. K. Busby, and L. Scotti, Am. Indust. Hyg. Assoc. J., 27, 278 (1966).
[76] A. L. Reeves, D. Deitch, and A. J. Vorwald, Cancer Res., 27, 439 (1967).
[77] A. L. Reeves and N. D. Krivanek, Trans. N.Y. Acad. Sci., 36, 78 (1974).
[78] A. L. Reeves, N. D. Krivanek, E. K. Busby, and R. H. Swanborg, Intern. Arch. Occup. Health, 29, 209 (1972).
[79] A. L. Reeves, R. G. Smith, and A. J. Vorwald, Federation Proc., 17, 1785 (1958).
[80] A. L. Reeves, R. H. Swanborg, E. K. Busby, and N. D. Krivanek, Inhaled Particles III (W. H. Walton, ed.), Unwin Bros. Ltd. Old Woking (Surrey), 1971, p. 599.

[81] A. L. Reeves and A. J. Vorwald, J. Occup. Med., 3, 567 (1961).
[82] A. L. Reeves and A. J. Vorwald, Cancer Res., 27, 446 (1967).
[83] F. R. Robinson, F. Schaffner, and E. Trachtenberg, Arch. Environ. Health, 17, 193 (1968).
[84] R. Rothe and H. Minden, Intern. Arch. Gewerbepathol. Gewerbehyg., 21, 161 (1965).
[85] C. L. Sanders, W. C. Cannon, G. J. Powers, and R. R. Adee, "Toxicology of Inhaled Low-Fired and High-Fired Beryllium Oxides in Rat and Hamster" Batelle NW Lab Rept. No. 1818, Richland, 1974.
[86] G. W. H. Schepers, Progr. Exptl. Tumor Res., 2, 203 (1961).
[87] G. W. H. Schepers, T. M. Durkan, A. B. Delahant, and F. T. Creedon, Arch. Indust. Health, 15, 32 (1957).
[88] J. Schubert and A. Lindenbaum, J. Biol. Chem., 208, 359 (1954).
[89] R. G. Smith, A. J. Boyle, W. G. Fredrick, and B. Zak, Anal. Chem., 24, 406 (1952).
[90] H. C. Spencer, J. C. Jones, S. E. Sadek, K. B. Dodson, and A. H. Morgan, Toxicol. Appl. Pharmacol., 7, 498 (1965).
[91] J. H. Sterner and M. Eisenbud, Arch. Indust. Hyg. Occup. Med., 4, 123 (1951).
[92] H. E. Stokinger (ed.), Beryllium—Its Industrial Hygiene Aspects, Academic, New York, 1966.
[93] V. H. Sussman, J. Lieben, and J. G. Cleland, Am. Indust. Hyg. Assoc. J., 20, 504 (1959).
[94] L. B. Tepper, H. L. Hardy, and R. I. Chamberlin, Toxicity of Beryllium Compounds, Elsevier, Amsterdam, 1961.
[95] T. Y. Toribara and R. E. Sherman, Anal. Chem., 25, 1594 (1953).
[96] R. Truhaut, B. Festy, and J. Y. LeTalaer, Compt. Rend. Acad. Sci., 266, 1192 (1968).
[97] J. Vacher, J. Med. Microbiol., 5, 91 (1972).
[98] J. Vacher, R. Deraedt, and J. Benzoni, Toxicol. Appl. Pharmacol., 24, 497 (1973).
[99] J. Vacher and H. B. Stoner, Biochem. Pharmacol., 17, 93 (1968).
[100] J. Vacher and H. B. Stoner, Br. J. Exptl. Pathol., 49, 315 (1968).
[101] C. D. VanCleave and C. T. Kaylor, Arch. Indust. Health, 11, 375 (1955).
[102] W. F. VanGanse, J. Oleffe, W. VanHowe, and C. Groetenbriel, Lancet, 1972-1, 1023.
[103] H. S. VanOrdstrand, R. Hughes, and M. G. Carmody, Cleveland Clin. Quart., 10, 10 (1943).
[104] L. N. Vauquelin, Ann. Chim., 26, 115 (1798).
[105] E. V. Vasil'eva, Byull. Eksp. Biol. Med., 67, 74 (1969).
[106] E. V. Vasil'eva, Vop. Med. Chim., 17, 361 (1971).

[107] E. V. Vasil'eva, Byull. Eksp. Biol. Med., 73, 76 (1972).
[108] G. A. Voisin, A. Collet, J. C. Martin, H. Daniel-Moussard, and F. Toullet, Rev. Franc. Et. Cein. Biol., 9, 819 (1964).
[109] A. J. Vorwald, Occup. Med., 5, 684 (1948).
[110] A. J. Vorwald, Pheumoconiosis—Leroy U. Gardner Memorial Volume (A. J. Vorwald, ed.), Paul B. Hoeber, New York, 1950, p. 391.
[111] A. J. Vorwald, Use of Nonhuman Primates in Drug Evaluation (H. Vagtborg, ed.), University of Texas Press, Austin, 1968, p. 222.
[112] A. J. Vorwald, P. C. Pratt, and E. J. Urban, Acta Unio Internat. Contra Cancrum, 11, 735 (1955).
[113] A. J. Vorwald and A. L. Reeves, Acta Unio Internat. Contra Cancrum, 15, 715 (1959).
[114] A. J. Vorwald and A. L. Reeves, Arch. Indust. Health, 19, 190 (1959).
[115] B. H. Waksman, Arch. Indust. Health, 19, 154 (1959).
[116] H. T. Walworth, Indust. Med. Surg., 18, 428 (1949).
[117] H. H. Weber and W. E. Engelhardt, Zbl. Gewerbehyg., 10, 41 (1933).
[118] M. R. White, A. J. Finkel, and J. Schubert, J. Pharmacol. Exptl. Therap., 102, 88 (1951).
[119] W. J. Williams, J. Grey, and E. Pioli, Brit. Med. J., 1972-4, 175.
[120] H. P. Witschi, Lab. Invest., 19, 67 (1968).
[121] H. P. Witschi, Biochem. J., 120, 623 (1970).
[122] H. P. Witschi and W. N. Aldridge, Biochem. J., 106, 811 (1968).
[123] F. Wöhler, Ann. Phys., 13, 577 (1828).
[124] H. Zorn and H. Diem, Zentr. Arbeitsmed. Arbeitsschutz, 24, 3 (1974).
[125] E. Zschunke and H. Folesky, Der Hautarzt, 20, 403 (1969).

XAD-2 Resin Drug Extraction Methods for Biologic Samples

ABRAHAM STOLMAN, Ph.D.

Connecticut State Department of Health
Toxicology Laboratory
Hartford, Connecticut

and

University of Connecticut
School of Medicine
Farmington, Connecticut

PATRICIA A. F. PRANITIS, B.A.

Connecticut State Department of Health
Toxicology Laboratory
Hartford, Connecticut

The compelling need for rapid mass screening techniques for drugs of abuse in urine samples stimulated the search for newer, rapid, efficient, and inexpensive extraction methods. The area of greatest promise has been the use of ion-exchange papers[1], ion-exchange resins, and nonionic resins with the nonionic resin Amberlite XAD-2 appearing to have the greatest overall potential for this purpose at the present time.

The toxicology laboratory today is required to analyze, in addition to autopsy material, multiple samples for drugs of abuse and patient samples when a drug overdose is suspected. The development of the XAD-2 resin column procedure has broadened the toxicologist's capabilities to perform rapid and accurate drug analyses with the advantage of economy.

DESCRIPTION OF XAD-2 RESIN

Amberlite XAD-2 nonionic resin is a synthetic crosslinked polystyrene polymer and is supplied as 20-50 mesh beads.* Because of its high surface area and nonionic character, it has the ability to adsorb many water soluble compounds mainly by van der Waals forces, hydrophobic bonding, and dipole-dipole interactions. During the process of adsorption, the hydrophobic portion of the molecule is preferentially adsorbed onto the surface of the resin while the hydrophilic portion of the molecule remains oriented in the aqueous phase. Recovery of the adsorbed substance is then accomplished without difficulty by elution with selected organic solvents. The XAD-2 resin can be regenerated by proper rehydration and can be reused repeatedly.

COLUMNS

Several types of commercial and "home made" columns have been described for XAD-2 chromatography. Brinkmann Instruments, Inc.† have prepared a Drug-Skreen kit containing an adsorbent cartridge with XAD-2 resin, buffer, and solvent. The columns are elaborately constructed with sample reservoir, cotton plugs, adsorbent cartridge, filter cartridge, and phase separating filters, all of which may contribute to drug loss. Pranitis et al. [4] describe glass columns 30 cm high and 1.5 cm in diameter. These columns are constructed so that the bottom end is funnel shaped with glass stem attached (4 cm × 0.5 cm). A plug of glass wool inserted in the bottom of the column retains the XAD-2 bed and helps to control the flow rate. These investigators used resin beds 15 to 20 cm high (12 to 20 gm XAD-2), whereas most others report using much shorter columns [5-7]. In general, the drug-containing fluid is passed through the XAD-2 resin bed where the drug adsorption process takes place. The drugs are then eluted from the resin bed with an appropriate organic solvent. In most instances the resin bed is then washed with sufficient water to regenerate it for further use.

---

*Rohm and Haas, Philadelphia, Pa.
†Westbury, N.Y.

RESIN PREPARATION

Prior to use in the extraction of biologic materials, XAD-2 resin should be washed thoroughly to remove any extraneous organic material that may interfere with TLC. Several different procedures for washing the resin have been used by various investigators, all of which are suitable and give good results.

1. Fujimoto and Wang [2] first rinsed the resin with 5% sodium chloride and 1% sodium carbonate solution to control bacteria and mold growth. Before use the XAD-2 was washed with at least four bed volumes of distilled water.
2. Wislocki et al. [5] placed approximately 150 gm of resin in a 4000-ml beaker and rinsed it repeatedly with 150 ml of methanol until clear. The resin was then rinsed twice with 150 ml of 5% sodium chloride solution followed by two washes with 150 ml of 1% sodium carbonate solution. Finally the XAD-2 was rinsed three times with a volume of distilled water equal to ten times the bed volume of the resin. The resin was then stored under methanol and water (30:70) in a refrigerator.
3. In the Mulé et al. [6] method, the resin was washed, with stirring, four times with four bed volumes of acetone, three times with three volumes of methanol, and three times with three volumes of distilled water.

DRUG SCREENING IN URINE

Fujimoto and Wang [2] were one of the first investigators to describe a simple procedure for the extraction of narcotic analgesics from urine with XAD-2 resin. The method consisted simply of pouring the urine sample through a column bed of XAD-2 resin on which adsorption of drug(s) takes place and then eluting the drug(s) from the resin with methanol. The organic solvent was then evaporated and the residue analyzed by thin layer chromatography. Their early work showed that urinary pigments were also adsorbed onto the resin and were eluted in the same fraction as the drugs and their metabolites. Thus, the peak in color intensity also corresponded to the fraction containing the greatest amount of drugs and their metabolites.

Urine samples from patients on therapeutic doses of narcotic analgesics were analyzed for meperidine, codeine, methadone, morphine, levorphanol, pentazocine, and dihydromorphinone. All urines examined were shown to contain alkaloids, although there was a 23% error of incorrect identification. Sensitivity of the method was determined only for morphine and was shown to detect 6 μg of morphine per 10 ml of urine.

Mulé et al. [6] further developed the resin column method for drugs

TABLE 1. Percent Recoveries of Drugs from XAD-2 Resin by Several Elution Techniques

Drug	Elution solvents employed				
	$CHCl_3$: isopropanol (3:1) [6]	Acetone-$CHCl_3$:methanol (3:1) [8]	Ethylacetate-methanol [4]	Ethylacetate:1,2 dichloroethane (6:4) [9]	$CHCl_3$:isopropanol (3:1) [11]
Acetylsalicylic acid		3.0[a]			
Amitriptyline					73[b]
Amobarbital		89.2	93.0[c]	89.0[d]	
Amphetamine	49.3[e]	90.5			
Caffeine	91.3	75.5	88.7		
Cocaine	91.6	90.6			
Codeine		88.9		100.0	
Colchicine			96.0		
Diphenylhydantoin					63
Imipramine					64
Meperidine	88.9	88.9			
Meprobamate	74.4	83.8			
Mescaline	72.9	83.0			
Methadone	55.5	93.2		93.0	
Methaqualone			90.0		
Morphine	64.0	85.0	92.0	93.0	63

Nalorphine		91.1			
Naloxone		86.9			
Nicotine	29.0				
Pentobarbital	88.4	86.4			
Phenobarbital	83.1		98.7	73.0	
Propoxyphene					76
Quinine					64
Secobarbital		92.4			60
Thioridazine			78.6		

[a] 1 to 30 μg of drug/ml of urine. A 25-ml aliquot of urine was processed.
[b] 0.05 to 2.50 mg of drug were added to a 60-ml sample of stomach contents.
[c] 2 to 5 μg of drug/ml of blood. Ten milliliters of blood was used. Six to 250 μg of drug per 20 gm of tissue were processed.
[d] 100 μg of drug were added to 25 ml of water.
[e] 2 μg of drug/ml of urine. A 20-ml sample of urine was processed.

of abuse in urine. These investigators used commercially prepared columns with a flow control apparatus. Elution of the resin was accomplished with chloroform:isopropanol (3:1). The organic solvent was then shaken with 1 ml of a saturated sodium bicarbonate solution. The aqueous phases were removed and the solvent evaporated for TLC. Extensive recovery studies were done, including most drugs of abuse (Table 1). It was also found that increasing the volume of eluting solvent increased the percent recovery as did controlling the flow rate of the columns.

Wislocki et al. [5] utilized the XAD-2 resin for drug screening in urine with an additional step for the removal of urinary pigments from the extract. Buffered urine (approximately pH 8.0) was passed through the resin for adsorption of drugs. The resin was then washed with 10 ml of 15% ethanol in water. This wash removed most of the urinary pigments, which occasionally made identification of the drugs on the TLC plate difficult. Although the ethanol wash reduced drug recovery, these investigators felt that the improved TLC selectivity and sensitivity more than compensated for this fact. This judgment may be valid for analysts involved in qualitative aspects of toxicologic analysis; however, if quantitation of patient samples is important, the ethanol wash should be eliminated. If the final residue from the column eluate appears to be unsuitable for analysis, a simple "clean up" procedure described by Pranitis, Milzoff, and Stolman [4] may be included before any chromatographic or instrumental analysis is undertaken.

DRUG ANALYSIS IN BIOLOGIC FLUIDS AND TISSUE

Until now, utilization of the XAD-2 resin extraction procedure was limited to analysis of urine. Recently Missen and Lewin [3, 10] extended the XAD-2 resin method to extracting drugs from blood. In their procedure a 5-ml sample of blood was diluted to 20 ml with water and then stirred with 3 ml of an XAD-2 resin slurry for 1 hr. The mixture was then filtered and the drugs eluted from the resin with 3 × 10 ml redistilled acetone. The solvent was then evaporated for analysis. The drug recovered by the XAD-2 procedure was compared with solvent extraction and protein precipitation methods. Recovery studies with amobarbital, methaqualone, and amitriptyline were done by gas chromatography. Results showed that the XAD-2 procedure gave the most efficient recovery of all three drugs, gave the cleanest extract, and offered the least complicated technique.

Further extension of this method was described by Pranitis et al. [4] who applied the XAD-2 resin method for drug extraction from all biologic fluids such as blood, serum, urine, bile, gastric contents, and all tissues. The procedure is simple and rapid, and gives recoveries such that even therapeutic doses of drugs, which are reflected in the blood and urine levels, can be detected by thin layer chromatography procedures. Biologic samples were prepared for analysis as follows.

Urine—Five to 20 ml samples were adjusted to pH 7.5-8.0 with 10% NaOH.
Blood—Ten milliliters or more of blood were mixed with five volumes of water and this mixture agitated for 1 min to lyse the blood cells. The diluted blood was then filtered through Whatman No. 40 filter paper with suction.
Serum—Serum required no special preparation prior to analysis. After measuring the sample available, the pH was adjusted to 7.5-8.0 if necessary.
Bile—A 10-ml sample was mixed with one-tenth its volume of concentrated HCl and then autoclaved at 15 psi for 30 min. After cooling, the sample was filtered through Whatman No. 40 filter paper and the pH adjusted to approximately 7.5-8.0.
Gastric contents—To a 5-gm sample, 25 ml of distilled water were added and the mixture was homogenized for 30 sec in a blender. The homogenate was then filtered and the pH adjusted to 7.5-8.0.
Tissues—Fifty grams of tissue and 150 ml of water were homogenized in a blender for 30-45 sec. The homogenate was transferred to a beaker and 2 ml of concentrated HCl were added. The mixture was then placed on a steam table for 30 min. After cooling, the pH of the homogenate was adjusted to 7.5 to 8.0 with saturated and 10% NaOH. The sample was then centrifuged at 20,000 rpm for 10 min. The supernatant (water extract) was filtered through glass wool to remove any particulate matter. A second extract was prepared by suspending the tissue pellets in 100 ml of water and the suspension shaken vigorously in a 250-ml stoppered Ehrlenmeyer flask. This was then centrifuged again, filtered through glass wool, and combined with the first water extract.

The samples were poured through XAD-2 resin columns followed by a water wash. Elution of drugs was accomplished by washing the resin with 60 ml ethyl acetate followed by 60 ml methanol. Some biologic samples presented a problem in that the final extract was not suitably clean for immediate qualitative analysis. Hydrolyzed bile and urine and occasionally tissue extracts were therefore subjected to a simple "clean up" procedure. The residue was taken up in 3-5 ml of water and extractions at pH 3 and pH 8.5-9 were performed with chloroform and chloroform:isopropanol (3:1), respectively.

A comparison of recoveries from the XAD-2 tissue method and several solvent extraction procedures are shown in Table 1. The XAD-2 procedure gave drug recoveries ranging from 50 to 493% greater than the other methods. In addition, a mild steam table hydrolysis of the tissue before XAD-2 extraction resulted in higher drug yields varying from 30 to 206%.

TABLE 2. Effect of Dilution on Recovery of Drugs from Bile (% recovered)[a]

	Volume of water added, ml				
Drug	0	10	20	40	80
Morphine	58	72	81	78	70
Codeine	55	68	73	80	79
Methadone	21	44	53	70	93
Amobarbital	29	57	72	95	104
Phenobarbital	57	84	100	110	113

[a]All drugs studied in 5-ml bile containing 100 μg drug. Recoveries corrected for determined XAD-2 and TLC losses.

Additional research was reported by Caplan [9] who modified the method for drug analysis of bile by XAD-2 extraction. Five to 10 ml of bile were diluted to 25 ml with water, 1.25 ml of concentrated H_2SO_4 were added, and the mixture autoclaved for 20 min (15-18 psi, 120°C). After autoclaving, the sample was filtered; the filtrate was buffered to pH 8-8.5 with 40% NaOH and solid $NaHCO_3$. The sample was then passed through a column of XAD-2. Drugs were eluted with a mixture of ethylacetate:1,2 dichloroethane (6:4). The recoveries from bile were shown to be dependent on the volume of water added to the sample and varied by as much as 70% (see Table 2).

The most recent application of the XAD-2 resin procedure was formulated by Ibrahim et al. [11]. The method involves a basic application of the Stas-Otto [15] procedure for tissue samples and the incorporation of a dialysis procedure for stomach contents.

A tissue sample of 500 gm was homogenized with 500 ml water; the slurry was acidified with 3 ml of saturated tartaric acid solution and the steam distilled. The distillate was reserved for the analysis of volatile poisons, and the remaining tissue slurry was filtered through filter paper. The residue was washed with 500 ml acetone, which was combined with the aqueous fraction; the mixture was filtered and evaporated to a volume of approximately 100 ml. This fraction was further processed for the analysis of pesticides. The filtrate from the distillation residue was evaporated to about 100 ml. Proteins were precipitated by the addition of 95% ethanol and the alcohol-water solution evaporated to remove excess alcohol. The residue was taken up with 100 ml hot water, adjusted to pH 8.5-9.0, and passed through the XAD-2 resin column. Drugs were eluted with 2 × 10 ml chloroform: isopropanol (3:1). Ten milliliters of methanol were passed through the column for the elution of drugs of high polarity.

Stomach Contents and Blood

Stomach contents or blood were diluted to about twice their volume with distilled water. The solution was acidified, placed on a steam bath for 15 min, cooled, and filtered. The filtrate was adjusted to pH 8.5-9.0 and passed through the XAD-2 column. When the stomach contents contained large amounts of solid food, the contents were dialyzed against distilled water for 1.5 hr. twice. The sample was then adjusted to pH 8.5-9.0 and dialyzed twice again. The dialysates were combined, adjusted to pH 8.5-9.0, and passed through the XAD-2 column. The authors' data show that most of the drugs were recovered in the first two acid dialysates. Total recoveries of drugs after dialysis and XAD-2 extraction varied from 60-76%.

The above procedure seems to be more tedious and complicated than that of Pranitis et al. [4]. The method involves some very time-consuming steps, such as dialysis and protein precipitation, which undoubtedly involve drug loss, thus low recoveries.

DIFFERENTIAL ELUTION OF XAD-2 RESIN

All the methods described up to this point elute all classes of drugs (acid, basic, and neutral) in the same fraction. Thin layer chromatography of the residue necessitates the use of a spray sequence to detect all or nearly all types of drugs. With this technique the analyst must be especially competent in the utilization of a long sequence of sprays, particularly when drug concentrations approach the limits of detection. An alternative would be to spot several plates with the same unknown and thus reduce the number of sprays applied to each plate. The alternative to general desorption and sequential spray reagents was a differential elution technique presented by Bastos et al. [12] in which the acid and basic drugs were desorbed from the column in separate fractions. After passing urine through the XAD-2 column, the resin was treated with 10 ml of isopropyl ether, which was collected in a centrifuge tube containing 0.1 N hydrochloric acid. The tubes were shaken, and after freezing the aqueous layer the solvent remained. The ether was evaporated and the residue contained primarily acid and neutral drugs. The column was then eluted with two 10-ml aliquots of chloroform:isopropanol (3:1), which was collected in the tube containing the frozen acidic aqueous phase. One milliliter of 0.125 M borax was then added, the tube shaken, and the organic solvent separated and evaporated. This residue contained basic and some neutral drugs. This fraction contained mostly basic drugs except for some meprobamate and small amounts of barbiturates.

A different type of differential elution technique without any extraction steps was developed by Pranitis and Stolman [13]. After the sample was passed through the column, the drugs were eluted in four consecutive steps. First, 30 ml of 0.05 M sodium acetate buffer, pH 4.5, was run through the resin bed and discarded. Then acid and neutral drugs were eluted with 5 × 20 ml of chloroform. The column was then washed with 30 ml of 0.1 M potassium carbonate, pH 11.6, which was discarded. Basic drugs were then eluted from the column with 5 × 20 ml of chloroform:isopropanol (3:1). The sensitivity of detection by thin layer chromatography was 0.5 μg/ml for all drugs tested.

ADDITIONAL STUDIES AND MODIFICATIONS

Miller et al. [14] carried out some extensive studies on the efficiency of XAD-2 resin extraction of morphine from urine. Urine spiked with radioactive morphine was adjusted to pH 9 with NH_4Cl buffer and passed through the resin column followed by a wash with distilled water. The urine and water were analyzed for radioactivity. The resin was then eluted with ethyl acetate/1,2-dichlorethane (3:2), which was also analyzed for radioactivity. Several parameters were then varied and studied with the following results:

1. Both adsorption and desorption of morphine was found to vary with urinary pH. A pH of 8.5 ± 1.0 was found to be optimal for overall morphine extraction from urine.
2. The effect of urine flow rate on morphine adsorption was studied by passing the urine through the resin column at flow rates varying from 0.74 to 7.5 ml/min. Maximum adsorption of morphine by the resin occurred when flow rates were less than 2 ml/min.
3. It was found that as the volume of urine passing through the resin column increased, the efficiency of morphine adsorption decreased.
4. The desorption of morphine from the resin varied with eluant volume and flow rate. Maximal elution of morphine from the resin occurred when the eluant to resin ratio was greater than 10 ml/gm.

Further similar studies on the extraction of amphetamine and phenobarbital from XAD-2 resin were done by Kullberg et al. [7]. The XAD-2 resin columns were wetted before use with NH_4Cl buffer and passed through the column followed by a wash with distilled water. Amphetamine was eluted with isopropanol/ethyl acetate/dichloroethane (25:45:30) and phenobarbital was eluted with ethyl acetate/dichloroethane (3:2). The extraction of both amphetamine and phenobarbital with XAD-2 resin was found to vary with urinary pH. Maximum extraction efficiency for amphetamine was achieved between pH 6.5 and 12.5 and for phenobarbital between pH 2.5 and 5.0. Maximum adsorption efficiency for amphetamine occurred for flow rates between 0.75 and 4 ml/min and for phenobarbital only at a rate less than 0.5 ml/min. Adsorption of amphetamine was not affected by varying urine (ml) to resin (gm) ratios. However, adsorption of phenobarbital proved to be greatly dependent on this parameter. By varying the amount of eluting solvent it was found that elution efficiency of both amphetamine and phenobarbital was increased with increased solvent volume and decreasing solvent flow rate.

It is clear from these studies that variation of many parameters is possible when extracting drugs with XAD-2 resin. Adsorption and desorption efficiency of different drugs may be highly dependent on certain conditions, whereas other drugs may behave in nearly the same manner even when these conditions are changed significantly. However, maximal overall extraction efficiency for all types of drugs can possibly be attained by utilizing appropriate flow rates, urine volume, eluting solvent volume, and a recommended urine pH of 8.5 ± 1.0.

SUMMARY

The XAD-2 resin extraction procedure is rapidly becoming an important tool for both the clinical and forensic toxicology laboratory. Although different investigators use different elution solvents and techniques, the basic procedure is to adsorb drugs onto the XAD-2 resin and then elute these drugs with an appropriate organic solvent. A number of parameters have been shown to be involved in obtaining good results. These include pH of sample, flow rate, type and volume of eluting solvent. These parameters can be adjusted so that maximum overall drug recoveries are obtained.

Since XAD-2 extraction of urine by Fujimoto and Wang [2] was introduced, the procedure has been extended to all types of biologic specimens. Various elution techniques have been reported [12, 13], namely, the differential elution of drugs from the resin into acid and neutral, and basic drug fractions. Overall, the techniques vary from rapid simple procedures for drugs of abuse in urine to more elaborate methods of extraction of autopsy material. The extraction procedure itself is flexible enough so as to suit the needs of almost any toxicology laboratory.

REFERENCES

[1] V. P. Dole, W. Kyun Kim, and I. Eglitis, Detection of narcotic drugs, tranquilizers, amphetamines, and barbiturates in urine, JAMA, 198, 115 (1966).

[2] J. M. Fujimoto and R. I. H. Wang, A method of identifying narcotic analgesics in human urine after therapeutic doses, Toxicol. Appl. Pharmacol., 16, 186 (1970).

[3] A. W. Missen and J. F. Lewin, A non-ionic resin extraction of drugs in blood, Clin. Chim. Acta, 53, 389 (1974).

[4] P. A. F. Pranitis, J. R. Milzoff, and A. Stolman, Extraction of drugs from biofluids and tissues with XAD-2 resin, J. Forensic Sci., 19, 917 (1974).

[5] A. Wislocki, P. Martel, R. Ito, W. S. Dunn, and C. D. McGuire, A method for the detection of drugs of abuse in urine, Health Lab. Sci., 11, 13 (1974).

[6] S. J. Mulé, M. L. Bastos, D. Jukofsky, and E. Saffer, Routine identification of drugs of abuse in human urine. II. Development and application of the XAD-2 resin column method, J. Chromatogr., 63, 289 (1971).

[7] M. P. Kullberg, W. L. Miller, F. J. McGowan, and B. P. Doctor, Studies on the single extraction of amphetamine and phenobarbitol from urine using XAD-2 resin, Biochem. Med., 7, 323 (1973).

[8] M. P. Kullberg and C. W. Garodetzky, Studies on the use of XAD-2 resin for detection of abused drugs in urine, Clin. Chem., 20, 177 (1974).

[9] Y. H. Caplan, personal communication, April, 1975.

[10] A. W. Missen and J. F. Lewin, A non-ionic resin extraction of drugs in glood, Clin. Chim. Acta, 53, 389 (1974).

[11] G. Ibrahim, S. Andryouskas, and M. L. Bastos, Application of Amberlite XAD-2 resin for general toxicological analysis, J. Chromatogr., 108, 107 (1975).

[12] M. L. Bastos, D. Jukofsky, and S. J. Mulé, Routine identification of drugs of abuse in human urine. III. Differential elution of the XAD-2 resin, J. Chromatogr., 81, 93 (1973).

[13] P. A. F. Pranitis and A. Stolman, The differential elution of drugs from XAD-2 resin, J. Forensic Sci., 20, 726 (1975).

[14] W. L. Miller, M. P. Kullberg, M. E. Banning, L. D. Brown, and B. P. Doctor, Studies on the quantitative extraction of morphine from urine using non-ionic XAD-2 resin, Biochem. Med., 7, 145 (1973).

Safety Testing of Fragrances: Problems and Implications

DONALD L. J. OPDYKE, Ph.D.

Research Institute for Fragrance Materials, Inc.
Englewood Cliffs, New Jersey

INTRODUCTION

Fragrance materials have been a part of the skin's environment since before recorded history. The materials themselves change somewhat with the times, but many of the currently employed fragrance materials date from the third millenium B.C. and Biblical references abound.

Not only have fragrances been used by human beings for much of our life's history but they are ubiquitous. From the baby products that are our first exposure, to the embalming fluids and cosmetics used at death, humans are exposed to fragrance materials. Cosmetics, indeed, are not the only exposure. In addition, fragrances are found in household and garden sprays, room fresheners, floor waxes and furniture polishes, insect repellents, bathroom cleansers, scouring powders, oven cleaners, shoe polish, incense, sachets, pommanders, and tobacco.

When one considers the long history of the use of fragrances, their broad distribution, and our length of exposure to them, one is impressed with the very few examples of injury to humans that can be attributed to these materials. The only problems reported have been occasional rashes on the skin and even more specifically, light-induced rashes.

And yet there is a persistent myth in the cosmetic industry that any problem encountered in the safety testing of a new cosmetic must be attributed to the fragrance component. Only by a systematic screening of all the materials used in fragrances by an independent scientific body and the systematic and voluntary zealous response by the industry to eliminate potential offenders can dispel this myth.

The Research Institute for Fragrance Materials, Inc., an international nonprofit organization, was established in 1966 by the industry to carry out research on the many ingredients employed in perfumery. At present, RIFM is supported by 48 of these companies, representing nearly 97% of the industry in the United States, Europe, and Japan. The sole purpose of RIFM is to assure the safety of perfumery raw materials.

The Board of Directors is composed of the chief executive officers of the member companies, elected at an annual meeting. In order to ensure an independent scientific status for the Institute, it is structured so that the only link between the administrative branches and the scientific arms is the president, who performs a dual role as scientist and administrator. The president has available to him the advice of a Scientific Advisory Committee composed of perfumers, research scientists, and analytical chemists drawn from the fragrance industry. Judgments in matters pertaining to the evaluation of safety are made completely independently by a panel of experts, who are toxicologists, pharmacologists, or dermatologists drawn from the academic world and have no connection whatever with the fragrance industry.

MATERIALS

Fragrance raw materials are derived from many geographical, natural, and chemical sources. Any program of safety evaluation has to consider the origin of the materials, types of uses, and the concentrations used.

First of all, some definitions. This is necessary because some of the terminology as used in the fragrance industry is different from that used elsewhere. Every industry has its own jargon.

Fragrance Material

1. An essential oil produced by solvent extraction or distillation of a plant or flower—or of an animal part or product. Example: anise oil.

2. A part of that essential oil, e.g., an absolute which is the alcohol extractable part or other fraction called an "isolate." Example: orange flower absolute. Citral ex-lemongrass oil.

3. A gum, a natural exudation of a plant—usually acidic solids. Example: olibanum or frankincense.

4. Something made in an organic chemistry plant—an aroma chemical. These constitute the bulk of the raw materials used in perfumery. Example: cyclohexyl acetaldehyde.

Fragrance Specialty

A combination by a perfumer, an artist, as a basic working tool. This may consist of 80 to 150 raw materials and is characterized as a specific company's woodsy, mossy, or floral, or oriental, or rose, or muguet, tabac, leather, etc. Usually, the composition of these compounds is a closely guarded secret—arrived at only after years of creative expertise. They are rarely sold.

Fragrance Oil

A fragrance oil is a finished fragrance that might be made from various admixtures of these specialties to produce a desired fragrance. This would later be diluted with alcohol to produce a perfume, diluted more for a cologne or toilet water, and especially adapted for use in soaps, aerosols, etc. It would not be the same formulation for all these applications—to smell the same in each use; it has to be adapted for the particular vehicle.

An elegant perfume that one might purchase at a boutique is a very complex mixture of natural and synthetic materials and may easily contain as many as 600 raw materials, many of which are also components of flavors.

The Research Institute for Fragrance Materials is conducting its program only on the starting raw materials. These are carefully selected by a Scientific Advisory Committee consisting of perfumers, analytical chemists, and research directors—all drawn from the fragrance industry.

The raw materials are selected on the basis of the following criteria: (a) they must be representative of the material in actual use by the industry; (b) they must conform to the specifications and standards, if any, of the Essential Oil Association of the United States (EOA), or of the International Fragrance Association (IFRA); (c) they must be supplied to the RIFM without indication of the supplier, with name and an identification number only; (d) they must be accompanied by gas-chromatographic, ultraviolet or infrared curves to "thumb-print" the materials.

The specifications and standards in the monographs will be those of the EOA, where available. The levels of usage reported are the result of an industry-wide survey.

METHODS

The chief parameters selected for toxicological screening of all of these materials include tests for allergenicity and phototoxicity on human skin; tests for general toxicity in animals by the oral and dermal route, and other procedures where required by a panel of experts drawn from outside the industry.

Doctor Leon Golberg has made the following comment with respect to the methodologies involved.

"Close relationships have traditionally existed between the use in fragrances of essential oils, balsams and spices and the therapeutic and even culinary applications of many of these same ingredients. During the past century, the introduction of many synthetic, often nature-identical, components has maintained the links between flavorings for foods and drugs on the one hand and fragrances for personal and household use on the other. Despite these similarities in regard to the use of certain basic components, the fragrances differ in many important respects. The most obvious of these is the predominance of skin contact in the case of fragrances, with the attendant issues of primary irritation, percutaneous absorption, and immediate and delayed hypersensitivity, as well as the possibilities of phototoxic and photoallergic responses. On a long-term basis, the question of skin carcinogenesis has been raised, although no evidence is apparent for such a potential hazard stemming from this source. Beyond the local effects at the sites of skin contact, fragrance components that are absorbed through the skin are, of course, capable of exercising systemic effects. Conceivably, systemic action may result from absorption through the respiratory system.

"In theory, therefore, the attainment of that Nirvana-like state of perfection—demonstration of virtually absolute safety—demands an immense effort, embracing not only each individual fragrance ingredient but also each finished product that incorporates a fragrance containing that component. The complexities of fragrances are not the outcome of a conspiracy to 'soak' the consumer: they are an essential basis of a highly skilled art that seeks to create aromatic loveliness appropriate to the particular circumstances of use, while satisfying the exacting technical requirements that have to be met in a wide variety of products. As long as we seek to pander to our aesthetic susceptibilities, and not to outrage them, highly complex fragrances are inescapable and, indeed, play a most important role in a wide range of consumer goods.

"Facing up to the facts of real life, one has to establish priorities for safety evaluation in regard to the fragrance components being tested and the tests that are most necessary." [1]

When each raw material arrives at the Institute, a retain sample is taken and the rest is sent out to various commercial laboratories for testing. A sample in petrolatum is prepared by the Institute for repeated insult patch testing [2], or maximization testing [3, 4] on human skin using, where feasible, a tenfold exaggeration of the maximum use level to which human skin could be exposed.

Acute oral and acute dermal LD_{50}s are determined as a general measure of toxicity and, wherever pertinent, a test for phototoxicity to human skin is included. The results of these preliminary data are reviewed by the panel of experts, who decide whether additional work is indicated. The panel of experts consists of internationally recognized dermatologists, pharmacologists, and pathologists having interests in toxicology.

In the course of testing these materials, it was found that the Kligman Maximization Test gave more uniformly reproducible and consistent results in the hands of two testing facilities than the repeated insult patch procedure. Consequently, this was chosen as the preferred test for potential allergenicity. In this procedure four materials are tested on each subject. It was learned the hard way that each of these materials had to be completely unrelated; that is, one cannot test two essential oils, two acetate esters, etc., in the same group.

Typical test groupings might be:

Group I	Group II
Citronella oil (Java)	Citronella oil (Ceylon)
Aldehyde C-11 undecylic	Aldehyde C-11 undecylenic
Allyl caproate	Allyl cyclohexyl propionate
Musk xylol	Musk tibetene

All of these materials would be tested at a ten times highest use level. For example, if a material has the following concentrations in final products that can come into contact with human skin, it will be the highest one multiplied by ten, where feasible, that determines the level used for maximization testing. For example:

Concentration in final product (%):

	Soap	Detergent	Creams, Lotions	Perfume
Usual	0.01	0.002	0.005	0.09
Maximum	0.15	0.024	0.03	0.20

In this case, 20%. This gives a considerable exaggeration of exposure. When tested in this fashion, the test becomes a pass or fail test, any positive result is taken to disqualify a material from further use.

Tests are also carried out for potential phototoxicity to human skin by testing undiluted materials on the skin of hairless mice, swine, and humans by the procedures used by Urbach, using natural sunlight and the solar ultraviolet simulator [5].

ETHYL VANILLIN

Synonyms: 3-Ethoxy-4-hydroxybenzaldehyde; protocatechuic aldehyde-3-ethyl ether.
Structure:

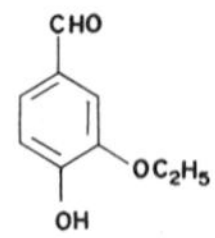

Description and physical properties: *Givaudan Index* (1961).
Occurrence: Has apparently not been reported to occur in nature.
Preparation: By ethylation of protocatechualdehyde (Bedoukian, 1967).
Uses: In public use since the 1930s. Use in fragrances in the USA amounts to less than 28,000 lb/yr.

Concentration in final product (%):

	Soap	*Detergent*	*Creams, lotions*	*Perfume*
Usual	0·01	0·003	0·003	0·12
Maximum	0·10	0·025	0·06	0·20

Analytical data: Gas chromatogram, RIFM no. 70–11; infra-red curve, RIFM no. 70–11.

Status

Ethyl vanillin was granted GRAS status by FEMA (1965) and is approved by the FDA for food use (GRAS). The Council of Europe (1970) listed ethyl vanillin, giving an ADI of 10 mg/kg. The *Food Chemicals Codex* (1972) and the *National Formulary* (1970) each has a monograph on ethyl vanillin and the Joint FAO/WHO Expert Committee on Food Additives (1967) has published a monograph and specifications for ethyl vanillin giving an unconditional ADI of 0–10 mg/kg.

Biological data

Acute toxicity. The acute oral LD_{50} value in rats was reported as >2000 mg/kg (Jenner, Hagan, Taylor, Cook & Fitzhugh, 1964) and the acute oral LD in rabbits as 3000 mg/kg (Deichmann & Kitzmuller, 1940). The sc LD in rats was reported as 1800 mg/kg (Deichmann & Kitzmuller, 1940). The ip LD_{50} was reported as 750 mg/kg in mice and as 1140 mg/kg in guinea-pigs, while the iv LD in dogs was reported as 760 mg/kg (Caujolle & Meynier, 1954).

Long-term toxicity. In feeding studies, 20 mg/kg body weight/day fed to rats for 18 wk produced no effects, while rats fed 64 mg/kg/day for 10 wk showed a reduction in growth rate and myocardial, renal, hepatic, lung, spleen and stomach injuries (Deichmann & Kitzmuller, 1940).

Neither 20,000 and 50,000 ppm fed to male rats in the diet for 1 yr nor 5000, 10,000 and 20,000 ppm fed to male and female rats in the diet for 2 yr produced any effects (Hagan, Hansen, Fitzhugh, Jenner, Jones, Taylor, Long, Nelson & Brouwer, 1967).

Irritation. Ethyl vanillin tested at 2% in petrolatum produced a mild irritation after a 48-hr closed-patch test in 25 human subjects (Kligman, 1970).

Sensitization. A maximization test (Kligman, 1966) was carried out on 25 volunteers. The material was tested at a concentration of 2% in petrolatum and produced no sensitization reactions (Kligman, 1970).

References

Bedoukian, P. Z. (1967). *Perfumery and Flavoring Synthetics.* 2nd ed., p. 344. Elsevier Publishing Co., New York.
Caujolle, F. & Meynier, D. (1954). *C.r. hebd. Seanc. Acad. Sci., Paris.* **238,** 2576.
Council of Europe (1970). Natural and Artificial Flavouring Substances. Partial Agreement in the Social and Public Health Field. List A(1), Series 1, no. 109, p. 54. Strasbourg.
Deichmann, W. & Kitzmuller, K. (1940). *J. Am. pharm. Ass.,* **29,** 425.
Flavoring Extract Manufacturers' Association (1965). Survey of flavoring ingredient usage levels. No. 2464. *Fd Technol., Champaign* **19**(2), part 2, 155.
Food Chemicals Codex (1972). 2nd ed. Prepared by the Committee on Specifications, Food Chemicals Codex, of the Committee on Food Protection. p. 303. National Academy of Sciences–National Research Council Publ. 1406, Washington, D.C.
Givaudan Index (1961). *Specifications of Synthetics and Isolates for Perfumery.* 2nd ed., p. 155. Givaudan-Delawanna, Inc., New York.
Hagan, E. C., Hansen, W. H., Fitzhugh, O. G., Jenner, P. M., Jones, W. I., Taylor, Jean M., Long, Eleanor L., Nelson, A. A. & Brouwer, J. B. (1967). Food flavourings and compounds of related structure. II. Subacute and chronic toxicity. *Fd Cosmet. Toxicol.* **5,** 141.
Jenner, P. M., Hagan, E. C., Taylor, Jean M., Cook, E. L. & Fitzhugh, O. G. (1964). Food flavourings and compounds of related structure. I. Acute oral toxicity. *Fd Cosmet. Toxicol.* **2,** 327.
Joint FAO/WHO Expert Committee on Food Additives (1967). Toxicological Evaluation of Some Flavouring Substances and Non-nutritive Sweetening Agents. *F.A.O. Nutr. Mtg Rep. Ser. no.* 44A, Geneva. p. 39. WHO/Food Add./68.33.
Kligman, A. M. (1966). The identification of contact allergens by human assay. III. The maximization test. A procedure for screening and rating contact sensitizers. *J. invest. Derm.* **47,** 393.
Kligman, A. M. (1970). Report to RIFM. 2 December.
National Formulary (1970). 13th ed. Prepared by the National Formulary Board. p. 303. American Pharmaceutical Association, Washington, D.C.

FIG. 1. Monograph on ethyl vanillin. Reprinted from Food and Cosmetic Toxicology by permission of the publisher.

RESULTS

Monographs on the individual fragrance raw materials are being published in alphabetical order as a regular feature of Food and Cosmetics Toxicology. A characteristic monograph showing its format is shown in Fig. 1.

The monographs with unfavorable results are published along with the favorable ones. Prepublication copies go to the FDA, CTFA, and member companies. To date, over 348 of these monographs, favorable and unfavorable, have been published or accepted for publication [7]. Among them are:

Abies alba oil from cones
Abies alba oil from needles
Acetaldehyde diethyl acetal
Acetaldehyde-ethyl-trans-3-hexenyl acetal
Acetate C-7
Acetate C-8
Acetate C-9
Acetate C-10
Acetophenone
Acetyl carene
5-Acetyl-1,1,2,3,3,6-hexamethyl indan
Alcohol C-6
Alcohol C-7
Alcohol C-8
Alcohol C-9
Alcohol C-10
Alcohol C-11
Alcohol C-12
Alcohol C-14 myristic
Aldehyde C-6
Aldehyde C-7
Aldehyde C-8
Aldehyde C-9
Aldehyde C-10
Aldehyde C-11 undecylenic
Aldehyde C-11 undecylic
Aldehyde C-12 lauric
Aldehyde C-12 MNA
Aldehyde C-14 myristic
Allyl caproate
Allyl cyclohexyl propionate
Allyl-alpha-ionone
Allyl phenoxy acetate
Ambrette seed oil
Ambrettolide
Amyl benzoate
Amyl cinnamate
alpha-Amyl cinnamic alcohol
Amyl cinnamic aldehyde
Amyl cinnamic aldehyde diethyl acetal
alpha-Amyl cinnamic aldehyde dimethyl acetal
4-tert-Amyl cyclohexanone
Amyl salicylate
Amyris oil acetylated
Anethole
Angelica root oil
Angelica seed oil
Anis star oil
Anise oil
Anisic aldehyde
Anisyl alcohol
Anisyl propionate
Anisylidene acetone
Armoise oil
Artemisia oil (wormwood)
Basil oil, sweet
Bay oil
Benzoin (resinoid)
Benzophenone
Benzyl acetate
Benzyl alcohol
Benzyl benzoate
Benzyl butyrate
Benzyl cinnamate
Benzyl formate
Benzylidene acetone
Benzyl isobutyrate
Benzyl isoeugenol
Benzyl isovalerate
Benzyl phenylacetate
Benzyl propionate
Benzyl salicylate
Bergamot oil expressed
Bergamot oil rectified
Birch tar oil
Bisabolene
Bois de rose acetylated
laevo-Bornyl acetate
Bornyl isovalerate
Bromstyrol
n-Butyl anthranilate
4-tert-Butyl cyclohexanol
p-t-Butyl cyclohexanone
Butyl isobutyrate
p-t-Butyl phenol
Cade oil
Cadinene
Camphene
Camphor oil white
Camphor oil yellow

Cananga oil
Caraway oil
Cardamom oil
delta-3-Carene
1-Carveol
1-Carvone
Caryophyllene
Caryophyllene acetate
Caryophyllene alcohol
Cassia oil
Castoreum
Cedar leaf oil
Cedarwood oil Virginia
Cedrenol
Cedrenyl acetate
Cedrol
Cedryl acetate
Celery seed oil
Chamomile oil German
Chamomile oil Roman
Cinnamic alcohol
Cinnamic aldehyde dimethyl acetal
Cinnamon bark oil
Cinnamon leaf oil
Cinnamyl acetate
Cinnamyl anthranilate
Cinnamyl cinnamate
Cinnamyl isovalerate
Cinnamyl propionate
Citral dimethyl acetal
Citronella oil
Citronellal
Citronellol
Citronellyl acetate
Citronellyl n-butyrate
Citronellyl formate
Citronellyl oxyacetaldehyde
Citronellyl propionate
Civet absolute
Clary sage oil
Clove bud oil
Clove stem oil
Cognac oil
Copaiba oil
Coriander oil
Costus root, essential oil, absolute and concrete
Coumarin
p-Cresol
p-Cresyl acetate
p-Cresyl isobutyrate
p-Cresyl methyl ether
p-Cresyl phenylacetate
Cumin oil
Cuminaldehyde
Cuminyl alcohol
Cyclamen aldehyde
Cyclohexanol
2-cyclohexyl cyclohexanone
Cyclohexyl ethyl acetate
Cyclohexyl ethyl alcohol
Cyclopentadecanolide
para Cymene
Cyste absolute
Decahydro-beta-naphthol
Decylenic alcohol
Diethyleneglycol monoethyl ether
Diethyleneglycol monomethyl ether
Dihydro anethole
Dihydrocoumarin
Dihydro jasmone
Dihydro myrcenol
Dihydrosafrole
Dihydro-alpha-terpineol
Dihydroterpinyl acetate
Dimethyl anthranilate
Dimethyl benzyl carbinol
Dimethyl benzyl carbinyl acetate
Dimethyl heptanal
Dimethyl heptenol
3,6-Dimethyl-3-octanol
3,7-Dimethyl-1-octanol
3,6-Dimethyl-3-octanyl acetate
Dimethyl phenyl ethyl carbinol
Dipentene
Diphenyl methane
Diphenyl oxide
Estragon oil
Ethyl acetate
Ethyl acetoacetate
Ethyl acrylate

Ethyl amyl ketone
Ethyl benzene
Ethyl benzoate
Ethyl butyrate
Ethyl cinnamate
Ethylene brassylate
Ethyl laurate
Ethyl maltol
Ethyl methyl phenyl glycidate
Ethyl octine carbonate
Ethyl phenyl acetate
Ethyl phenyl glycidate
Ethyl vanillin
Eucalyptol NF
Eucalyptus oil
Eugenol
Eugenyl acetate
Fennel oil
Fir balsam (Canadian)
Fir needle oil Canadian
Fir needle oil Siberian
Geraniol
Geranium oil Bourbon
Geranium oil Moroccan
Geranyl acetate
Geranyl benzoate
Geranyl butyrate
Geranyl crotonate
Geranyl formate
Geranyl isobutyrate
Geranyl phenylacetate
Geranyl propionate
Geranyl tiglate
Ginger oil
Grapefruit oil expressed
Guaiacwood acetate
Guaiacwood oil
Heliotropin
2-n-Heptyl cyclopentanone
Hexadecanolide
cis-3-Hexenol
trans-2-Hexenol
cis-3-Hexenyl acetate
Hexen-2-al
Hexyl acetate
Hexyl cinnamic aldehyde
n-Hexyl ethyl acetoacetate
Hexyl salicylate
Ho leaf oil
Hydratropic alcohol
Hydratropic aldehyde
Hydroabietyl alcohol
Hydroxycitronellal
Hydroxycitronellal dimethyl-acetal
Hydroxycitronellal-methyl anthranilate
Hydroxycitronellol
Indole
Ionone
alpha-Irone
Isoamyl acetate
Isoamyl propionate
Isobornyl acetate
Isobornyl propionate
Isobutyl benzoate
Isobutyl phenyl acetate
Isobutyl salicylate
Isoeugenol
Isoeugenyl acetate
Isopropyl quinoline
Isopulegol
Lemon oil distilled
Lemon oil expressed
Lime oil distilled
Lime oil expressed
d-limonene
Linalool
Linalyl formate
Linalyl isobutyrate
Linalyl methyl ether
Linalyl propionate
Maltol
Mentha arvensis oil
p-Methoxyacetophenone
o-Methoxy cinnamic aldehyde
4-(p-Methoxyphenyl)butan-2-one
Methyl abietate
p-Methylacetophenone
Methyl n-amyl ketone
Methyl anthranilate
Methyl benzoate
Methyl cinnamate
alpha-Methyl cinnamic alcohol

alpha-Methyl cinnamic aldehyde
Methyl diphenyl ether
Methyl ester of rosin
(partially hydrogenated)
Methyl eugenol
Methyl heptenone
Methyl hexyl ketone
Methyl ionone
Methyl isoeugenol
beta-Methyl naphthyl ketone
Methyl nonyl ketone
Methyl octine carbonate
Methyl phenylacetate
Mimosa absolute
Musk ambrette
Musk ketone
Musk tibetene
Musk xylol
beta-Naphthyl methyl ether
Nerolidol
Nerolin
gamma-Nonalactone
Nopyl acetate
Oakmoss concrete
Octyl isobutyrate
Orange oil expressed
Bitter orange oil
Origanum oil
Orris absolute
Palmarosa oil
Parsley seed oil
Pennyroyal oil Eurafrican
Peru balsam
Peru balsam oil
Phenethyl phenyl acetate
Phenoxyethyl isobutyrate
Phenyl acetaldehyde dimethyl
acetal
Phenyl acetic acid
Phenylethyl acetate
Phenylethyl alcohol
Phenylethyl benzoate
Phenylethyl formate
Phenylethyl isovalerate
Phenylethyl propionate
Phenylethyl tiglate
Phenylpropyl acetate
Phenylpropyl aldehyde
Phenylpropyl cinnamate
Pimenta leaf oil
Piperonyl acetate
Rhodinyl acetate
Rosemary oil
Rose absolute French
Rose oil Bulgarian
Rose oil Moroccan
Oil, rose otto, Turkish
Rue oil
Safrole
Sage oil Dalmatian
Sandalwood, oil, East Indian
alpha-Santalol
Santalyl acetate
Styrallyl alcohol
Terpineol
Terpinyl acetate
Terpinyl propionate
Thyme oil, red
Tonka absolute
Treemoss concrete
Trichloromethyl phenyl
carbinyl acetate
3,5,5-Trimethyl cyclohexanol
3,5,5-Trimethyl hexyl
acetate
gamma-Undecalactone
Veratraldehyde
Vetiver acetate
Vetiver oil
Ylang ylang oil

To date, all of the large volume items have been tested as well as those whose past reputations were questionable. Reprint lists are huge with copies going to health ministries worldwide and to the National Clearinghouse for Poison Control Centers. Out of 553 materials tested thus far, 21 have been found to be sensitizers and seven to have phototoxic properties. All of these are being investigated further and, if not already published, the results will be published as soon as feasible.

Among the allergens are:

Alantroot oil
Anisylidene acetone
Benzylidene acetone
p-t-Butyl phenol
Cassia oil
Cinnamon bark oil
Costus oil
Diethyl maleate
Dihydrocoumarin
Ethyl acrylate
Fennel oil, bitter
Hydroabietyl alcohol
Peru balsam

Among the phototoxic oils are to be found:

Angelica root oil
Bergamot expressed
Cumin oil
Lemon oil expressed
Lime oil expressed
Orange oil bitter
Rue oil

Maximization testing is not without its difficulties, one of which we call the "spillover effect." While others have referred to this before [4, 10], it becomes striking in its effect in the maximization procedure. In this test, four unrelated materials are tested on each of 25 human subjects. In the event one of the four test materials turns out to be an overwhelming sensitizer, false weak positive results may occur with the other three materials. When these three materials are subsequently retested out of the context of the serious allergen and in the same or different group of subjects, they prove to be negative.

For example, this was one result:

Material and concentration tested	Subjects sensitized
Costus oil, 4%	25/25
Jasmine absolute, 3%	2/25
Hydroxycitronellol, 10%	0/25
Amyris oil, high gravity, 10%	0/25

When the jasmine sample was retested out of the potent sensitizer context, it was found to be negative.

In another instance,

Material and concentration tested	Subjects sensitized
Phenylacetaldehyde, 2%	11/25
Phenylacetaldehyde dimethyl acetal, 2%	2/25
Butyl methyl hydrocinnamic aldehyde, 5%	9/25
Lemon oil, 10%	0/25

When the phenylacetaldehyde dimethyl acetal and butyl methyl hydrocinnamic aldehyde were repeated separately, they were unequivocally negative.

In another instance, one of the investigators doing maximization testing relocated his laboratories, going from a prison population of predominately male blacks to a university student population of mixed male and female—white, black, and Oriental individuals. The result was an increased susceptibility on the part of the new test subjects to the irritating effects of sodium lauryl sulfate (SLS) used as a pretreatment. Some false positive results were obtained which proved to be negative in repeated tests using lower concentrations of the SLS. Although considered insignificant, in the interest of completeness, these results are included in the pertinent monographs. This observation is explained in detail in a recent publication [4].

UNEXPLAINED OBSERVATIONS

In the course of maximization testing, three instances have arisen in which a pure aldehyde, isolated from a natural source, has proved to be a strong sensitizer. Upon examining the essential oil from which it was isolated, the oil did not induce sensitization even though the aldehyde was present in concentrations as high as 85%. It appeared that something in the natural oil was inhibiting the induction of sensitization. As a test of this hypothesis, several terpenes and alcohols, found along with the aldehyde in the natural composition were combined with the aldehydes in question. It appears now to be a consistent finding that these three aldehydes, although potent sensitizers per se, do not sensitize in selective 1:1 mixtures.

There is no suggestion at this point that this is anything more than an unexplained observation. The implications are that there may be materials that abort the induction of the allergic condition in the human. Do these key materials combine with aldehydes to form a new compound? Do they work with all aldehydes? Do they inhibit the penetration of the allergen through human skin? All allergens? Do they compete for binding sites on the cells responsible for the sensitization manifestation? Do they prevent the formation of haptens? The work in this fascinating area continues, and the results will be published as soon as available.

DISCUSSION

Marzulli and Maibach [8] have published a scholarly paper on the phototoxicity of perfumes and perfume ingredients. They attribute the phototoxic properties of bergamot oil to a single material—bergapten, or 5-methoxypsoralen. Now phototoxicity is related to primary irritation, and consequently, should produce the same response with every individual exposed. In fact, this is the case if all of the conditions are met for eliciting the phototoxic reaction: The stratum corneum must be adequately exposed to the material in order to allow opportunity for saturation, the material must contain an adequate concentration of phototoxic agent, and the skin must then be exposed to adequate intensity and frequency of ultraviolet light for an adequate length of time. Usually, this means exposure to solar radiation for an hour at least one-half hour after the application of the material but not longer than three hours after. If all of these conditions are met, 100% of the subjects should respond with the characteristic erythema, swelling, and subsequent hyperpigmentation.

We know that phototoxicity, like primary irritation, is concentration dependent and consequently, levels could be found for each of these materials for safe application to human skin. But it is not known if their individual properties in a given mixture are additive. Marzulli and Maibach conclude that levels of bergamot oil below 0.3% might be considered harmless. This would provide levels less than 0.001% of bergapten.

If these phototoxic materials are to be used at levels in which they do not evoke phototoxic skin responses, it would seem the only way to be assured of safety from possible additive phototoxicity in the finished compound or mixture would be to test the final product for phototoxicity. Probably the answer lies with the perfumer whether to employ them and test the end product, or to formulate with safer forms of the oils, that is, furocoumarin-free oils or distilled versions that have been shown to be free of the phototoxic agent.

Allergenicity is another problem, and it is difficult to predict. The methods for predictive testing in the human are not entirely satisfactory; but those in animals are completely unsatisfactory in our experience to date. The maximization test has provided the Research Institute more consistent, reliable, reproducible results than those of the repeated insult patch test. For fragrance materials, it is by far the method of choice. In addition, it minimizes the number of subjects at risk who may be made allergic to a material, 25 as compared with 200 in the repeated insult procedure.

Allergenicity is not as much a function of concentration as primary irritation or phototoxicity are. Certainly, many familiar with the methods of skin testing have observed that reducing the concentration of an offender may enable a negative test response to be obtained. However, if one repeats the exposure at the lower concentration for enough times, the same allergenic response will be observed. It appears that the number of exposures to an allergen is of greater significance than the actual concentration used. This was observed originally by Kligman [9], and we have confirmed this observation.

It would appear then that the only satisfactory program for dealing with known allergenic materials is to eliminate them completely from formulations that come into contact with the skin, or to use them only with extreme caution and continuous watchfulness over the complaint track record.

It is of interest here to note that both "natural" and "synthetic" materials are found among the allergens detected thus far.

Elimination of any single material from fragrances already made and sold, most of which have good safety records, is a considerable hardship to an industry. Certainly, these items can be eliminated from the palette of the artist in new creations. However, with an industry that has close to 5000 materials in its armamentarium, eliminating the few potential troublemakers is only good insurance.

The fact that the fragrance industry has been so relatively trouble-free may in part be attributable to the fact that many fragrance materials are also used in flavors. In sensitizing guinea pigs to dinitrochlorobenzene (DNCB), it has been observed that the development of cutaneous reaction may be effectively aborted by the prior administration of the DNCB as a component of the animal's diet.

This has also been observed in the human. This phenomenon of immunosuppression has been extensively reviewed by Lowney [11, 12]. Perhaps there would be more fragrance allergies if these same materials had not been used in flavors over the years. It is an interesting point for conjecture.

RIFM is pin-pointing fragrance materials with a potential for causing severe cutaneous reactions in a given segment of the population. It is not known how predictive predictive-testing is. We do know that the repeated insult procedure, which is based on 200 subjects, does not give as many positives, consistently and reproducibly, as the maximization test does on 25 subjects. What we have done is select the more severe screening method. Certainly, there is no proof that these materials will cause difficulty in actual use, but certainly their elimination is well advised.

There is no way of screening out by any presently known test methodology those materials to which the rare individual, who has idiosyncrasies and cannot eat strawberries or who has a cat, may become sensitized.

We hope to eliminate the general sensitizers. We know we cannot eliminate all reactions to cosmetics attributable to the fragrance moiety; we will reduce them to a minimum.

CONCLUSION

The Research Institute for Fragrance Materials, Inc., is the largest repository of safety data on fragrance raw materials anywhere in the world. In its ongoing program, it has tested 553 materials and has published, or submitted for publication, monographs on 349 of them.

The ubiquity of fragrances as such, and in cosmetics, household goods, insect repellents, etc., makes the responsibility of such an Institute a significant one, and it is hoped that in time, this ingredient approach, responded to zealously by the industry, will eliminate potential offenders from fragrances worldwide.

REFERENCES

[1] L. Golberg, Foreward, Fd. Cosmet. Toxicol., 12, 807 (1974).

[2] H. A. Shelanski and M. V. Shelanski, Modified repeated insult patch test, Proc. Sci. Sect. TGA, 19, 46 (1953).

[3] A. M. Kligman, The identification of contact allergens by human assay. III. The maximization test. A procedure for screening and rating contact sensitizers, J. Invest. Derm., 47, 393 (1966).

[4] A. M. Kligman and W. L. Epstein, Updating the maximization test for identifying contact allergens, Contact Dermatitis, 1(4), (1975) in press.

[5] P. D. Forbes and F. Urbach, Photocarcinogenesis: Lack of Enhancement by Three Fluorescent Lightening Agents, Environmental Quality and Safety (F. Coulston and F. Korte, eds.), Academic, New York, and Georg Thiene, Stuttgart, Germany, 1974.

[6] D. L. J. Opdyke, Monographs on fragrance raw materials—ethyl vanillin, Fd. Cosmet. Toxicol., 13, 91 (1975).

[7] D. L. J. Opdyke, Monographs on fragrance raw materials, Fd. Cosmet. Toxicol., 11, 95, 477, 855, 1011 (1973); 12, 385, 517, 703, 807 (1974); 13, 91 (1975).

[8] F. N. Marzulli and H. I. Maibach, Perfume phototoxicity, J. Soc. Cosmet. Chem., 21, 695 (1970).

[9] A. M. Kligman, The SLS provocative patch test in allergic contact sensitization, J. Invest. Derm., 46(6), 573 (1966).

[10] A. Björnberg, Skin reactions to primary irritants in patients with hand eczema. An investigation with matched controls. Oscar Isacsons Tryckerc Ab, Götesborg, Sweden, 1968.

[11] E. D. Lowney, Immulogical unresponsiveness, J. Invest. Derm., 54, 355 (1970).

[12] E. D. Lowney, Suppression of contact sensitizer in man by prior feeding of antigen, J. Invest. Derm., 61, 90 (1973).

In Vitro Mutagenesis Assays as Predictors of Chemical Carcinogenesis in Mammals

DAVID J. BRUSICK, Ph.D.

Director, Department of Genetics
Litton Bionetics, Inc.
Kensington, Maryland

INTRODUCTION

It was noted by the Millers in 1966 [1] that the association between mutagenicity and carcinogenicity, if present at all, was certainly confusing and was not significantly altered from earlier conclusions drawn by Burdette in 1955 [2]. Only a relatively small group of chemical carcinogens were clearly established as mutagens at this time, and they consisted almost entirely of highly reactive alkylating agents, which under most circumstances were relatively weak carcinogens. A later review by the Millers published in 1971 presented clearly different conclusions, suggesting the empirical correlation between the mutagenic and carcinogenic properties of chemicals has increased dramatically [3-16]. The difference between the correlations observed in 1966 and today can be accounted for by improvements in mutagenic screening methodology. As more biochemical and pharmacologic information accumulated from animal carcinogenesis bioassays, it became obvious that many chemical carcinogens were not themselves the ultimate carcinogenic molecule, but they produced intermediates with neoplastic activity following metabolic biotransformation in the treated animal [17-20]. The failure to detect mutagenic activity in many of the early tests using carcinogens could be directly attributed to the fact that most genetic assays were conducted in microbial species which lacked many of the appropriate enzymes required to activate the chemical to its biologically active form. Mutagenicity tests employing either chemically pure carcinogenic metabolites or host-mediated activation techniques, such as the Gabridge and Legator Host-Mediated Assay [21-31], were able to demonstrate that many additional carcinogens were also potent mutagens when examined as biologically active metabolites.

The ability to examine synthetic or purified metabolites of chemical carcinogens has been limited because for many agents the ultimate carcinogenic form was either not known or too unstable to be isolated. The use of host-mediated techniques was also limited because the methodology was suited only to chemicals which were metabolized and easily dispersed throughout the whole animal. Metabolites which were prohibited from distribution to the peritoneal cavity by physical, permeability, or chemical barriers would not be detected as active mutagens [22, 32, 33]. Aromatic amine and polycyclic hydrocarbon carcinogens have been consistently negative in host-mediated type tests.

More recent methodology employing in vitro microbial mutagenesis assays coupled with fortified microsomal metabolic activation systems prepared from mammalian tissues has generated a large data base demonstrating that a significant correlation exists between carcinogenicity and mutagenicity [7, 12, 14, 33, 34]. Carcinogens of all classes have been examined in these systems, and except for steroid and hormonal chemicals, some carcinogenic metals, and certain physical carcinogens such as asbestos, all types of synthetic and natural carcinogen molecules have exhibited mutagenic activity. Molecular events considered to be premutational in nature, such as DNA repair processes [14, 35] and mitotic recombinational phenomena [36], have also been used as indicators in similar in vitro activation assays but have not contributed significantly more to the data base than that which has been derived from bacterial mutagenesis assays using a series of histidine-requiring mutants. The fact that many chemical carcinogens are also mutagens is not particularly surprising since the initiation of both biologic end points appears to act through an electrophic attack on DNA by either the parental or metabolite form of the chemical. The highly reactive electrophilic form of these chemicals will react with many nucleophilic sites such as proteins or nucleic acids upon entering the cell [37]. If the active molecules bind to the DNA, producing breaks, deletions, or base changes, mutations may be induced. Figure 1 illustrates a working model which interrelates several features of chemical mutagenesis and carcinogenesis. The central component of the scheme is the reactive electrophilic agent. If this molecule can be demonstrated to be either the parental form or one of the metabolic products of a chemical, the potential for carcinogenic activity may be present. This type of thinking forms the rationale behind the utilization of mutagenicity

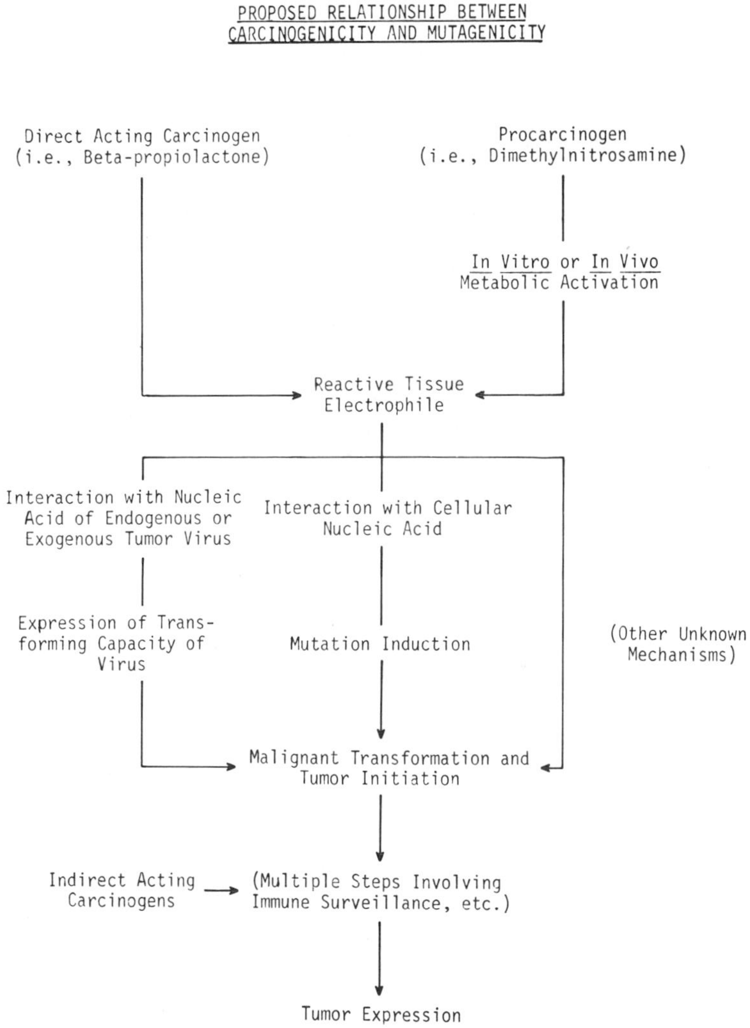

FIG. 1. Mutagenicity assays are designed to identify the reactive electrophile, which is also hypothesized to be involved in tumor initiation. According to this scheme only carcinogens that have a reactive electrophilic state are expected to be detected by mutagenicity assays. Carcinogens, such as hormones, which act indirectly and which promote tumor development following initiation steps will probably not exhibit mutagenic activity.

assays in screening for potential carcinogens. If chemical carcinogens or their electrophilic metabolites induce genetic changes which directly or in association with other cellular dysfunctions result in the malignant transformation of normal cells to potential tumor cells, then by the detection of mutagenic activity, potential carcinogens can be identified. The proposed scheme also explains the lack of mutagenic properties in steroids, hormones, and other chemicals that do not produce electrophilic forms. These agents probably act during the steps following initiation of transformed cells, possibly by altering the effectiveness of the immune surveillance system in clearing spontaneously transformed cells from the host [38, 39].

Several hypotheses for chemical induction of cancer in animals have attributed the tumor initiation to activation of oncornaviruses or their genomes already present in the host [40-42]. Such hypotheses are even more appealing in light of the cocarcinogenic enhancement of in vitro transformation by combined virus-chemical treatments [43-45]. However, biochemical and immunologic comparisons of chemical- and virus-induced tumors in mammals strongly suggest that the mechanisms for initiation by the two agents are distinct from each other [46-49].

Although the chemical mechanisms related to the initiation of cancer in animals may be diverse and not well comprehended at this time, in vitro methods that accurately identify compounds that are likely candidates for exhibiting carcinogenic activity in animals have considerable value from several standpoints. A sneak preview into the likely outcome of animal bioassay studies via short-term mutagenicity screens would enable many time and cost-saving decisions to be programed early in the development of any industrial chemical or drug. The information would be helpful in determining safe occupational exposures or selecting among an array of chemicals possessing equal efficacy, one with the lowest probability of exhibiting deleterious effects in later phases of product development. Mutagenicity screens might also act as components of a quality control system in the manufacture of bulk chemicals to detect the presence of a potential carcinogenic contaminant formed during synthesis or as an oxidation product produced during storage.

At a time when more and more evidence is pointing to the conclusion that most human cancer is initiated by exposure to environmental chemicals, rapid and reliable methods of identifying potentially carcinogenic materials are becoming increasingly important in overall chemical safety evaluation programs.

TECHNIQUES

Certainly the most widely employed methodology for the detection of mutagenic chemicals or metabolites is that developed by Ames and co-workers at the University of California, Berkely. Their assay employs a series of histidine-requiring auxotrophs of Salmonella typhimurium that has been adapted, by specific mutations, for use in screening chemicals to detect agents capable of inducing base-pair substitution of frameshift point mutations. The specific mutations incorporated into the strains TA-1535, TA-1537, and TA-1538 in addition to the histidine mutations consist of a deletion of the gal-bio-uvrB region of the chromosome altering the ability of the cell to undergo excision repair and a deep rough (rfa) mutation increasing the permeability of the cell to large molecules that would normally be excluded by the presence of a complete lipopolysaccharride component of the cell wall [6]. Strain TA-1535 is a missense mutant and reverts by base-pair substitution mechanisms, whereas strains TA-1537 and TA-1538 are frameshift mutants with long GC base sequences at the mutant sites [6, 8]. All three strains appear to be easily reverted "hot spots" responding to an extremely wide range of chemical mutagens [4-9]. More recently two additional Salmonella testing strains TA-98 and TA-100 have been introduced by Ames. These two strains (frameshift and base-pair substitution, respectively) carry an R factor plasmid which increases the sensitivity of the strains to some compounds, and the mutants have responded to several carcinogens not detected with the original three tester strains [10].

Chemicals are examined for reverse mutation induction in one or more of the five indicator organism by incubating the bacteria cells, a fortified microsome preparation, and various dose levels of the compound in aliquots of semisolid overlay agar containing trace amounts of histidine. The aliquots, each containing a separate indicator strain and dose level of the chemical, are poured over the surface of a plate of selective medium and incubated at 37°C for two days after which the number of revertant colonies on each plate is counted. Figures 2 and 3 illustrate the type of data generated in these assays using several classes of chemical carcinogens.

Ames and his co-workers have standardized the mammalian activation system (S9) used in their procedures so as to function with a wide range of procarcinogens. The S9 mixture consists of a 9000 × g supernatant fraction prepared from liver tissue removed from rats that have been pretreated with the polychlorinated biphenyl Aroclor 1254 (a general microsomal enzyme inducer) combined with TPN, glucose-6-phosphate, $MgCl_2$, and phosphate buffer [7]. The use of induced microsome preparations appears to be beneficial in amplifying the responses of many polycyclic hydrocarbon and aromatic amine mutagens. Microsomal enzyme induction in mammals can also be accomplished by phenobarbital treatment or dietary changes [50, 51]. Some comparisons of mutation induction responses using induced and noninduced tissue are shown in Fig. 4. With some chemicals the use of induced tissue may mean the difference between obtaining a clear-cut or an equivocal mutagenic response. In other cases, no differences may be observed.

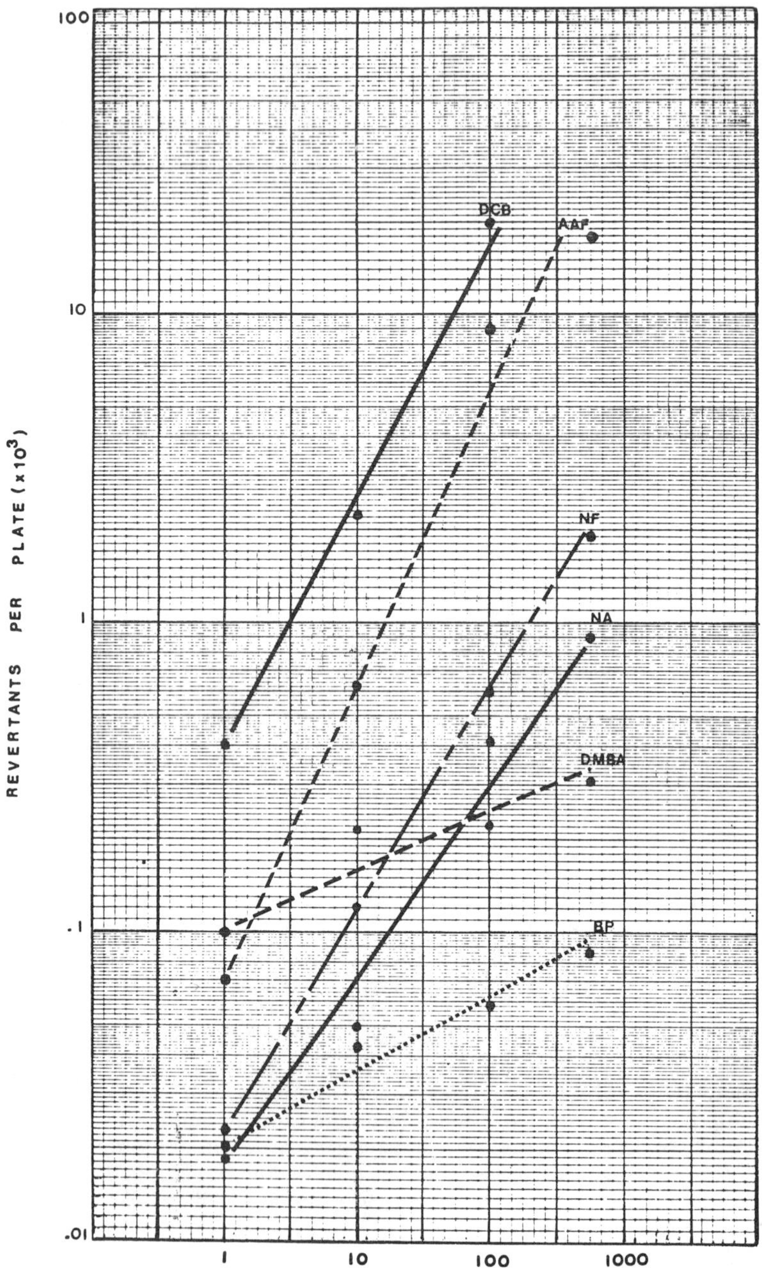
100
10
1
.1
.01
REVERTANTS PER PLATE (x10^3)
1
10
100
1000
DCB
AAF
NF
NA
DMBA
BP

The results depend on the species and tissues employed in the assay. For instance, phenobarbital and Aroclor 1254 can both reduce the activation of DMNA in some tissues of mice [52].

It has been suggested that human autopsy material should be used in the bacterial screening systems to make the results more relevant. Although human liver tissue has been used, the large number of variables encountered might prohibit confidence in some test results. Diet, previous medication, age, sex, length of time following death, genetic background, and innumerable other variables, all of which influence metabolic reactions, could produce completely erroneous or nonreproducible results, and reproducibility is an essential feature of any screening assay. However, the inclusion of human tissue in a battery of tests comparing the mutagenicity of a chemical with rodent and other mammalian activation systems might be a productive approach to answer some questions of extrapolation.

Although the in vitro microsomal activation systems were initially developed for use in screening programs, modified procedures in which a single compound is examined for activation to a mutagen by tissues obtained from several animal species can yield a wealth of information about the likely metabolic fate of the compound in each of those species. This approach can also be used to compare age, diet, and sex-related differences in metabolism. For example, in vitro mutagenicity assays with activation mixtures prepared from male and female kidney microsomes from mouse, rat, dog, and monkey were compared using the carcinogen dimethylnitrosamine (Fig. 5). The results show that for the two rodent species, the females have very little activation potential compared with the males. For the two nonrodent species, however, the females show considerably higher activity than males. It is not known whether the tumor sus-

---

FIG. 2. The mutagenic responses of six chemical carcinogens in plate tests using S. typhimurium. The activation system utilized a $9000 \times g$ supernatant fraction from rat liver obtained from phenobarbital-induced animals. All points were corrected for the spontaneous background [84]. Concentrations in micrograms per plate.

DCB, dichlorobenzidine: indicator strain TA-1538 (no activation required). AAF, N-2-fluorenylacetamide: indicator strain TA-1538. NF, 2-nitrofluorene: indicator strain TA-1538 (no activation required). NA, 2-naphthylamine: indicator strain TA-1535. DMB, 7,12 dimethylbenzathracene: indicator strain TA-98 (tested with rat liver from aroclor induced animals). BP, benzo(a)pyrene: indicator strain TA-1538.

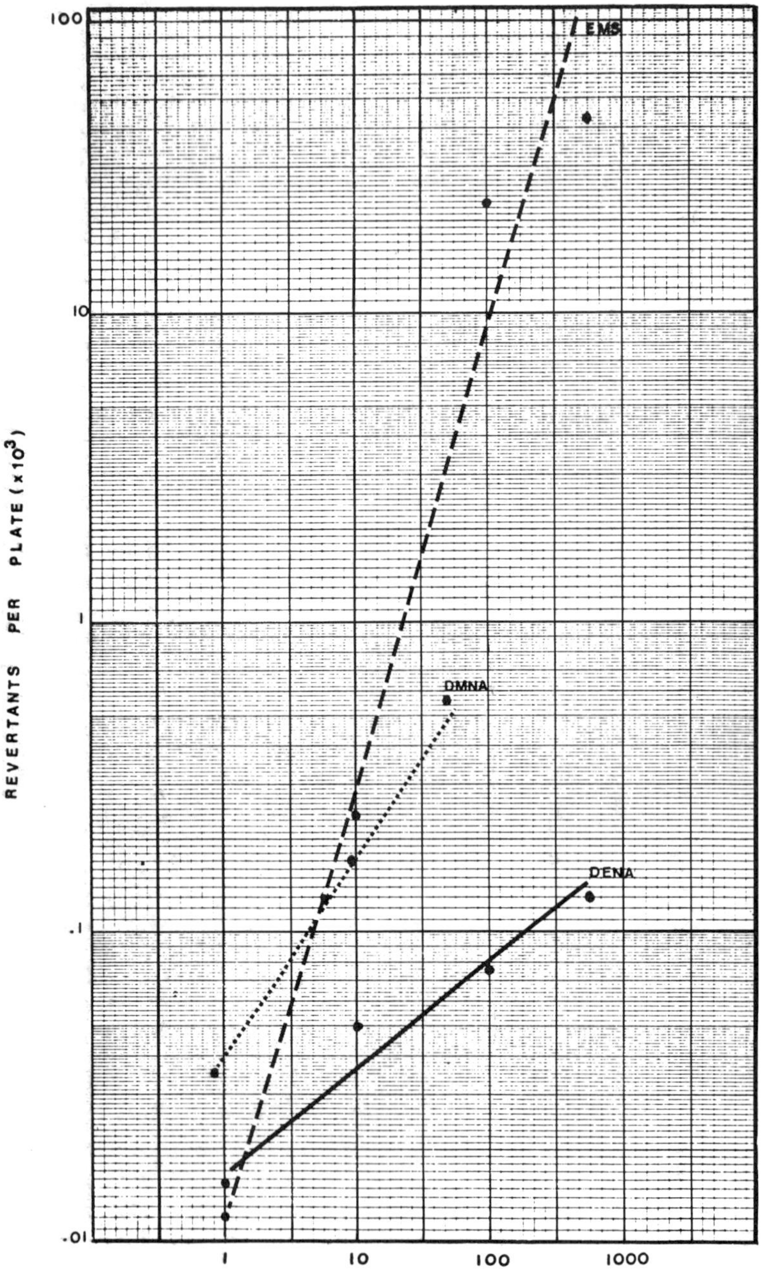

REVERTANTS PER PLATE (x10^3)
100
10
1
.1
.01
1
10
100
1000
EMS
DMNA
DENA

ceptibility of male and female animals to DMNA is different, but the data suggest male rodents may be more susceptible to renal tumors than females. It has been reported that exposure of mice to levels of carbon tetrachloride that have little or no effect on female animals produce acute kidney necrosis in male animals [53]. The data also indicate that if sex-related renal effects were found in rodent tests, the extrapolation of such effects to primates, for example. might be completely erroneous because of the reversed sex effects.

Other microbial mutation, repair, and recombination assays have also been used in chemical screening. A repair test in E. coli proposed by Rosenkranz and co-workers at Columbia University has been used extensively in chemical screening [14]. It compares the relative survivals of strains W3110 (pol A^+) and p3478 (pol A^-) following exposure to chemicals spotted on lawns of each strain. If the chemical interacts with DNA and induces a lesion that is repairable, the pol A^+ strain will exhibit less sensitivity than the pol A^- strain, which lacks a functional repair enzyme [54]. Other forward and/or reverse mutations, as well as DNA repair systems in strains of E. coli, have been described by Bridges [55], Nakajima and Iwahara [34], Kada et al. [35], Kondo [56], and Mohn and Ellenberger [57]. The data base for carcinogenicity-mutagenicity correlation established with these strains is relatively limited at this time.

The yeast Saccharomyces cerevisiae has been used extensively to study the recombinogenic properties of chemicals. Several diploid strains of S. cerevisiae developed by Zimmermann have been employed in chemical screening programs [58]. The purpose of including yeasts in genetic screening programs was to have at lease one eukaryotic cell type among the array of microbial indicator organisms. Mitotic recombination is a nonmutational genetic alteration that can result in the phenotypic expression of heterozygous alleles by the production of a homozygous state following recombination and cell division. This type of an event may be operative in the production of genetic abnormalities or diseases during prenatal development. A recom-

---

FIG. 3. The mutagenic responses of two chemical carcinogens in plate tests using S. typhimurium. The activation system utilized a 9000 × g supernatant fraction from rat liver tissue. All points were corrected for the spontaneous background [84]. Concentrations in micromoles per plate.

DMNA, dimethylnitrosamine: indicator strain TA-1535. DENA, diethylnitrosamine: indicator strain TA-1535. EMS, ethyl methanesulfonate: indicator strain TA-1535 (no activation required).

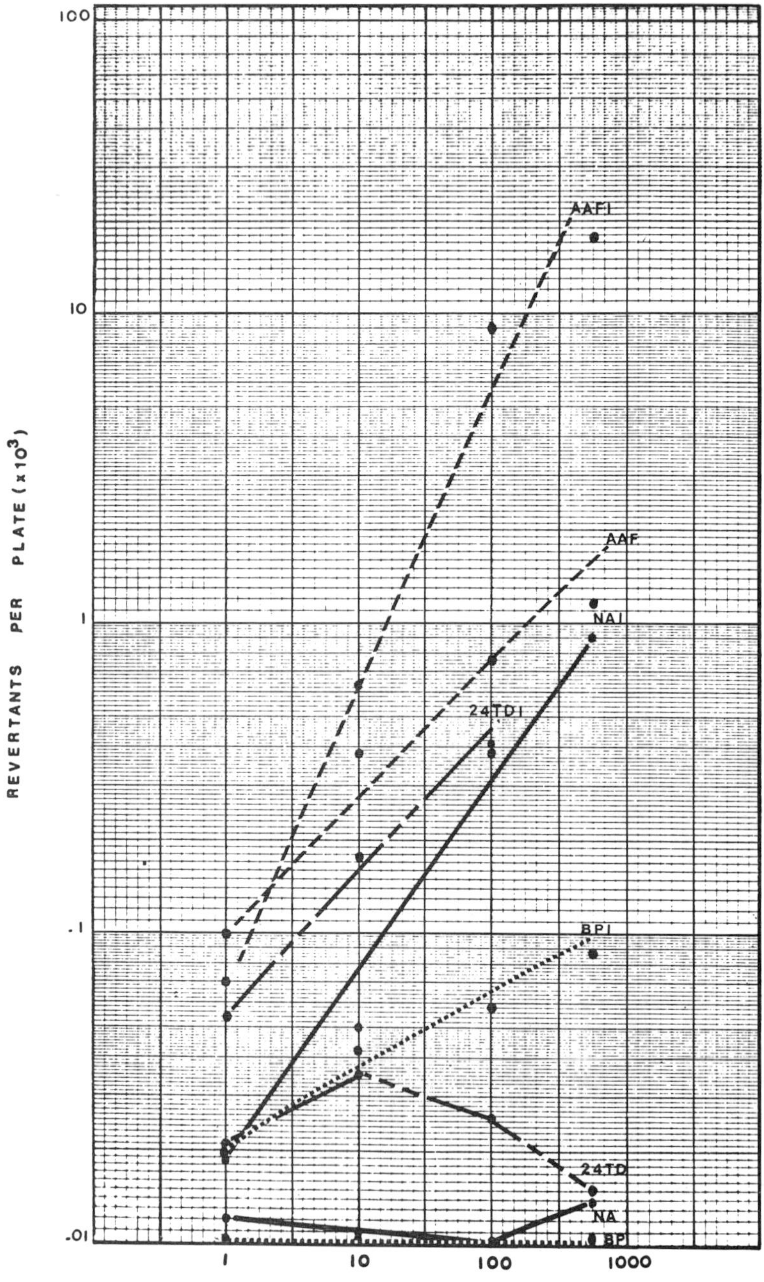
REVERTANTS PER PLATE (x10³)
100
10
1
.1
.01
1
10
100
1000
AAFI
AAF
NAI
24TDI
BPI
24TD
NA
BP

binogenic mechanism for the initiation of neoplastic transformation has also been proposed by Zimmermann [59]. The data that have been generated by various yeast systems have shown that in general most direct-acting carcinogens are active in yeast [60, 61], but that only relatively few of the procarcinogens (requiring metabolic biotransformation) have been detected in yeast in vitro activation assays [36, 61]. It has been proposed that cell wall and nuclear membrane barriers and efficient repair systems all interact to considerably reduce the overall sensitivity of yeast to a wide variety of chemical carcinogens [36]. One cannot too easily dispel this lack of sensitivity since most eukaryotic cells would be expected to respond similarly and thus yeast may represent the typical eukaryotic cell sensitivity.

Mutagenicity assays using Neurospora [62], Drosophilia [63], and cultured animal cells [64] as indicators are widely used to examine test chemicals but are not usually considered to be screening assays. Each of these assay systems has its own advantages and disadvantages enabling it to work in certain instances where others fail. This fact has often been criticized as a weakness in the proposed use of mutagenicity screening. It has been felt that if it is necessary to utilize many, and often exotic, types of mutagenicity assays to ensure total reliability, how is the industrial toxicologist who is concerned with proper safety evaluation procedures to know which of the tests to use and when to use them? In many respects this criticism is not easy to answer because of the newness of the concept of using mutagenesis as a screen for potential carcinogens. One has little past published experience to use in selecting the best test for a particular agent. This is also the motivating factor behind the extensive development and

---

FIG. 4. The mutagenic response of four chemical carcinogens for S. typhimurium using activation systems from phenobarbital-induced and noninduced rats. The activation systems utilized a 9000 × g supernatant fraction from rat liver tissue. All points were corrected for the spontaneous background [84]. Concentrations in micrograms per plate.

AAFI, N-2-fluorenylacetamide: induced tissue (TA-1538). AAF, N-2 fluorenylacetamide: noninduced tissue (TA-1538). NAI, 2-naphthylamine: induced tissue (TA-1535). NA, 2-naphthylamine: noninduced tissue (TA-1535). 24TDI, 2,4-diaminotoluene: induced tissue (TA-1538). 24TD, 2,4-diaminotoluene: noninduced tissue (TA-1538). BPI, benzo(a)pyrene: induced tissue (TA-1538). BP, benzo(a)pyrene: noninduced tissue (TA-1538).

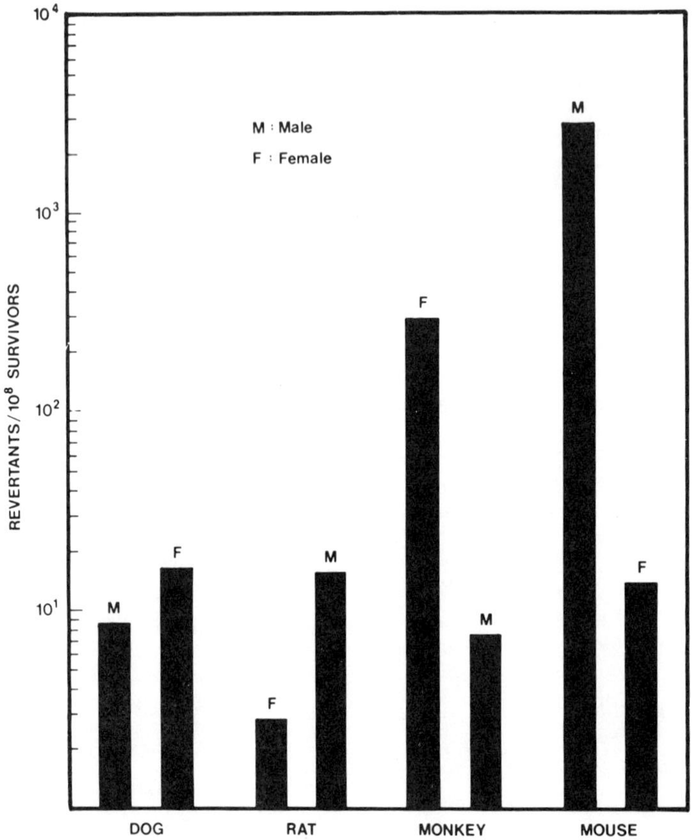

FIG. 5. Sex-related differences in the in vitro activation of DMNA (100 μM/ml) to a mutagen by kidney microsomal fractions from male and female BALB/c mice, Sprague-Dawley rats, mixed breed dogs, and rhesus monkeys. The treatment period for each test was 60 min at 37°C. Each point was corrected for the spontaneous frequency. The data were taken from Jagannath [52].

validation studies with the Ames assay. The Salmonella test system appears presently, at least, to be the most generally applicable screen when little or no information is available regarding the biologic activity of the chemical in question. No other mutagenesis assay has been shown to respond to such a wide group of chemical types as the Salmonella mutants described earlier.

Some general suggestions, however, can be given regarding the selection of a screening procedure:

1. Select the procedure to be employed in response to the question that is being asked. If one simply wishes to determine the capability of a chemical to produce mutations, in vivo assays such as the Dominant lethal test or cytogenetic analysis are not appropriate. A simple microbial assay would adequately suffice. Dominant lethal and heritable translocation assays are not designed as screening procedures but rather to assess germ cell risk from proven mutagens. There are little or no data indicating a correlation between responses in these in vivo assays with chemical carcinogenesis.

2. Chemicals that have antibiotic properties may prove to be difficult to screen in bacteria assays unless certain resistant strains are employed. It may be advisable with such compounds to run complementary tests using fungal, Drosophila, or cultured animal cell assays to ensure that the indicator organisms are exposed to sufficient dose levels to produce some biologic activity.

3. Bacterial reverse mutation assays screen only for point mutations. Chemicals which react with DNA primarily by inducing chromosomal alterations and producing only few point mutations may appear as a weak or nonmutagen in reversion tests. Simple chromosome screens such as the micronucleus test [65] might be valuable as complementary assays as would E. coli repair or S. cerevisiae recombinational tests. Some of the known carcinogens presently not found to be mutagenic in point mutation assays may produce high frequencies of chromosomal aberrations and would therefore only be detected with chromosome techniques.

4. Occasionally, there is a desire to rank a group of compounds for their mutagenic activity with respect to each other. If the chemicals are all of a closely related structure, it may be possible to utilize reverse mutation tests for the ranking; however, forward mutation systems would be preferable. For a similar comparison among structurally unrelated compounds, the use of a forward mutation assay is essential. The reason being that reverse mutation assays present a "restricted target" for the chemical while forward mutation assays present a relatively "unrestricted target" for the chemical. For example, if two frameshift mutagens with equal activity were evaluated in a reverse mutation assay in which the mutant site of the tester strain contained only GC base sequences and if one of the chemicals has a high affinity for reaction with G or C bases while the other had an affinity for A or T bases, the chemical with affinity for the G or C bases would appear to be a potent mutagen, whereas the other compound would appear to be negative or weakly mutagenic. A better comparison of the two chemicals would be obtained in assays where a whole gene is the "target" since it can be assumed that both AT and GC base pairs would be available for reactions between the chemical and DNA.

ADVANTAGES AND LIMITATIONS OF USING MUTAGENICITY SCREENS AS PREDICTORS OF CHEMICAL CARCINOGENS

The advantages of using mutagenicity screens to identify potential chemical carcinogens are usually obvious. Certainly the short time and small expense involved are two outstanding features of these in vitro tests when compared with standard bioassay procedures, but of equal importance is the continually increasing correlation between the mutagenic and carcinogenic properties of different groups of chemicals. The real value of any assay, no matter how rapid and inexpensive, depends upon the reliability of the results it generates. If mutagenicity assays gave no better than a 50:50 prediction of neoplastic activity their worth would be less than their cost, but for each increase in correlation toward the surely unattainable 100% predictability, the value of the assay grows exponentially. The reliability estimate at the present time for bacteria assays ranges between 85% and 95% predictability depending upon the bias of the individual giving the rating or reviewing the data. Compilations of the carcinogenicity and mutagenicity correlations for a large group of chemicals are presently in preparation and will be published elsewhere [83]. Until all of the available data are reviewed and published, correlation values will have to remain as generalized figures. Results on many chemicals can be compiled from the literature, and the correlation range mentioned previously appears to be consistent. A true 95% predictability ascertainment is very impressive, but even 85% correlation would be valuable. What, then, about the 10-15% of known carcinogens not identified by the tests (false negatives) and to what extent are compounds regarded to be noncarcinogens found to have mutagenic properties ("false positives")? These questions immediately arise when correlation estimates are discussed. Since it is unusual for investigators to spend much time publishing negative results, the mutagenicity literature appears to suggest that almost everything tested is mutagenic. However, a large group of chemicals (>200) generally regarded as noncarcinogenic have been screened with the microbial assays and only a very low percentage (2-3%) exhibit mutagenic activity [84, 85]. Whether that 2-3% represents potential carcinogens is only conjecture at this point. The frequency of "false positives" increases slightly if one selects chemicals with structural similarities to known carcinogens. Many compounds of this latter class have been tested for carcinogenicity and have not exhibited any significant response; however, at this point it should be noted that the standard bioassay using 50 male and 50 female animals at each dose level as well as in the control groups has a built-in insensitivity such that chemicals showing slight increases in tumor frequencies cannot be assessed with reasonable confidence. Mutagenicity assays, however, are sensitive enough to demonstrate that increases of two or three times the spontaneous level can be significant and thus may well be more adept at identifying very weak carcinogens than our animal models. In vivo assessment of extremely weak carcinogens would require enormous animal populations that would be prohibitively expensive.

Retrospectively, it could also be argued that certain chemical carcinogens might not have been positive in animal bioassay programs if only a single test species had been employed (i.e., N-2-fluorenylacetamide in the guinea pig or 2-naphthylamine in the mouse). Species differences, in most cases, have been attributed to an inability of the nonsusceptible animal to form the carcinogenic metabolite. Selection of species for animal carcinogenesis studies, however, it generally predicated on considerations of time and expenses and therefore normally limited to small rodents. An overlooked advantage of the bacterial mutagenicity assays coupled with mammalian activation systems is the potential to screen a given chemical with the bacteria using activation preparations from many different mammalian species, including human [7, 66]. Mutagenicity screens with microsomal fractions from several species including rodent and nonrodent may help identify erroneous conclusions of "no response" based on data from only mice and rats, and additionally may be used as an aid in the selection of an appropriate test species for carcinogenesis bioassays.

The bulk of disadvantages associated with microbial mutagenesis screening for chemical carcinogens is related to toxicologic and pharmacologic parameters. The in vitro mutagenicity approach is most often criticized because the route of chemical administration is irrelevant; there is no assurance that the in vitro metabolic systems accurately represent in vivo activation and detoxification processes; the dose levels have little relationship to animal exposures; compound drug distribution and elimination from the exposed animal cannot be studied; and, of course, mutation in bacteria cells is not cancer in animal cells. All of these facts are true, but mutagenicity assays should not be viewed as definitive tests for carcinogenicity in mammals. They are proposed as short-term screens for potential carcinogens and rely almost exclusively on the empirical correlation established with respect to mutagenic and carcinogenic properties of test compounds. Whether routes of administration or detoxification processes play a role in the expression of that potential can only be determined, in the final analysis, with appropriate animal models. But this does not lessen the role prescreening techniques can play in chemical safety evaluation programs.

Another disadvantage of mutagenesis screens has already been mentioned with respect to Fig. 1. Carcinogens that act by indirect mechanisms and are not direct initiators of malignant transformation via an electrophilic attack on cellular nucleophiles will most likely not demonstrate mutagenic activity. It is doubtful, as well, that metal carcinogens or physical carcinogens will be identified in mutagenesis screening. This is clearly a deficiency since much attention has recently focused on the carcinogenic effects of certain hormones [67, 68] and physical agents [38].

Finally it should not be forgotten that the mutagenesis-carcinogenesis correlation is being constructed retrospectively using carcinogenesis bioassay data primarily from mice and rats as the reference point for the mutagenesis responses, and any attempt to directly extrapolate data from bacterial assays to humans must take the following facts into consideration.

1. It is still totally unknown whether the animal carcinogenesis bioassay model system acting as the template to which the microbial model system is being correlated has any relevance to the human cancer experience. Until the question of animal extrapolation can be more adequately answered, the microbial mutagenesis assays are actually most applicable as predictors of rodent carcinogens.

2. There is always the danger of bias entering into the evaluation of data when one knows in advance the carcinogenic properties of a reference chemical. As a result, known carcinogens may get a more thorough examination for mutagenic activity than noncarcinogens during comparative investigations. A better approach in correlation development would be to examine chemicals for mutagenic activity prior to the determination of their bioassay evaluation and thus preclude all forms of bias. A program of this nature is currently in progress [84].

3. A tendency may develop to think of mutagenic potency as an indication of carcinogenic potency. Actually there may be no relationship between the two. If a chemical is a carcinogen and a mutagen, its mutagenic potency in reverse mutation assays will be a reflection of its affinity for the DNA base sequence at the mutant site in the tester organism and may have little or no quantitative relationship to carcinogenic activity in vivo. Caution, therefore, should be introduced in evaluating data from mutagenicity assays. A compound which appears as a weak mutagen in reverse mutation tests cannot be regarded with any less concern for potential carcinogenicity than a potent mutagen.

THE FUNCTIONAL RELATIONSHIP BETWEEN CARCINOGENESIS AND MUTAGENESIS

The development of a good correlation between the mutagenic and carcinogenic properties of chemicals suggests the intriguing possibility that a molecular event may be shared by the two phenomena. Somatic mutation theories for cancer induction have been proposed in one form or another by several investigators [3, 7, 59]. Other indirect evidence supporting a functional relationship comes from the properties of in vitro transformed rodent cells. Mutation produced transmissable alterations in phenotypic traits of cells such as morphologic, biochemical, and immunologic properties. The induction of malignant transformation by chemical treatment of a population of normal animal cells follows the characteristics expected of mutational alterations. It is known, in addition, that mutant cells can undergo spontaneous and induced reverse mutation, depending upon the nature of the original lesion. Often the reverse mutation response following chemical treatment can be of assistance in identifying the type of mutational lesion induced [69]. Transformed animal cells also undergo reverse transformation, which would be expected if the transformation event were mutational in origin [70]. Thus, the indirect evidence accumulated during the past several years is beginning to implicate the role of mutations in chemically induced malignant transformation.

There are numerous hypotheses linking mutational alterations to the initiation of malignant transformation. Two commonly discussed working hypotheses are:

Mutational Alterations That Affect Genes Controlling Differentiation

It may be that during the developmental process in organogenesis regulator genes cause the cessation in cell division of differentiated tissues. Mutations induced in these regulator genes by chemical carcinogens might then result in a loss of cellular control and a de-differentiation process. The unregulated cells lose their differential phenotypes and acquire properties of nondifferentiated, rapidly dividing cell masses. Biochemical and morphologic changes also occur, giving the cells different antigenic and growth characteristics typical of transformed cells.

Mutational Alterations That Affect Expression of Oncogenes

Because of the viral implications in certain types of mammalian cancer, it has been suggested that chemical carcinogens might act by mutating oncogenes or their regulators located in the host cell [40]. The oncogenes would be of viral origin and contain information essential for cellular transformation. The mutation may act directly on the transformation-specific gene or on a regulator gene producing a repressor of the transformation gene. Induction, activation, or expression of the oncogene could, therefore, be initiated by mutational alterations produced by chemical carcinogens (Fig. 1).

To conclusively demonstrate that a mutation is a required step in the initiation of malignant transformation, studies of the mutagenesis of the cellular gene or genes responsible for transformation would have to be performed. Current work with in vitro transformation and mutation methods using cultured rodent cells may provide some information concerning the feasibility of this approach [31].

There are however, other indirect data demonstrating both a functional and empirical correlation between mutagenesis and carcinogenesis. The data comes from investigations of the in vitro activation of procarcinogens to mutagenic intermediates using microsome preparations from organs of animals that are both susceptible and resistant to the carcinogenic activity of the compound studied. The rationale behind this approach is that if the active intermediate produced during metabolism is both carcinogen and mutagen, then it would be expected that a relationship should exist between the amount of mutagen (carcinogen) produced and the level of tumor initiation observed. For example, if chemical X were metabolically activated to a mutagen (carcinogen) in species A but not in species B, then one might predict that species A but not species B would develop tumors. If the relationship between the mutagen and carcinogen was not functional but only circumstantial, the prediction of carcinogenicity susceptibility would be incorrect as often as it is correct.

Application of this rationale to studies of the carcinogenic and mutagenic relationship of dimethylnitrosamine (DMNA) has been quite successful. DMNA is both mutagenic and carcinogenic following metabolic activation in vivo [71] and mutagenic following activation in vitro [12]. The in vitro studies demonstrate that metabolic capacity for biotransformation of DMNA is present in several different tissues of rodent species [33]. The hypothesized mechanism for DMNA activation includes the formation of a shortlived alkylating intermediate [72], and it is this intermediate which is believed to produce mutagenic and neoplastic changes in cells [33, 73]. In vitro microsomal activation of DMNA to a mutagen was initially reported by Malling using S. typhimurium G-46 and mouse liver microsomes [12]. Subsequent studies by Nakajima and Iwahara [34] and Gletten et al. [66] reported in vitro microsomal activation of DMNA to a mutagen by several species including human. Using similar in vitro methods, Czygan et al. [73] demonstrated that the rate of mutagen formation was linked to the rate of enzymatic conversion of DMNA. This information permitted the mutation assay to be used as an indirect assay for the enzymatic activity of a particular tissue to biotransform DMNA into a mutagenic (carcinogenic) intermediate. Weekes and Brusick used this approach to compare the relationship between target organ susceptibility for DMNA-induced tumors and in vitro metabolic activation of DMNA to a mutagen [33]. In mice, DMNA induces predominantly liver and lung tumors with low frequencies of kidney tumors and rarely, if ever, tumors of the spleen or gonads [71, 74-76]. The activation of DMNA to a mutagenic intermediate by microsome preparations from these organs of BALB/cJ, RF/J, and C57B1/6J mice show the same ranking (liver>

lung > kidney > spleen > testes) suggesting that at least for this chemical carcinogen, the level of metabolic activation of a tissue may be directly related to the susceptibility of the organ as a target for tumor induction [33]. The results of these studies stimulated additional comparisons between mouse strains demonstrating different spectra of target organ susceptibility. While the liver and lung tumor susceptibilities of most mouse strains to DMNA are roughly similar, there are some striking differences with respect to the incidence of renal tumors. C3H and Swiss mouse strains exhibit high susceptibility, exhibiting renal tumor incidences of approximately 16 and 11%, respectively, while BALB/c and RF mice are resistant showing renal tumor frequencies lower than 4% [74-76]. When microsome preparations from the kidneys of these four strains were compared for their ability to activate DMNA to a mutagen (Fig. 6), the relationship between carcinogenic susceptibility and mutagen production was excellent. The data for liver and lung tissues from all four strains are similar as expected (Figs. 7 and 8). Examination of kidney size and protein content of the microsome preparations from the four strains did not show any substantial differences [77], and it was assumed that the metabolic activity of the enzymes obtained from the kidney cells of the susceptible and resistant strains were in some way different. The differences might be related to qualitative variations in specific enzyme molecules or quantitative variations in the amount of specific enzyme molecules produced per cell. Data obtained by Jagannath [52] from crosses between the susceptible (Ha/ICR Swiss) and resistant (BALB/c) strains demonstrate that the metabolic differences are inherited and that for both the C3H/HeJ and Ha/ICR Swiss albino strains the gene(s) associated with high levels of DMNA metabolism is recessive to the gene(s) of the BALB/cJ strain. From crosses between the Ha/ICR Swiss albino susceptible strain and the BALB/cJ resistant strain, F_1 selfings were made and F_2 progeny were examined for distribution of high and low metabolic activity. The results, although preliminary in nature, suggest that only a single gene product may be involved in the different susceptibilities.

It has been reported that injection of newborn BALB/c mice with DMNA gives rise to tumors of the liver and lung but no kidney tumors, whereas DMNA administered to adult BALB/c mice did produce a low incidence of kidney tumors [64]. When the capacities of liver and kidney microsome preparations to metabolically convert DMNA to a mutagen were examined beginning at birth, it was seen that the activation capacity of the liver of newborns to convert DMNA was almost at the adult level, but that the kidney enzymes were not functional (Table 1). In fact the kidney demethylase activity appears not to function until five weeks following birth. Similar results were obtained with C3H/HeJ male mice [52]. These results may represent a hormonally influenced regulation of enzyme production. The gradual increase in male kidney activity starting between the fourth and fifth week might

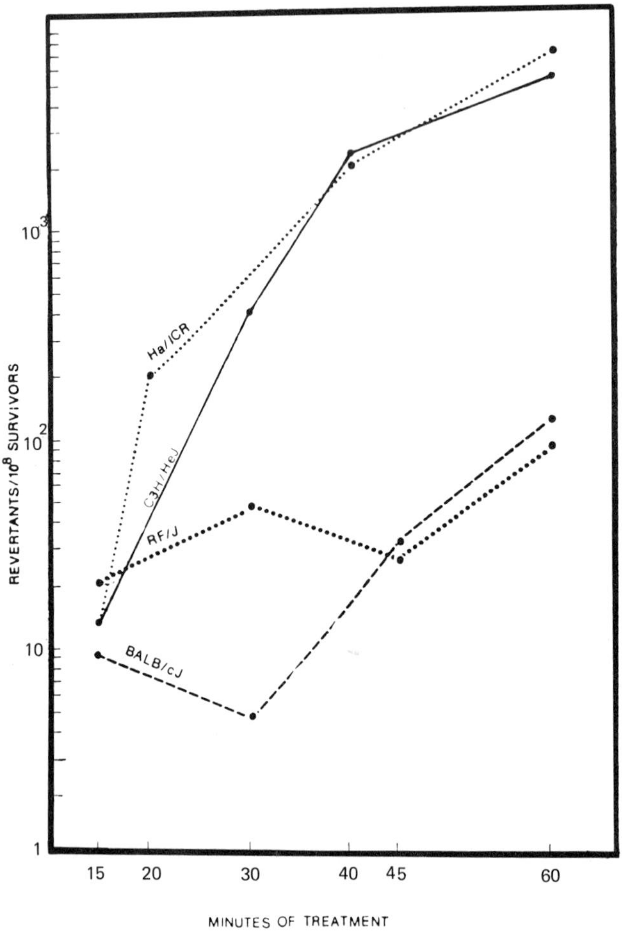

FIG. 6. The in vitro activation of DMNA (100 μM/ml to a mutagen by purified kidney microsomes from Ha/ICR Swiss albino, C3H/HeJ, RF/J, and BALB/cJ male mice during a 60-min incubation period at 37°C. The indicator strain was S. typhimurium G-46. The spontaneous frequency was approximately 1×10^{-8} for each experiment. The data were taken from Weekes [77].

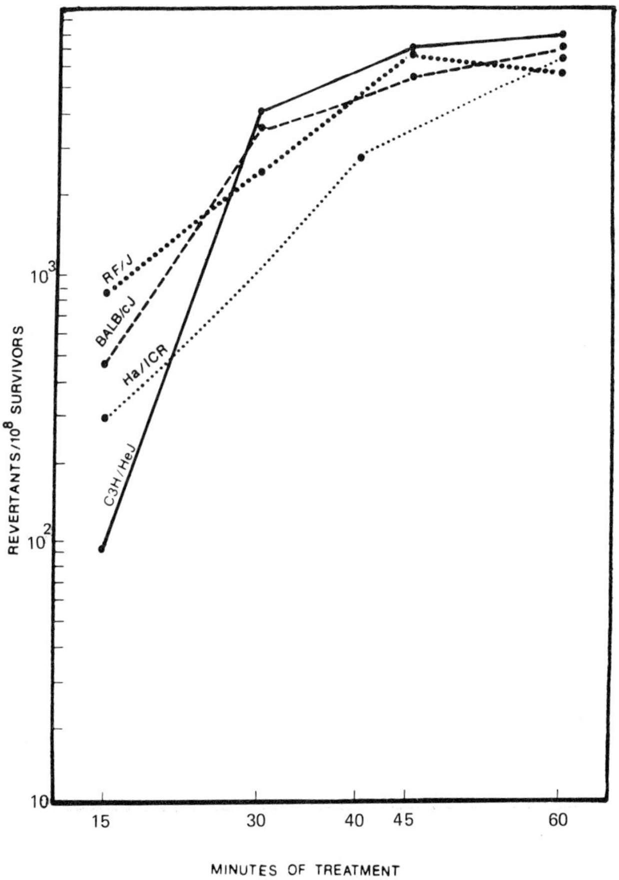

FIG. 7. The in vitro activation of DMNA (100 μM/ml) to a mutagen by purified liver microsomes from Ha/ICR Swiss albino, C3H/HeJ, RF/J, and BALB/cJ male mice during a 60-min incubation period at 37°C. The indicator strain was S. typhimurium G-46. The spontaneous frequency was approximately 1×10^{-8} for each experiment. The data were taken from Weekes and Brusick [33].

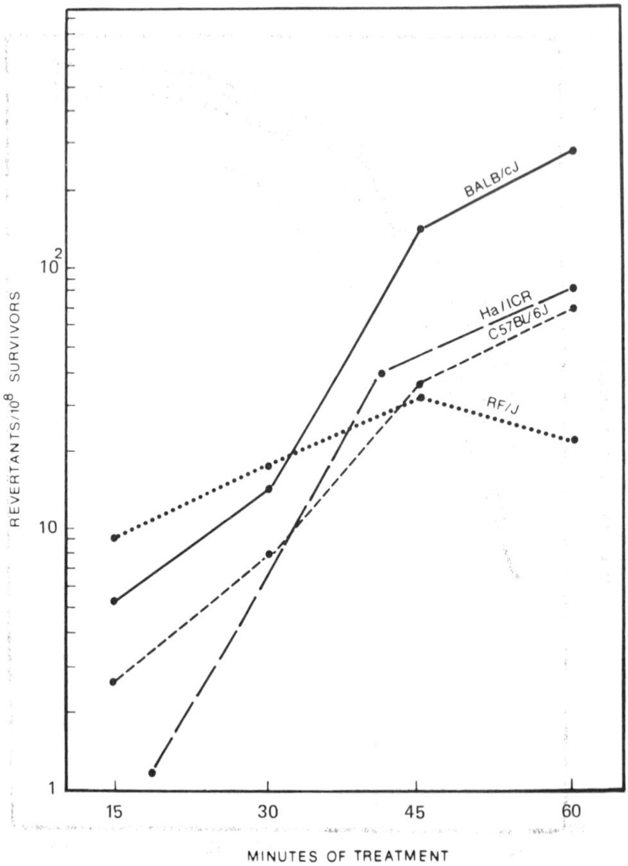

FIG. 8. The in vitro activation of DMNA (100 μM/ml) to a mutagen by purified lung microsomes from Ha/ICR Swiss albino, C3H/HeJ, RF/J, and BALB/cj male mice during a 60-min incubation period at 37°C. The indicator strain was S. typhimurium G-46. The spontaneous frequency was approximately 1×10^{-8} for each experiment. Data were taken from Weekes and Brusick [33].

be due to increasing production of male hormones. This observation was consistent with the in vivo tumorigenic effects produced by DMNA and again supported the belief that the active DMNA metabolite is both the ultimate mutagen and carcinogen. In female mice, the kidney enzymes never become active even in adult animals [33, 52].

TABLE 1. Conversion of DMNA to a Mutagenic Metabolite 9000 × g Supernatant Fractions from the Kidneys and Livers of Male BALB/cJ Mice at Various Ages[a]

Age days postpartum	Liver activation	Kidney activation
Spontaneous	1.1[b]	2.1[b]
1	133.8	–
11	13,270.4	–
14	6,456.1	0.7
21	13,259.7	0.0
28	15,148.9	0.0
35	11,085.3	41.0
42	16,378.9	180.0
49	2,562.7	895.5
56	15,813.9	1,493.3

[a]Data from Jagannath [52].
[b]Revertants of S. typhimurium, strain G-46, per 10^8 surviving cells following exposure to DMNA at 100 μM/ml for 60 min at 37°C.

The functional relationship between carcinogenesis and mutagenesis for DMNA appears to be excellent. In fact it may be possible to predict not only species of animals that will be susceptible to DMNA, but even the potential target organs.

A similar but less extensive approach was taken with the well-defined carcinogen N-2-fluorenylacetamide (AFF). Data shown in Table 2 represent the mutagenic activity of AAF for S. typhimurium TA-1538 using noninduced 9000 × g supernatant fractions from six mammalian species as components of the in vitro activation system. Among the six species represented, four (mouse, rat, dog, and rabbit) are susceptible to the carcinogenic effects of AAF. The guinea pig is resistant to AAF presumably because it cannot form the N-hydroxy-AAF metabolite believed to be one of the ultimate carcinogens [79]. N-Hydroxy-AAF itself, however, is carcinogenic for the guinea pig [80]. Monkeys fed AAF for up to eight years have not developed tumors nor have autopsied animals exhibited any lesions suggestive of developing neoplasia [81]. The mutagenesis data are consistent with the carcinogenic responses in all cases except the guinea pig. Other investigators have reported similar results for guinea pig liver

TABLE 2. Comparative Mutagenesis for AAF[a] Using Activation Tissues (9000 × g Fractions) from Six Mammalian Species [84]

Species[b]	Strain	Organ	Revertants of TA-1538 per 10^8 surviving cells ($\times 10^{-8}$)[c]
Mouse	ICR random bred	Liver	27.4
		Kidney	587.5
		Lung	3.2
Rat	Sprague-Dawley	Liver	39.9
		Kidney	3.5
		Lung	1.0
Guinea pig	Strain 13 Inbred	Liver	272.3
		Kidney	43.5
		Lung	5.1
Rabbit	New Zealand White	Liver	222.1
		Kidney	3.3
		Lung	0.5
Dog	Mixed breed	Liver	160.37
		Kidney	11.15
		Lung	5.81
Monkey	Rhesus	Liver	11.0
		Kidney	14.3
		Lung	0.7

[a]AAF concentration for all assays was 800 μg/ml. Treatment was at 37°C for 60 min.

[b]All animals were males.

[c]The spontaneous frequencies were subtracted from each value.

[82]. In fact, the guinea pig liver microsomes appear to be more active than the liver microsomes of any of the other five mammals; yet, studies have demonstrated that the active metabolite (N-hydroxy-AAF) is not formed by this species in vivo or in vitro [79]. One is

left with the conclusion that guinea pig liver enzymes must form a mutagenic intermediate (other than N-hydroxy-AAF) that has no carcinogenic properties. A hydroxylamine derivative has been found in the urine [79]. The results with this species are inconsistent with the current hypothesis relating mutagenesis and carcinogenesis and will be extensively investigated, but they serve to illustrate that many biologic parameters are involved in the development of neoplasia.

One additional positive point from Table 2 worth noting is the fact that mouse kidney microsomes are more active than any other tissue for metabolic activation of AAF to a mutagen. This is especially interesting since AAF produces a higher incidence of urinary bladder tumors in mice compared with other susceptible species [79, 80].

SUMMARY

In vitro microbial mutagenesis assays coupled with mammalian activation systems offer a promising technique to screen chemicals for their potential carcinogenic activity. The correlation between mutagenic and carcinogenic properties for a large array of chemicals is approximately 0.9. The best correlation exists for those carcinogens which are themselves highly electrophilic or produce electrophilic metabolites. Correlation between mutagenicity and carcinogenicity for hormonal, metallic, or physical carcinogens has been disappointing but not unexpected based on their proposed mechanisms of action.

In addition to the application of in vitro mutagenesis techniques to screening chemicals for the identification of potential carcinogens, they are useful tools for investigating genetic, biochemical, and pharmacologic properties of different animal species. Studies with the chemical carcinogen dimethylnitrosamine have been conducted and show a functional relationship between mutagenesis and carcinogenesis. The assays can also be conducted using activation systems prepared from the tissues of any mammalian species. This permits a direct assessment of phylogenic extrapolation by comparing the metabolic activation capabilities of tissues from several mammalian species, including human samples. The advantages of mutagenicity testing are the short period of time required for results, the high sensitivity of the assay (microgram or nanogram quantities of chemicals can be used), and the fact that the ultimate agent can be detected biologically without first necessitating chemical identification and isolation.

It appears from current studies that in vitro mutagenesis techniques may well open new avenues of investigation into some old toxicologic problems.

ACKNOWLEDGMENTS

Portions of the work cited in this article were supported by research grants to the author from the U.S. Food and Drug Administration (No. IRO1 FD 00521) and the National Cancer Institute (No. IPO1 CA 14718). The author would also like to thank Dr. D. R. Jagannath for permission to use unpublished data.

REFERENCES

[1] J. A. Miller and E. C. Miller, A survey of molecular aspects of chemical carcinogenesis, Lab. Invest., 15, 217 (1966).

[2] W. J. Burdette, The significance of mutation in relation to the origin of tumors: a review, Cancer Res., 15, 201 (1955).

[3] E. C. Miller and J. A. Miller, "The Mutagenicity of Chemical Carcinogens: Correlation, Problems, and Interpretations" in Chemical Mutagens: Principles and Methods for Their Detection (A. Hollaender, ed.), Plenum, New York and London, 1971, p. 83.

[4] B. N. Ames, "The Detection of Chemical Mutagens with Enteric Bacteria" in Chemical Mutagens: Principles and Methods for Their Detection, Vol. 1 (E. A. Hollaender, ed.), Plenum, New York and London, 1971, p. 267.

[5] B. N. Ames, "A Bacterial System for Detecting Mutagens and Carcinogens" in Mutagenic Effects of Environmental Contaminants (M. E. Sutton and M. I. Harris, eds.), Academic, New York, 1972, p. 57.

[6] B. N. Ames, F. D. Lee, and W. E. Durston, An improved bacterial test system for the detection and classification of mutagens and carcinogens, Proc. Natl. Acad. Sci., U.S., 70, 782 (1973).

[7] B. N. Ames, W. E. Durston, E. Yamasaki, and F. D. Lee, Carcinogens are mutagens: A simple test system combining liver homogenates for activation and bacteria for detection, Proc. Natl. Acad. Sci., U.S., 70, 2281 (1973).

[8] K. Isono and J. Yourno, Chemical carcinogens as frameshift mutagens: Salmonella DNA sequence sensitive to mutagenesis by polycyclic carcinogens, Proc. Natl. Acad. Sci., U.S., 71, 1612 (1974).

[9] L. D. Kier, E. Yamasaki, and B. N. Ames, Detection of mutagenic activity in cigarette smoke condensates, Proc. Natl. Acad. Sci., U.S., 71, 4159 (1974).

[10] J. McCann, N. E. Spingarn, J. Kobori, and B. N. Ames, The detection of carcinogens as mutagens: Bacterial tester strains with R factor plasmids, Proc. Natl. Acad. Sci., U.S., 72, 979 (1975).

[11] F. Kao and T. T. Puck, Genetics of somatic mammalian cells XII: Mutagenesis by carcinogenic nitroso compounds, J. Cell. Physiol., 78, 139 (1971).

[12] H. V. Malling, Dimethylnitrosamine: Formation of mutagenic compounds by interaction with mouse liver microsomes, Mutation Res., 13, 425 (1971).

[13] D. R. Stolz, L. A. Poirier, C. C. Irving, H. E. Stich, J. H. Weisburger, and H. C. Grice, Evaluation of short-term tests for carcinogenicity, Toxicol. Appl. Pharmacol., 29, 157 (1974).

[14] E. E. Slater, M. D. Anderson, and H. S. Rosenkranz, Rapid detection of mutagens and carcinogens, Cancer Res., 31, 970 (1971).

[15] T. Yahagi, M. Nagao, K. Hara, T. Matsushima, T. Sugimura, and G. T. Bryan, Relationships between the carcinogenic and mutagenic or DNA-modifying effects of nitrofuran derivatives, including 2-(2-furyl)-3-(5-nitro-2-furyl) acrylamide, a food additive, Cancer Res., 34, 2266 (1974).

[16] K. Teranishi, K. Hamada, and H. Watanabe, Quantitative relationship between carcinogenicity and mutagenicity of polyaromatic hydrocarbons in Salmonella typhimurium mutants, Mutation Res., 31, 97 (1975).

[17] P. N. Magee and P. F. Swann, Nitroso compounds, Brit. Med. Bull., 26, 240 (1969).

[18] D. V. Parke and R. T. Williams, Metabolism of toxic substances, Brit. Med. Bull., 25, 256 (1969).

[19] A. H. Conney and J. J. Burns, Metabolic interactions among environmental chemicals and drugs, Science, 178, 576 (1972).

[20] H. R. Gutmann, D. Malejka-Giganti, E. J. Barry, and R. E. Rydell, On the correlation between the hepatocarcinogenicity of the carcinogen, N-2-fluorenylacetamide, and its metabolic activation by the rat, Cancer Res., 32, 1554 (1972).

[21] M. G. Gabridge and M. S. Legator, A host-mediated assay for the detection of mutagenic compounds, Proc. Soc. Exptl. Biol. Med., 130, 831 (1969).

[22] M. S. Legator and H. V. Malling, "The Host-Mediated Assay, a Practical Procedure for Evaluating Potential Mutagenic Agents in Mammals" in Chemical Mutagens: Principles and Methods for Their Detection (A. Hollaender, ed.), Plenum, New York and London, 1971.

[23] P. Propping and W. Buselmaier, The influence of metabolism on mutagenic activity in the host-mediated assay, Arch. Toxikol., 28, 129 (1971)

[24] E. Zeiger and M. Legator, Mutagenicity of N-nitrosomorpholine in the host-mediated assay, Mutation Res., 12, 469 (1971).

[25] W. J. Martone and F. H. Mukai, Bacteriophage T4 as an indicator organism for the host-mediated assay, Proc. Am. Assoc. Cancer Res., 13, 113 (1972).

[26] B. N. Ames, P. Sims, and P. L. Grover, Epoxides of polycyclic hydrocarbons are frameshift mutagens, Science, 176, 47 (1972).
[27] B. N. Ames, F. G. Gurney, J. A. Miller, and H. Bartsch, Carcinogens as frameshift mutagens: Metabolites and derivatives of acetylaminofluorene and other aromatic amine carcinogens, Proc. Natl. Acad. Sci., U.S., 69, 3128 (1972).
[28] S. Belman, W. Troll, G. Teebor, and F. Mukai, The carcinogenic and mutagenic properties of N-hydroxyaminonaphthalenes, Cancer Res., 28, 535 (1968).
[29] F. Mukai and W. Troll, The mutagenicity and initiating activity of some aromatic amine metabolites, Ann. N. Y. Acad. Sci., 163, 828 (1969)
[30] E. Huberman, L. Aspiras, C. Heideberger, P. L. Grover, and P. Sims, Mutagenicity to mammalian cells of epoxides and other derivatives of polycyclic hydrocarbons, Proc. Natl. Acad. Sci., U.S., 68, 3195 (1971).
[31] E. Huberman, P. J. Donovan, and J. A. DiPaolo, Mutation and transformation of cultured mammalian cells by N-acetoxy-N-2-fluorenylacetamide, J. Natl. Cancer Inst., 48, 837 (1972).
[32] H. V. Malling, Mutagenic activation of dimethylnitrosamine and diethylnitrosamine in the host-mediated assay and the microsomal system, Mutation Res., 26, 465 (1974).
[33] U. Weekes and D. J. Brusick, In vitro activation of chemical mutagens. II. The relationships among mutagen formation, metabolism and carcinogenicity for dimethyl- and diethylnitrosamine in the liver, kidneys and lungs of GALB/cJ, C57BL/6J and RF/J mice, Mutation Res., 31, 175 (1975).
[34] T. Nakajima and S. Iwahara, Mutagenicity of dimethylnitrosamine in metabolic processes by rat liver microsomes. Mutation Res., 18, 121 (1973).
[35] T. Kada, K. Tutikawa, and Y. Sadaie, In vitro and host-mediated "rec-assay" procedures for screening chemical mutagens: and phloxine, a mutagenic red dye detected, Mutation Res., 16, 165 (1972).
[36] D. J. Brusick and H. Andrews, Comparison of the genetic activity of dimethylnitrosamine, ethylmethane sulfonate, 2-acetylaminofluorene and ICR-170 in Saccharomyces cerevisiae strains D3, D4 and D5 using in vitro genetic assays with and without metabolic activation, Mutation Res., 26, 491 (1974).
[37] H.-G., Neumann, Ultimate electrophilic carcinogens and cellular nucleophilic reactants, Arch. Toxicol., 32, 27 (1974).
[38] A. L. Reeves, H. E. Puro, and R. G. Smith, Inhalation carcinogenesis from various forms of asbestos, Environmental Res., 8, 178 (1974).
[39] R. T. Prehn, Function of depressed immunologic reactivity during carcinogenesis, J. Natl. Cancer Inst., 31, 791 (1963).

[40] G. J. Todaro and R. J. Huebner, The viral oncogene hypothesis: New evidence, Proc. Natl. Acad. Sci., U.S., 69, 1009 (1972).
[41] H. M. Temin, On the origin of the genes for neoplasia: G. H. A. Clowes Memorial Lecture, Cancer Res., 34, 2835 (1974).
[42] R. E. Benveriate and G. J. Todaro, Evolution of C-type viral genes: Inheritance of exogenously acquired viral genes, Nature, 252, 456 (1974).
[43] N. Ledinko and M. Evans, Enhancement of adenovirus transformation of hamster cells by N-methyl-N'-nitro-N-nitrosoguanidine, caffeine and hydroxylamine, Cancer Res., 33, 2936 (1973).
[44] L. Diamond, R. Knorr, and Y. Shimizu, Enhancement of simian virus 40-induced transformation of Chinese hamster embryo cells by 4-nitroquinoline 1-oxide, Cancer Res., 34, 2599 (1974).
[45] B. C. Casto, W. J. Pieczynski, and J. A. DiPaolo, Enhancement of adenovirus transformation by treatment of hamster embryo cells with diverse chemical carcinogens, Cancer Res., 34, 72 (1974).
[46] G. Klein and E. Klein, Antigenic properties of other experimental tumors, Symposia Quant. Biol., 27, 463 (1962).
[47] G. Klein, H. O. Sjogren, E. Klein, and K. E. Hellstrom, Demonstration of resistance against methylcolanthrene-induced sarcomas in the primary autochthonous host, Cancer Res., 20, 1561 (1960).
[48] L. J. Old, E. A. Boyse, D. A. Clarke, and E. A. Carswell, Antigenic properties of chemically-induced tumors, Ann. N.Y. Acad. Sci., 101, 80 (1962).
[49] H. O. Sjogren, I. Hellstrom, and G. Klein, Transplantation of polyoma virus-induced tumors in mice, Cancer Res., 21, 329 (1961).
[50] H. Remmer, Induction of drug metabolizing enzymes in the liver, Europ. J. Clin. Pharmacol., 5, 115 (1972).
[51] T. C. Campbell and J. R. Hayes, Role of nutrition in the drug-metabolizing enzyme system, Pharmacol. Rev., 26, 171 (1974).
[52] D. R. Jagannath, "In vitro biotransformation of chemical carcinogens to mutagenic intermediates by kidney microsomal fractions of male and female mice," Ph.D. Thesis, Howard University, Washington, D.C., 1975.
[53] P. G. Gyorgy, J. Siefter, R. M. Tomarelli, and H. G. Goldblatt, Influence of dietary factors and sex on the toxicity of carbon tetrachloride in rats, J. Exptl. Med., 83, 449 (1946).
[54] P. DeLucia and J. Cairns, Isolation of an E. coli strain with a mutation affecting DNA polymerase, Nature, 224, 1164 (1969).
[55] B. A. Bridges, Simple bacterial systems for detecting mutagenic agents, Lab. Pract., 21, 413 (1972).
[56] S. Kondo, Environmental mutagen testing in Escherichia coli and phage lambda, Mutation Res., 26, 235 (1974).

[57] G. Mohm and J. Ellenberger, Mammalian blood-mediated mutagenicity tests using a multipurpose strain of Escherichia coli K12, Mutation., 19, 257 (1973).
[58] F. K. Zimmermann, Procedures used in the induction of mitotic recombination and mutation in the yeast Saccharomyces cerevisiae, Mutation Res., 31, 71 (1975).
[59] F. K. Zimmermann, Genetic aspects of carcinogenesis, Biochem. Pharmacol., 20, 985 (1971).
[60] F. K. Zimmermann, R. Schwaier, and U. V. Laer, Mitotic recombination induced in Saccharomyces cerevisiae with nitrous acid, diethylsulfate and carcinogenic alkylating nitrosamides, Z. Vererbungsl., 98, 230 (1966).
[61] D. J. Brusick and V. W. Mayer, New developments in mutagenicity screening techniques using yeast, Environ. Health Perspectives, 6, 83 (1973).
[62] F. J. deSerres and H. V. Malling, "Measurement of Recessive Lethal Damage over the Entire Genome and at Two Specific Loci in the ad-3 Region of a Two-Component Heterokaryon of Neurospora crassa," in Chemical Mutagens, Principles and Methods for Their Detection (A. Hollaender, ed.), Plenum, New York, Vol. 2, 1971, p. 311.
[63] F. H. Sobels, The advantages of Drosophila for mutation studies, Mutation Res., 26, 277 (1974).
[64] D. Clive and J. F. S. Spector, Laboratory procedure for assessing specific locus mutations at the TK locus in cultured L5178Y mouse lymphoma cells, Mutation Res., 31, 17 (1975).
[65] W. Schmid, The micronucleus test, Mutation Res., 31, 9 (1975).
[66] F. Gletten, U. Weekes, and D. J. Brusick, "In vitro activation of chemical mutagens. I. Development of an in vitro mutagenicity assay using liver enzymes for activation dimethylnitrosamine, Mutation Res., 28, 113 (1975).
[67] P. Greenwald, J. J. Barlow, P. C. Nasca, and W. S. Burnett, Vaginal cancer after maternal treatment with synthetic estrogens, New Engl. J. Med., 285, 390 (1971).
[68] A. L. Herbst, H. Ulfelder, and D. C. Poskanzer, Adenocarcinoma of the vagina: Association of maternal stilbesterol therapy with tumor appearance in young women, New Engl. J. Med., 284, 878 (1971).
[69] E. Freese, Structure and function of the genetic elements on the molecular explanation of spontaneous and induced mutations, Brookhaven Symp. Biol., 12, 63 (1959).
[70] P. J. Fischinger, S. Nomura, P. T. Peebles, D. K. Haapala, and R. H. Bassin, Reversion of murine sarcoma virus transformed mouse cells: Varients without a rescuable sarcoma virus, Science, 176, 1033 (1972).
[71] S. Takayama and K. Oota, Malignant tumors in mice fed with N-nitrosodimethylamine, GANN, 54, 465 (1963).

[72] D. F. Heath, The decomposition and toxicity of dialkylnitrosamines in rats, Biochem. J., 85, 72 (1962).
[73] P. Czygan, H. Greim, A. J. Garro, F. Hutlerer, F. Schaffner, H. Popper, O. Rosenthal, and D. Y. Cooper, Microsomal metabolism of dimethylmitrosamine and the cytochrome P-450 dependency of its activation to a mutagen, Cancer Res., 33, 2983 (1973).
[74] S. Takayama and K. Oota, Induction of malignant tumors in various strains of mice by oral administration of N-nitrosodimethylamine and N-nitrosodiethylamine, GANN, 56, 189 (1965).
[75] B. Terracini, G. Palestro, M. R. Gigliard and R. Montesano, Carcinogenicity of dimethylnitrosamine in Swiss mice, Brit. J. Cancer, 20, 871 (1966).
[76] N. K. Clapp, R. L. Tyndall, and J. A. Otten, Differences in tumor types and organ susceptibility in BALB/c and RF mice following dimethylnitrosamine and diethylnitrosamine, Cancer Res., 31, 196 (1971).
[77] U. Weekes, Metabolism of dimethylnitrosamine to mutagenic intermediates by kidney microsomal enzymes and correlation with reported host susceptibility to kidney tumors, J. Natl. Cancer Inst., 5, 1199 (1975).
[78] B. Toth, P. N. Magee, and P. Shubik, Carcinogenesis study with dimethylnitrosamine administered orally to adult and subcutaneously to newborn BALB/c mice, Cancer Res., 24, 1712 (1964).
[79] J. H. Weisburger and E. K. Weisburger, Biochemical formation and pharmacological, toxicological and pathological properties of hydroxylamines and hydroxamic acids, Pharmacol. Rev., 25, 2 (1973).
[80] E. C. Miller, J. A. Miller, and M. Entomoto, The comparative carcinogenicities of 2-acetylaminofluorene and its N-hydroxy metabolite in mice, hamsters, and guinea pigs, Cancer Res., 24, 2018 (1964).
[81] R. W. O'Hara and R. H. Adamson, "Spontaneous and Induced Neoplasma in Nonhuman Primates," in Pathology of Simian Primates (R. N. T-W-Fiennes, ed.), Karger, New York, 1972, p. 190.
[82] D. McGregor, "The relationship of 2-acetamidofluorene mutagenicity in plate tests with its in vivo liver cell component distribution and its carcinogenic potential." A paper presented at the 14th Annual Meeting of the Society of Toxicology, Williamsburg, Virginia, 1975.
[83] J. McCann, E. Choi, E. Yamasaki, and B. Ames, Detection of carcinogens as mutagens in the Salmonella/microsome test: Assay of 300 chemicals, Proc. Natl. Acad. Sci. U.S., 72, 5135 (1975).
[84] F. J. deSerres, Report of the Conference on In Vitro Mutagenicity and Carcinogenicity Tests, Mutation Res., 1976, in press.
[85] H. S. Rosenkranz, unpublished results.

Necropsy of Animals for Scientific Research

MELVIN DWAINE REUBER, M.D.

11014 Swansfield Road
Columbia, Maryland

INTRODUCTION

Autopsies on human beings have been done for hundreds of years. The complete autopsy was first proposed by Rokitansky and has been referred to as the "Rokitansky dissection" [1]. Complete and precise autopsies on animals used for research are of more recent origin and have not been described in detail. The following is a procedure that has been useful for scientific research.

GROSS DESCRIPTION

The lesions in organs are described grossly at the time of removal from the body and weighing. This description is based upon the size, color, shape, and consistency. It is not a pathologic description or diagnosis (with the exception, perhaps, of an examiner trained in pathology).

The size is the weight in grams and measurements are made in centimeters. Color is self-explanatory. The shape is any distortion in the usual contour of an organ, such as a change in the surface from smooth to rough or nodular. Shape also includes the location of the

TABLE 1. Necropsy Record

Card for recording data at the time of necropsy. This particular card was designed primarily for the study of diseases of the liver; therefore, more space is available for weights and descriptions of the various lobes of the liver. There is space for a general description of the animal, and for weights of the various organs with a brief description. The back is blank and can be used either for drawing lesions of organs or for histologic notes. The cards are 4 in. by 8 in. and can be stored in files.

STRAIN	SEX	AGE (In Weeks) ☐ Killed ☐ Died	AUTOPSY NUMBER
ANIMAL NUMBER	GROUP	CARCINOGEN	EXPERIMENT NUMBER
INTACT	CASTRATED	ADRENALECTOMY	AGE AT START OF EXP. (In Weeks)
BODY WEIGHT	LIVER WEIGHT	DESCRIPTION	
LEFT LOBE			
MEDIAN LOBE		HEART	PITUITARY
		THYMUS	OVARY
RIGHT LOBE (Upper)		SPLEEN	UTERUS
RIGHT LOBE (Lower)		RIGHT KIDNEY	SEMINAL VESICLES
		LEFT KIDNEY	PROSTATE
CAUDATE LOBE (Anterior)		TESTES	ADRENAL
		BREAST	THYROID
CAUDATE LOBE (Posterior)		TUMOR	SALIVARY GLAND
		LUNGS	

NIH-970
6-66

LABORATORY BIOLOGY BRANCH, NCI

ANIMAL AUTOPSY RECORD

lesion within an organ. Consistency ranges from liquid to soft, and from firm to hard.

Detailed descriptions of the anatomical structure can be consulted [2-5].

RECORDS

Forms are best designed by the particular investigator to suit the situation. They include the gross description, body and organ weights, animal numbers, experiment numbers, dates, and other notes. An example is shown in Table 1.

THE FIXATIVE

The fixative that is most convenient and serves most purposes is 10% formalin (4% formaldehyde) [6]. Tissue can be preserved for days and weeks before transferring to alcohol. The ideal time is one week. Tissues such as bowel and pituitary can be placed on blotter before placing in fixative to prevent curling or loss and to aid in trimming later. The tissue and lesions can be readily recognized at the time of trimming. Stains for glycogen (periodic acid-Schiff), reticulum, bilirubin, cholesterol, lipid (oil red O), connective tissue, mucin (periodic acid-Schiff or mucicarmine), and even mitochondria (Hortega) can be done on the tissue [7-9]. If formalin pigment [9] is a problem, it can be avoided by using neutral buffered formalin—diluted formalin shaken with calcium carbonate and stored over a layer of this salt.

Formal Zenker's is also commonly used for fixation of tissues [6]. After 48 hr of fixation, the tissues must be washed by water for at least 24 hr. The tissue is harder and more difficult to identify at the time of trimming than that fixed in formalin. Stains for lipid cannot be done on the tissue.

A suitable amount of fixative must be used for proper fixation of tissues. Generally, the 100-cc container can be used for small animals and the 200-cc or larger container for rats or larger rodents.

DECAPITATION

Weigh the animal. The animal can be anesthetized with ether and killed by decapitation and exsanguination. This can be accomplished with a guillotine or with a pair of scissors. The head should be extended and the blood vessels and vertebrae severed near the clavicles and scapulae in order to avoid injury to the salivary glands and thyroid. If blood is needed for chemical studies the animal can be exsanguinated by puncture of the heart. Removal of the blood prevents dilution of the fixative. If exsanguination is not complete, the tissues can be rinsed with water and the bloody formalin replaced with clear formalin.

THE NECROPSY

The same procedure should be followed for each necropsy; otherwise some tissue may not be excised and examined. Obtain an autopsy number for the record and container for fixative and tissue. Record the gross description and weight of each organ when it is removed and placed in fixative.

External Examination

Record such measurements as tail, bone, or muscle length. Examine the skin for dermatitis or tumors. Remove the skin from the carcass and look for skin appendage tumors or subcutaneous lesions. A representative portion of skin and its appendages can be obtained from the back of the animal, preferably over the neck or anterior or posterior back after the hair has been removed with a clipper. For detailed studies of the skin or subcutaneous tissues, the entire skin can be pinned to a board and immersed in fixative (Fig. 1) [10]. If there are no gross lesions remove mammary gland tissue from one groin and from the opposite axilla. Place on blotter before fixation.

To facilitate handling, the animal may be pinned by the legs to an appropriate board.

Remove the anterior abdominal and thoracic wall so that the organs of the chest and abdomen are exposed (Fig. 2).

Remove the heart so that the blood from the atria and ventricles will drain before clotting. Weigh. Remove and weigh the thymus.

Remove the spleen and adjacent pancreas. Place the pancreas on blotter and into fixative. Weigh the spleen.

If the animal is male, remove the testes and epididymi. Weigh the testes separately and cut the right testis transversely near one end. Remove the urinary bladder, prostate gland, and seminal vesicles in one piece. If weights are needed, separate the prostate gland and seminal vesicles from the bladder.

In the female animal leave the ovaries, uteri, and urinary bladder intact. Remove all adipose tissue adjacent to the right ovary, but not from the left ovary. When taking weights of ovaries, place the right in a separate bottle with autopsy number labeled as R.

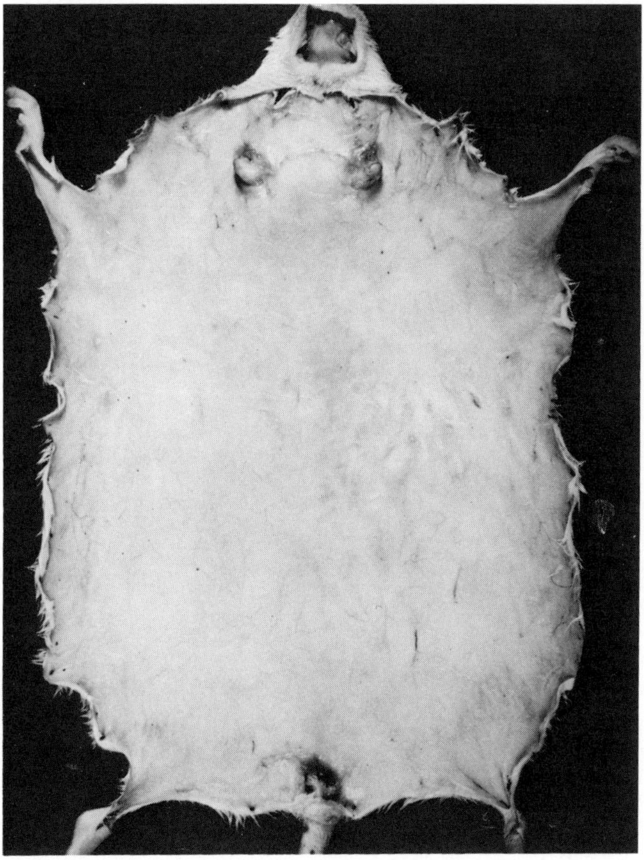

FIG. 1. Skin of a rat has been removed in one piece. This is useful for recording the precise location of skin or subcutaneous lesions. Small lesions will not be overlooked.

Cut the jejunum near the duodenum. Take the jejunum and apply pressure so that the small intestine down to the cecum separates from the mesentery. From the cecum to the rectum the large bowel can be more easily separated from the mesentery by cutting with a scissors. Spread the small and large intestines out on a large board. Rinse the cecum with water in order to remove the contents. Open and examine the mucosa. Take sections of lesions. If the bowel is not abnormal, section the jejunum, ileum, cecum, colon, and rectum

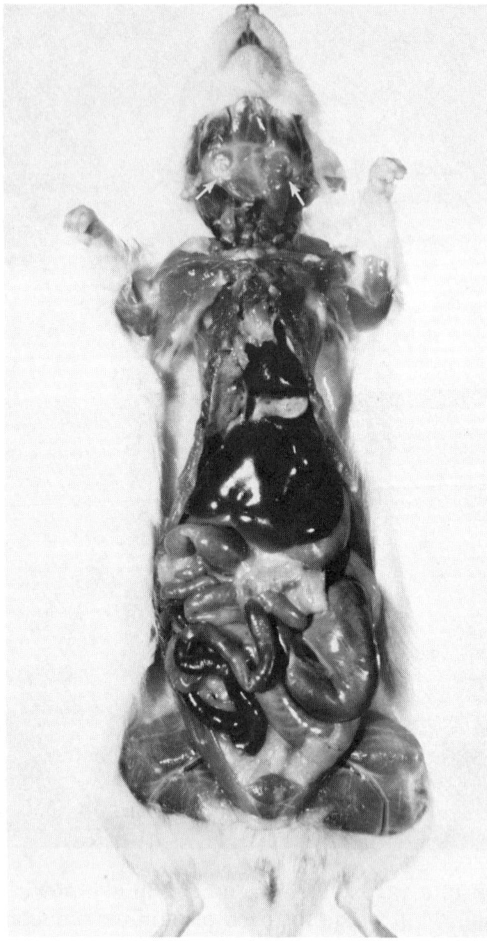

FIG. 2. Anterior abdominal wall has been removed. The organs can be easily removed. Notice the neck where the blood vessels have been severed for exsanguination. Arrows point toward salivary glands.

and place on blotter. (Opening and sectioning of bowel can be deferred until the remainder of the autopsy has been completed.)

Any part of the bowel, such as the cecum, can be placed on cork with straight pins and placed in fixative separately for 1 hr (Fig. 3); then remove pins and add to the bottle with the other tissues. The

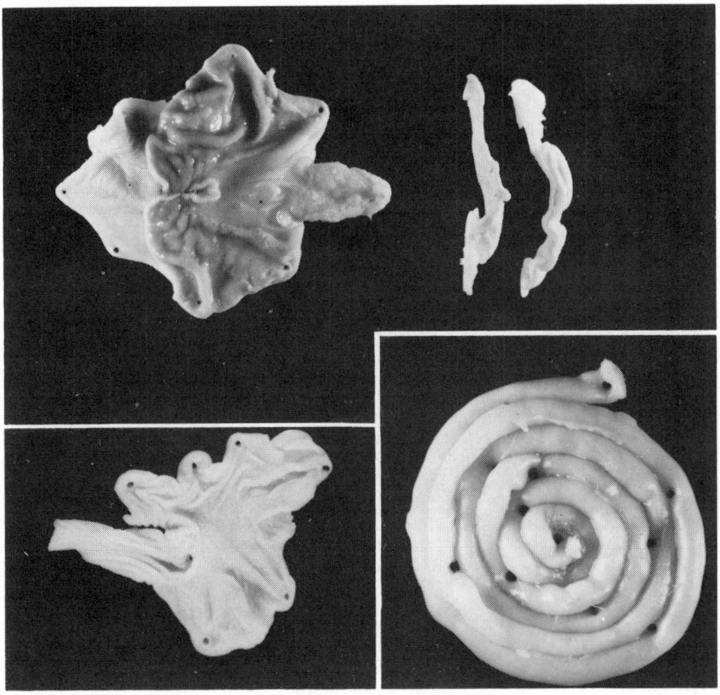

FIG. 3. The stomach is shown at the top after being pinned to cork and fixed. Longitudinal sections to be embedded in paraffin on edge are shown on the top right. Lower left: cecum fixed in a similar manner. Lower right: small intestine rolled, fixed, and ready for trimming and embedding.

entire intestines can be studied histologically. After the bowel has been opened on the board, it can be wrapped in a ball, tied with string, and fixed (Fig. 3).

Place the left adrenal without adipose tissue on blotter and weigh the left kidney. Transect the left kidney longitudinally in the flat plane into two similar parts. Place the right adrenal with some adherent adipose tissue on the blotter with the left adrenal. Weigh the right kidney and excise the upper pole (Fig. 4). Transect the right kidney in the first plane longitudinally. If adrenal weights are required, place the right adrenal in the bottle with the right ovary labeled with the autopsy number and R.

Excise a portion of the right psoas muscle. Remove enlarged

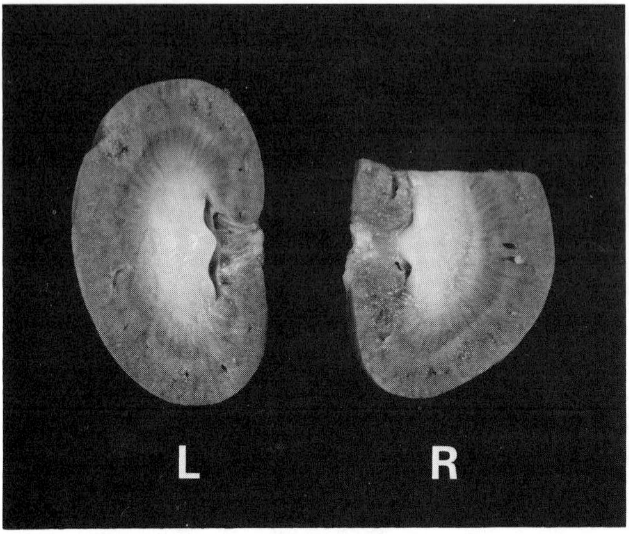

FIG. 4. R: right kidney; L: left kidney.

retroperitoneal lymph nodes. If there are lesions of the nodes, place in a separate bottle labeled RP.

Remove the esophagus, stomach, and duodenum with attached pancreatic tissue. Open the stomach along the greater curvature and rinse with water in order to remove gastric contents. If there are lesions of the stomach, pin the stomach on a cork with straight pins and place in fixative separately for 1 hr (Fig. 3). The same can be done for the esophagus. Remove pins and add to the bottle with the other tissues. Weigh the anterior caudate lobe of the liver and place in separate bottle labeled Ca. Weigh the posterior caudate lobe. Remove the portahepatic lymph nodes, and if there are lesions place in a separate bottle labeled PH. If nodes appear normal, place on blotter and into fixative.

Remove and weigh the remaining liver; weigh each lobe of the liver—right lower, right upper, left, and median—in that order. If there are lesions save all tissue; if not, save representative sections in the manner described under trimming (Fig. 5).

Remove the lungs intact and with thoracic aorta.

Remove the salivary glands, extraorbital lacrymal glands (Figs. 6 and 7), and the cricothyroid cartilage with thyroid and parathyroid glands. If there are lesions of the thyroid gland, weigh each lobe separately and place in the bottle with the pituitary gland; otherwise do not remove from the cricothyroid cartilage.

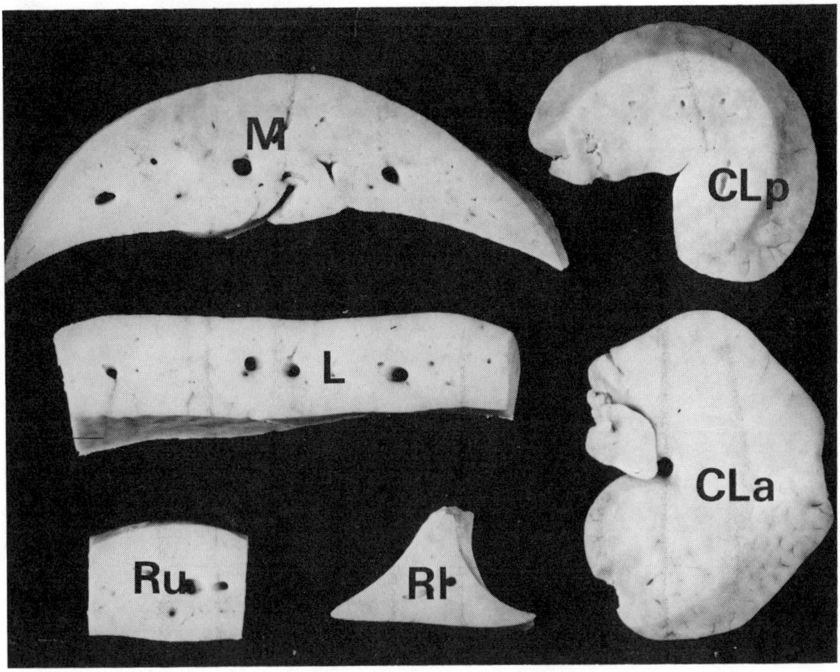

FIG. 5. Trimmed liver tissue. M, median lobe; L, left lobe; RU, right upper lobe; Rl, right lower lobe; CLa, anterior caudate lobe; and CLp, posterior caudate lobe.

Remove the maxillae with the tongue; excise the tongue.

Excise the top of the skull. Remove the brain with pressure, tearing the cranial nerves. Cut the membrane overlying the pituitary and place the pituitary on blotter in a separate bottle with label P. Remove both eyes intact with the Harderian glands (Fig. 8).

Save the skull so that the middle ear, snout, and sinuses can be examined [11, 12]. If microscopic sections of the skull are not obtained, a cut through the skull behind the eye sockets makes removal of the eyes and glands easier.

Save femur and sternum for bone marrow. Remove vertebrae if diffuse bone disease is present.

Thin sections of fresh tissue usually curl or warp after being placed in fixative and make trimming difficult. Warping can be prevented if the organs are slightly firm. Approximately 15 to 30 min after completion of the autopsy remove heart, spleen, brain, tongue, skeletal muscle, mammary tissue, liver, and tumors of other organs. Make cuts 4 or 5 mm apart in the long axis of each organ, but let the organs remain in one piece.

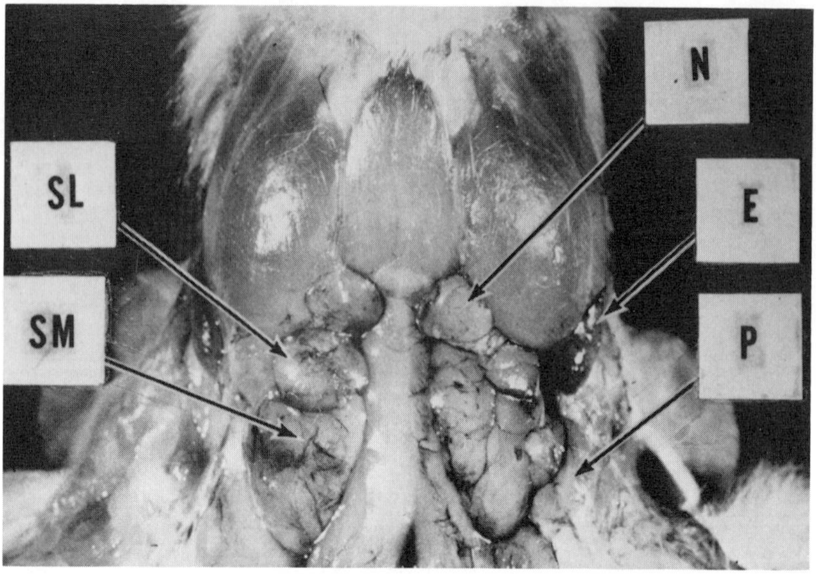

FIG. 6. Identification of the major exocrine glands in the neck. Ventral view shows the lobulated submaxillary gland (SM), the major sublingual gland (SL), the parotid gland (P), the extraorbital lacrymal gland (E), and lymph nodes (N). [Reproduced with permission of M. F. Stanton and the American Journal of Pathology.]

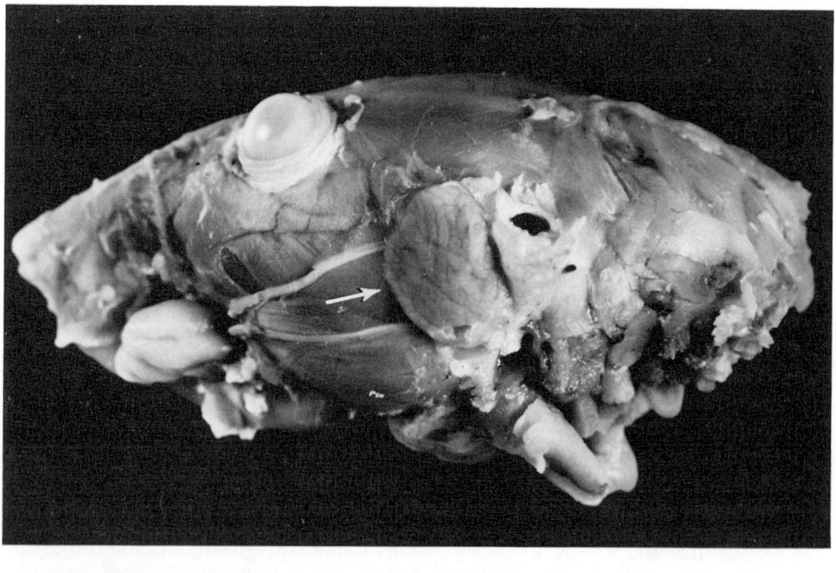

FIG. 7. Extraorbital lacrymal gland is designated by arrow.

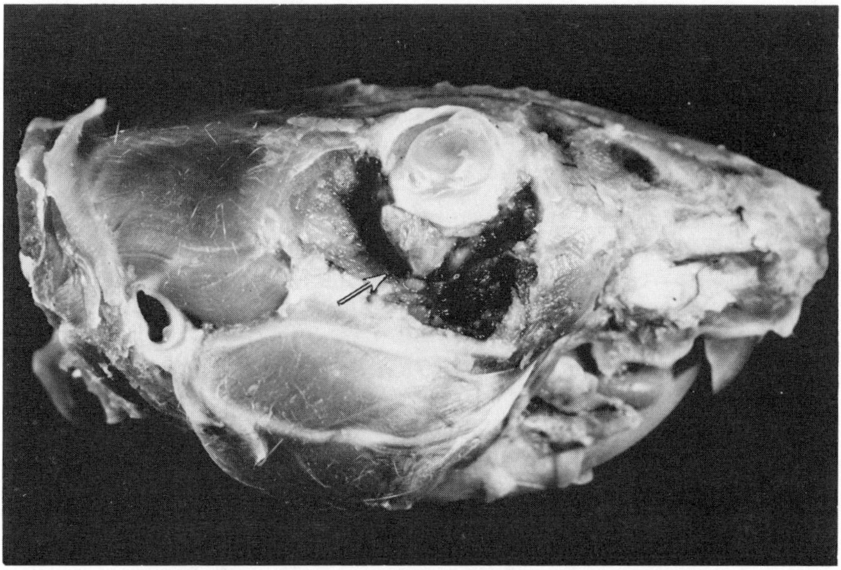

(a)

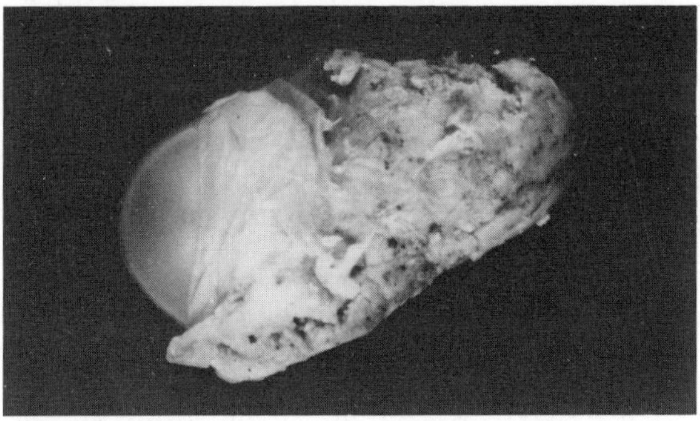

(b)

FIG. 8. (a) Harderian gland in situ (arrow) above. (b) Gland removed with eye.

Species Differences

There are very few differences in the organs of animals of the different species. Rats do not have a gall-bladder, whereas mice, hamsters, rabbits, and guinea pigs do have that organ. In hamsters the caudate lobes of the liver are rudimentary or absent.

SPECIAL PROCEDURES

If the lungs are being studied, the trachea can be injected with fixative after the thoracic cavity has been opened.

Hepatic parenchymal cell function can be studied by injecting Rose Bengal dye intravenously into the saphenous vein 30 min before the animal is killed. The liver stains dark pink. Dye is excreted into the intestines by way of the common bile duct. Hyperplastic and neoplastic lesions of the liver usually remained unstained by the dye [13].

Function of Kupffer cells can be studied by the injection of India ink 5 min before killing the animal. The ink can be injected into the leg vein or a laparotomy can be done and the ink injected directly into the portal vein. Grossly the vein will turn gray or black, depending upon the amount of ink injected. The pigment can be seen within the Kupffer cells on sections of the liver [20].

A smear of the blood or imprint of the spleen and/or lymph nodes are necessary when studying leukemia or other diseases of the blood. It must be done when the animal is killed. Tissues for histochemical procedures must be fixed in other fixatives or frozen [14].

TRIMMING

All sections should be 3 to 4 mm in thickness and the length and width should be such that the microscopic section can be mounted easily on the area on a glass slide 2.5×5.0 cm in size. Lesions of any organ should be trimmed so that the adjacent normal tissue is included in the section.

The periodic-acid Schiff-orange G stain can be requested on the pituitary when tissue is submitted for sectioning. This stain distinguishes between the various cell types of the pituitary. Special stains can also be requested on other organs when the tissue is submitted for sectioning. They can be done along with the hematoxylin and eosin, and will prevent relocating and cutting of the paraffin or paraplast block at a later time.

Rinse the formalin-fixed tissue in running water for several minutes. The following normal tissues can be placed in new 10% formalin (4% formaldehyde) without trimming: thymus, pancreas, portahepatic and other lymph nodes, lacrymal glands, and ovaries.

Section the skin with subcutaneous tissue and the mammary tissue. See that the hair is removed from the skin. It is extremely difficult to cut and causes dullness of the microtome knife. The mammary tissue, which is located in fat, should be no thicker than 3 mm. Fat fixes poorly in all fixatives and is not easily penetrated by paraffin.

Remove the aorta. Section the left lung in the flat plane. Make one cut through the periphery of the right lung without disturbing the

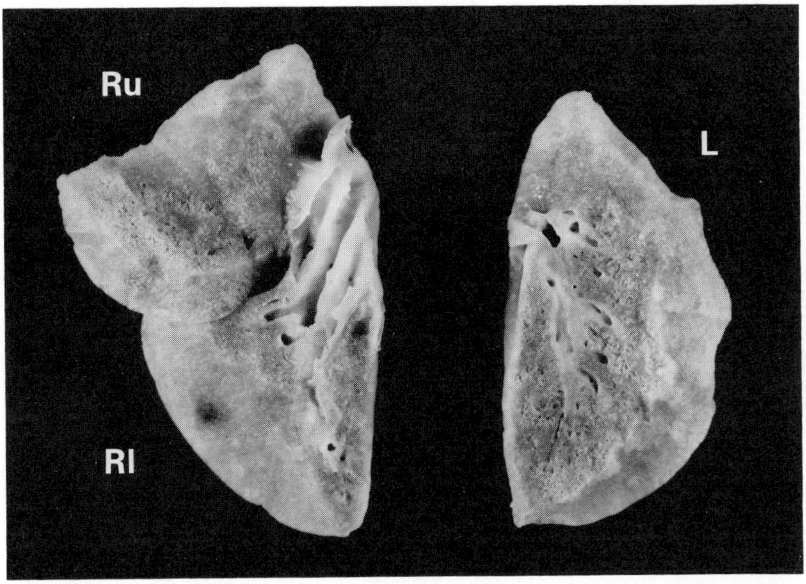

FIG. 9. Trimmed lung tissue. Ru, right upper lobe; Rl, right lower lobe; and L, left lobe. Right middle and lingual lobes are not shown.

bronchi. Then cut the bronchus so that the three lobes of that lung remain in one section attached to the bronchus (Fig. 9).

If the male genital organs have not been separated previously, separate the seminal vesicles from the prostate and urinary bladder in the male. One section can include the bladder and both sides of the prostate. Longitudinal and transverse sections can be made through the uteri. The section of urinary bladder can include the cervix in the female.

Cut the adrenal glands through the center. Trim the kidneys so they are the proper thickness. Submit the longitudinal sections of the right and left kidneys and the transverse section of the right. Use or save the additional sections of formalin-fixed kidney for lipid stains.

Trim a transverse and longitudinal section of skeletal muscle, and a transverse section of the diaphragm.

Previous cuts were made in the liver in order to make it possible to identify each lobe after trimming. Sections of the left lobe will be rectangular, right upper lobe square, right lower lobe rectangular, caudate lobes oval, and median lobe elliptical (Fig. 5). The gall bladder, when present, should be included in the section of the median lobe. If the individual lobes are distorted by tumors, place the tissue

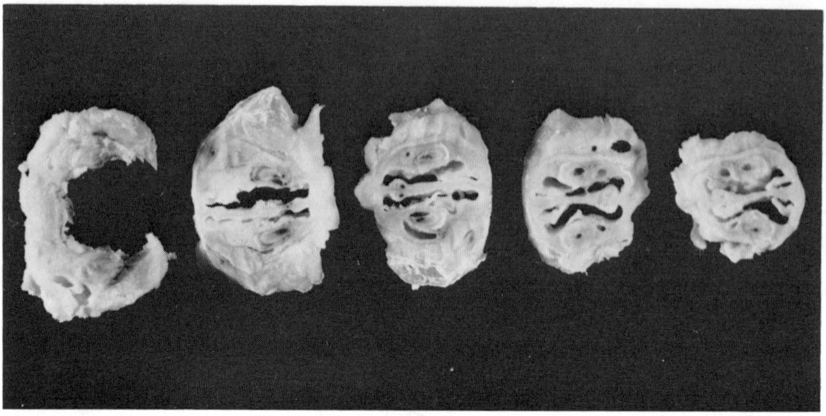

FIG. 10. Sections of trimmed skull after decalcification showing snout on the right and posterior skull on the left.

into separate bottles and put L, M, Ru, Rl, Ca, or Cp after autopsy number on the label.

The intestines are cut longitudinally in thin sections that can be embedded on edge (Fig. 3).

If the thyroid gland is attached to the cricothyroid cartilage, remove both sides. A transverse section can be made through the cartilage and gland when the gland is small. Place a cut through the center of each (right and left) salivary gland, without separating the submaxillary, parotid, or sublingual glands. If there is a lymph node, do not remove.

Calcium must be removed from the skull and other bones before sectioning. Acetic acid is commonly used and takes from 24 to 48 hr, depending upon the size of the tissue. The cells in the bone marrow are preserved more satisfactorily if a 10% solution of ethylenediaminetetraacetate is utilized. The latter solution requires approximately 1 week. In both instances the bone must be observed and when the tissue is soft enough for sectioning it should be removed, washed, and placed in 70% alcohol. Transverse sections are made through the length of the skull (Fig. 10). The long bones, vertebrae, and sternum are sectioned longitudinally.

TISSUE PROCESSING

Tissue sections in formalin are washed in running water for 3 to 6 hr depending on the amount of tissue. Tissue is then placed in 70%

alcohol. Zenker's-fixed tissue was washed previously and stored in 70% alcohol, so washing at this time is not necessary.

COMMENT

Special emphasis in the autopsy is given to any organ or organs that are being studied. If lesions of the mammary gland are of importance, all of the glands are dissected, weighed, and sectioned. If there are no lesions of the mammary tissue, routine sampling of one auxillary and one groin is usually adequate.

Likewise, emphasis is placed on the separate lobes of the liver in the study of hepatic disease. The different lobes of the liver are involved to varying degrees in studies of carcinogenesis and cirrhosis [13, 15-20].

Skin and subcutaneous tissue should be taken from the back of the animal because that is the site where dermatitis or tumors are most often observed. Routine sections of skin can otherwise be obtained from the abdomen.

Weigh the thymus because it is usually enlarged in leukemia. Enlarged lymph nodes are involved and should also be weighed. The spleen is enlarged in diseases of the liver, infections, and with carcinomas, as well as with leukemia.

The bone marrow is essential in the diagnosis of leukemia or other diseases of the blood. It must be well-fixed and processed in order to identify individual cells. In such cases a smear of blood and imprints of spleen, and/or lymph nodes are also required.

Weights of the organs of the urogenital system are useful if rats of specific or varying strains are used. One kidney can have hydronephrosis. One testis can be atrophic. Over 10% of ACI strain male rats have absence of or a cystic kidney on one side with atrophy of the seminal vesicle and testis on the same side [21]. In females of the same strain there is absence of the uterine horn on the side of the kidney abnormality. The endocrine organs vary also in the different strains. There may be adenomas of the pituitary, interstitial cell tumors of the testis, or variation in the size of the adrenal glands [22, 23].

Excellent gross and microscopic descriptions of the nasal cavities have been described by Keleman [11, 12], and microscopic description of the major exocrine glands in the neck by Innes and Stanton [24].

SUMMARY

Techniques for the necropsying of animals and the trimming of tissues for histologic sections have been described for scientific research. It has been helpful to refer to the description, records, fixatives, and to other special procedures. The comment explains the reasons for using some of the procedures.

REFERENCES

[1] R. D. Baker, Postmortem Examination; Special Methods and Procedures, Saunders, Philadelphia, 1962.
[2] E. C. Greene, "Gross anatomy" in The Rat in Laboratory Investigation (J. Q. Griffith, Jr. and E. J. Farris, eds.), Lippincott, New York, 1942, Chap. 3.
[3] J. Q. Griffith, Jr. and E. J. Farris (eds.), The Rat in Laboratory Investigation, Lippincott, New York, 1942.
[4] R. A. G. Wells, The Rat. A Practical Guide (A Dissection Manual), Dover, New York, 1964.
[5] E. L. Green, Biology of the Laboratory Mouse, 2nd ed., McGraw-Hill, New York, 1966.
[6] B. Saunders, Animal Histology Procedures, Government Printing Office, Washington, D.C., 1973.
[7] R. D. Lillie, Histopathologic Technic, Blakiston, Philadelphia, 1948.
[8] F. B. Mallory, Pathological Technique, Saunders, Philadelphia, 1944.
[9] G. Gomori, Microscopic Histochemistry: Principles and Practice, University of Chicago Press, Chicago, 1952.
[10] S. How and K. C. Snell, Skin tumors induced in rats by the dietary administration of N,N'-2,7-fluorenylenebisacetamide, J. Natl. Cancer Inst., 38, 408 (1967).
[11] G. Kelemen and F. Sargent, Non-experimental pathologic findings in laboratory rats, Arch. Otolaryngol., 44, 24 (1946).
[12] G. Kelemen, Junction of nasal cavity and pharyngeal tube in rat, Arch. Otolaryngol., 45, 159 (1947).
[13] M. D. Reuber, Development of preneoplastic and neoplastic lesions of the liver in male rats ingesting 0.025% N-2-fluorenyldiacetamide, J. Natl. Cancer Inst., 34, 697 (1965).
[14] A. G. E. Pearce, Histochemistry, Theoretical and Applied, Little Brown, Boston, 1972.
[15] M. D. Reuber and E. L. Glover, Cholangiofibrosis in the liver of Buffalo strain rats injected with carbon tetrachloride, Brit. J. Exptl. Pathol., 48, 319 (1967).
[16] M. D. Reuber and E. L. Glover, Thrombosis of hepatic veins accompanying cirrhosis in rats injected with carbon tetrachloride, Arch. Pathol., 83, 267 (1957).
[17] M. D. Reuber and E. L. Glover, Carbon tetrachloride-induced cirrhosis, Effect of age and sex, Arch. Pathol., 85, 275 (1968).

[18] M. D. Reuber, L. F. Dove, and E. L. Glover, Severe cirrhosis with hepatic vein thrombosis in rats given carbon tetrachloride and 3-methylcholanthrene, Pathol. Microbiol., 32, 314 (1968).

[19] M. D. Reuber, Hepatic vein thrombosis. Increased incidence in rats given methylcholanthrene and carbon tetrachloride, Arch. Environ. Health, 20, 458 (1970).

[20] M. D. Reuber, Evolution of hyperplasia, hyperplastic nodules and carcinoma of the liver induced in rats by N-2-fluorenyl-diacetamide, Gann Monograph Cancer Res., 17, 303 (1975).

[21] M. K. Deringer and W. E. Heston, Abnormalities of urogenital system in strain A x C line 9935 rats, Proc. Soc. Exptl. Biol. Med., 91, 312 (1956).

[22] K. C. Snell, "Spontaneous Lesions of the Rat" in The Pathology of Laboratory Animals (W. E. Riblein and J. R. McCoy, eds.), Charles C Thomas, Springfield, Ill., 1965, pp. 1-60.

[23] E. Cotchin and F. J. C. Roe (eds.), Pathology of Laboratory Rats and Mice, Blackwell, Oxford, 1967.

[24] J. R. M. Innes and M. F. Stanton, Acute disease of the submaxillary and harderian glands (sialo-dacryoadenitis) of rats with cytomegaly and no inclusion bodies, Am. J. Pathol., 38, 455 (1961).

Adverse Drug Reactions
The Scene Revisited—An Update

J. K. WESTON, M.D.

Department of Clinical Engineering
George Washington University School of Medicine
Washington, D.C.

KATHLEEN WESTON, M.D.

Purcellville, Virginia

INTRODUCTION

Our revised interest in revisiting the adverse drug reaction scene indepth was sparked by the Rather-Schorr broadcast nearly a year ago, entitled, "Prescription Drugs, Take With Caution."

We unfortunately did not listen to the original broadcast since we were unaware it was to appear. It was called to our attention, and we subsequently have had the opportunity to listen several times to the videotape of the broadcast and to discuss it in depth with other medically and scientifically interested and qualified persons.

*Address requests for reprints to: R. R. #1, Box 33, Purcellville, Virginia, 22132.

As we viewed and listened to this program, we found that it definitely promoted misinformation and misconceptions in the biomedical area generally. It was somewhat more blatant, in poor informational taste generally, and more inexcusable, at least in our opinion, than most media efforts in the biomedical field, especially in the therapeutic area. For many years we have been concerned about the apparent total disinterest most such media efforts demonstrate in even making a cursory bow in the direction of fair balance when dealing with biomedical matters. It was this aspect of the Rather-Schorr activity to which we took strong exception; the more so since we happened to know how readily available a great deal of published data was to them. The data sources concerning the other side of the coin were obviously unconsulted by them. The major distorted topic throughout the program which impressed us (and depressed us)—and on which we were moved to comment strongly—was the overemphasis on adverse drug reactions, especially the life-threatening ones. The repetition throughout the broadcast of the theme "hundreds of thousands of such adverse reactions," the "many hospital admissions related thereto," the "many deaths therefrom," and, along with that, the parallel suggestive themes that the physician is therapeutically incompetent and irresponsible—the tool of the detail man—therefore likely culpable, are continually pounded upon both overtly and covertly throughout the broadcast. Also the statement that 80% of such large numbers of adverse drug reactions are avoidable was noteworthy, the more so since no mention of specific means of avoiding them was made or the term "large numbers" defined.

Clearly, if the picture presented by Rather-Schorr to the large mass of television viewers has solid substance, this country is in a sad way therapeutically. Furthermore, those who listened to this unbalanced performance would be legitimately concerned as to whether they should pay any attention to the prescriptions their doctors give them and whether they should purchase, let alone take the prescribed product after buying it. Also, they might wonder whether the medical profession and the pharmaceutical industry are seriously culpable and possibly in league with each other to promote drug damage to patients, as some TV personalities and others allege.

None of the foregoing was even an approximation of the picture as we were aware of it—and we have been reasonably well aware for many years of the actual, published literature dealing with this important and involved matter of adverse drug reactions.

Let us go back to 1965-1968 when J. K. Weston, M.D., was Director of the Department of Drugs at the American Medical Association (AMA). In that capacity, he had direct responsibility for the, then, only program in existence (or which had ever existed) for some time attempting to obtain access to the physician's experience with adverse drug reactions. This program was known as the Blood Dyscrasia Registry of the AMA Department of Drugs. Later it was expanded to the

Adverse Drug Reaction Reporting Program of the AMA Department of Drugs. Thus in the later stages of its existence, it dealt generally with any sort of adverse reaction which it could induce any physician to report, with the assurance that such information would be held confidential.

During that time the AMA program had negotiated a cooperative arrangement with the Food and Drug Administration's recently established adverse drug reaction reporting program whereby both were to exchange information on a confidential basis and attempt to use similar formats for soliciting such information; the FDA had agreed to put it all into their computer for storage and retrieval.

The FDA had advanced to the point where they had instituted a hospital reporting program whereby they would pay staff residents or young physicians working in the hospitals a specific fee for each such adverse drug reaction reported fully on the standard FDA reporting form. This program was netting variable numbers of adverse drug reaction reports monthly. On the surface it looked good.

We, at AMA, had misgivings about the validity of the FDA reports as well as the manner in which they were being put into their computer from the standpoint of the likelihood that invalid data were going into the computer and, if this was established, that anything coming out of the computer would have no reliability whatsoever. AMA staff wanted to put the AMA total blood dyscrasia data into the AMA computer independently and add to it, to the degree possible, the reports currently obtained independently, together with those received from the Food and Drug Administration. Parenthetically, the AMA gave the FDA far more reports than they received from the FDA throughout the total AMA attempt to cooperate with them.

Having had some experience with the problems of computerization of biomedical data at that time and previously, we felt we should thoroughly evaluate the validity of the raw data in our own AMA files before even considering putting it into computers. Accordingly, one of our more experienced medical staff members reviewed this matter in depth and quite exhaustively. The report which he prepared and which was validated by independent checking, established clearly the fact that the quality of the data in the whole AMA Blood Dyscrasia file left a great deal to be desired, was not at all adequately validated to warrant computerization, and that substantial amounts of information based on the utilization of such material was already in the literature and was far from authoritative or capable of being validated, and therefore was probably misleading also. In short, the suspicion developed that the whole AMA Adverse Drug Reaction effort was, if not a travesty, certainly far from a strong or viable operation! And that the FDA program was no better, if as good.

It was about this time that the confidentiality of such information in the files of the Food and Drug Administration could no longer be assured. Staff, nonprofessional in character, of Senate Investigative

Committees were permitted access to the files despite Doctor Sadusk's opposition and strong protest. Breach of confidentiality put a whole new complication into the ball game of voluntary reporting on the part of the physicians in this country.

Since a good deal of the material most recently collected by AMA's program had already been passed on to the Food and Drug Administration in confidence, clearly the AMA Department of Drugs was not able to maintain such a cooperative relationship and still live up to their guarantee of confidentiality to physicians who cooperated with them and voluntarily reported their experience with adverse drug reactions.

This had to be of concern to the Department of Drugs and the Administration of the American Medical Association, and it became necessary for the AMA to discontinue its cooperation with the Food and Drug Administration in this area. We did this most regretfully and only after we made realistic proposals which could have maintained confidentiality of all such data in either the AMA or FDA files. Furthermore, AMA lawyers appeared to be reluctant to assure us and the administration of the AMA that, indeed, the material already in the AMA's files relative to adverse drug reactions, voluntarily reported by physicians under AMA's assurance that confidentiality would be maintained, could be maintained confidential; this properly caused considerable concern at all levels at the AMA. Our understanding is that an AMA administrative decision was subsequently made to destroy all such confidential material. This would seem to have been justified in view of the fact that the situation then obtaining was such that apparently the confidentiality we had assured those who had cooperated with us was no longer able to be maintained or guaranteed! Actually—and comfortingly—nothing real was lost because of the unsatisfactory quality of the majority of the reports.

Since that time, it is our impression that there have been a relatively small number of reports of adverse drug reactions to the Department of Drugs of the AMA and that the same is the situation with the FDA. However, we understand that sporadically, following appeals by them for such information, the FDA appears to have inconstantly obtained more adverse reports. (They, of course, by law receive all reports of adverse drug reactions forwarded to the manufacturer of any NDAed drug products.)

One of the ongoing studies in which both the AMA and the Food and Drug Administration were most interested and were encouraging was that of the greater Philadelphia group, headed by Marcus Reidenburg, M.D. It was a cooperative study utilizing five of the major teaching hospitals in the Greater Philadelphia area that was organized, mounted, carried on quite effectively for a period of two full years, and concluded during the close of J. K. Weston's tenure as Director of the Department of Drugs of the AMA.

The results of this study were published in the Journal of the American Medical Association for January 1, 1968 [1]. Along with this, the then editor of the Journal of the American Medical Association, Doctor John Talbot, requested J. K. Weston to write a commentary to appear concurrently with the report of the Greater Philadelphia study.

As a result of his personal experience in this area, both from the standpoint of having been in a responsible industry medical position for many years and having been in charge of, and responsible for this area in his tenure as Director of the Department of Drugs of the American Medical Association and Secretary of the Council of Drugs there, J. K. Weston produced such a commentary, which Doctor Talbot published [2]. It comprised essentially a state-of-the-art review.

In that commentary, the total published material available at that time dealing with adverse drug reactions was consulted and the picture brought up to date.

It is notable that few significant papers on adverse reactions have appeared in the United States since 1968. The contributions of the Tufts Drug Surveillance program and the Armed Forces Institute of Pathology program comprise most of the significant contributions. None of these have substantially modified the basic total situation existing at the time Reidenburg's report of the Philadelphia experience, and J. K. Weston's commentary thereon appeared. Despite that, the picture viewed by professional and layman today is one of gross overexaggeration of the incidence and severity of the adverse drug reaction aspect of the therapeutic use of drug products in the whole United States. Unfortunately, the same overexaggeration of the hazard to humans of all environmentally contacted substances appears to be mounting at express-train speed and with even less validated published data in support thereof. Some of the implications of this are more frightening and disconcerting than the alleged or potential hazards extrapolated from minimal animal data. For instance, the warning of a potential human carcinogenic hazard of trichloroethylene on the basis of one preliminary mouse experiment, despite its wide human industrial use for nearly 50 years in industry and its long use as an anesthetic agent in medicine with no hint of related human carcinogenesis! This was despite the fact that any chlorinated hydrocarbon that could replace TCE can boast nowhere near the relatively safe human use experience of TCE!

It appears that the data reported in 1968 by the Greater Philadelphia study, despite the fact that it was retrospective, was really valid, substantial, useful data under the conditions and the methods which they utilized to review the situation at the reporting hospitals. Furthermore, their conclusions were eminently justified, namely, that they had produced so little helpful adverse reaction information—and no new adverse reactions whatsoever—that they could no longer justify the apparent waste of the physician's time to continue that type of study. The commentary accompanying the publication of their results seems still a reasonably valid commentary on the factual state-of-the-art of adverse drug reaction reporting today. Certainly it was a valid commentary at that time. Also, just as certainly, the recent Medicine in the Public Interest (MIPI) report [3] differs little in substance. However, due partly to media efforts of the kind alluded to previously (the Rather-Schorr type of broadcast), a tremendous amount of public and professional misconception has been enhanced by most of the commentary in this area since those two papers were published in 1968. Some of the undesirable fallout noted as likely in the 1968 commentary has become much more obvious, namely, the worsening malpractice situation and the undeniable fact that, related to that worsening situation, an increasing number of physicians are unquestionably practicing "defensive" medicine, particularly in the therapeutic area.

In summary, the total available data on adverse drug reactions, which have appeared since the publication of the previous two papers on January 1, 1968, has become progressively more and more distorted, out of phase and out of context with the published total material dealing with the great mass of the data derived or derivable from all the studies carried out and reported in the literature. In our view, it has been clearly counter-productive.

It seems to have become a favorite pastime of some physicians--but more of nonphysicians—to extrapolate from selected data in the literature, or even unpublished data, the maximum possible number and kind of serious adverse drug reactions and to swamp the literature and the communications media with such extrapolations!

Those professionals culpable have been primarily in academia, in the regulatory agencies, and in or close to "consumer" organizations. Their extrapolations were picked up by legislators, and/or the communications media and others who like to "view with alarm" and given greater and greater currency and more and more exaggeration as time went on.

We would recommend to any reader really interested in the facts available concerning adverse drug reactions that he read the two papers previously referred to [1, 2] and the recently published "Medicine in the Public Interest" report, entitled "Adverse Drug Reactions in the United States" [3]. This is a reasonably accurate and objective picture of what the real facts are. The reader will, we are convinced, be appropriately horrified at the tremendous disparity between the real facts and the extrapolations which have been indulged in by individuals of the types noted above.

Let us actually see what we can derive objectively from the literature by reviewing the basic sources as well as these two attempts to lay out the state-of-the-art at two different points in time. It will be instructive to see what extrapolations have supervened in the interim and what the mistaken extrapolations are that seem to be firmly fixed in the minds of both professionals and nonprofessionals in far too great numbers today.

This matter is of extreme importance because it is human toxicology—human toxicology related to substances actually professionally prescribed in many instances for humans by the therapeutic experts of our society, the physicians. And please note that such substances have proven, in the experience of physicians, to be beneficial in treating disease when properly used; in short, their benefit-risk ratio sums on the side of benefit, not risk, overall. Actually, it can be considered that it is really the physician's controlled use of their toxic properties (which can and do result in adverse effects) which makes them helpful in disease control! If one keeps that in mind, it seem utterly incomprehensible that such therapeutic experts could possibly mistakenly over-prescribe or malprescribe for very many people substances which they know to be hazardous. Granting the preponderant use of proper dosage and admitting individual idiosyncrasies, are there a sufficient number of supportable cases reported to justify the claimed "hundreds of thousands" of deaths; or of hospital admissions; or of reactions developing while in the hospital and so on alluded to by Rather-Schorr and other "viewers with alarm"? Actually, if that be true, then it seems apparent that this professionally competent therapeutic segment of our society is somehow misinformed or actually criminal in its incompetence and neglect of its professional responsibilities. And close examination of those responsible for teaching therapeutics requires rigorous scrutiny if such reports be true.

DEFINITION OF ADVERSE REACTIONS

First let us define the term "adverse reaction." Here we immediately realize one of the reasons for the great variations in numbers in the figures encountered. The definitions of adverse drug reactions vary tremendously among those who publish in this area. Following are samples of some of the differences in the definitions of adverse drug reactions on the part of those who have actually attempted to make serious studies—primarily in hospitals—of the appearance of adverse drug reactions, to categorize them, to summarize them, and to arrive at some rationally supportable conclusions concerning them.

An adverse drug reaction is:

> "A response to a drug product that was unintended and undesired by the physician that prescribed it and which was severe enough to be commented upon in the progress notes" [1].
>
> "An Adverse Drug Reaction is any response to a drug which is noxious and unintended and which occurs at doses used in man for prophylaxis, diagnosis, or therapy, excluding therapeutic failures" [3].
>
> "In its broadest sense any undesirable effect produced by a drug" [3].

> "Any response to a drug which is noxious and unintended and which occurs in doses used in man for prophylaxis, diagnosis or therapy," WHO, reported in Ref. [3].

Relative to this matter, the following quotation from the Weston [2] commentary is still pertinent:

> "Likewise, in the studies which have been carried out by Cluff and others, where very high incidences of adverse reactions to drugs have been reported a very broad definition was employed; a great deal broader than that used by the Greater Philadelphia group. There is considerable question as to whether or not the incidences related chiefly to those cases in which the physiological or pharmacological effect of the drug in the individual patient reaches such a level that signs and symptoms, of course, result. In some of these it is these signs and symptoms which, before all this emphasis on adverse drug reactions, were looked for by the thoughtful physician and utilized in regulating the dose of the drug in the best interests of the individual patient."

Noteworthy in this area is that for the period from the mid 50s to the present there have been very few studies, Reidenburg's being one of the first and still one of the largest, attempting to obtain control values for adverse drug reactions as defined by those who work in this area. His limited study demonstrated quite clearly that a large number of purported adverse drug reactions—probably the largest number —the minor drug reactions, could be elicited in substantial numbers from patients who had no disease observable or clinically detectable and who were taking no drug products of any sort. Immediately this one study and the lack of any attempt on the part of those who work in this field to obtain additional such control data, if one wishes to use that term, let alone placebo data—casts substantial doubt on the numbers game which has been played with adverse drug reactions for all these many years. When the relatively large numbers of minimal adverse drug reactions—many of which on the basis of Reidenburg's study could be occurring without any relationship to drugs whatsoever—gets juggled into juxtaposition with severe adverse reactions, particularly life-threatening ones or those associated with fatalities, the picture is bound to get jumbled and, particularly in the minds of the nonprofessional who does not understand this clearly, becomes of frightening concern.

PURPORTED HOSPITAL ADMISSIONS RELATED TO ADVERSE DRUG REACTIONS

Let us consider the purported numbers of hospital admissions due to adverse drug reactions. Here, quite obviously, the minor reactions would scarcely be likely to be responsible for many, if any, hospital admissions. We can quite reasonably suspect or conclude that those which are truly responsible for the hospital admission of a patient are the more severe, possibly life-threatening types of adverse drug reactions. Let us contrast the comment made in the Rather-Schorr report of the "hundreds per week or per month admitted to hospitals because of adverse drug reactions" to the more modest and more substantial ones based on the available data figures which the MIPI report documents from the published literature. This is indeed quite a different kind of figure and relates back to the foregoing comment as to the therapeutic culpability of the therapeutic experts, the physicians, who would mistakenly and routinely give drugs to patients in manners which would threaten the health and well being of very many of those patients. Into this picture also comes hospital admissions for self-administered agents or those taken in a fashion other than as directed by the physician. Clearly these are neither the result nor the responsibility of the medical profession.

The MIPI report says, "In summary, adverse drug reactions have been reported to be responsible for 1.0-3.5% of admissions to general medical wards and for 0.3 to 1% of general hospital admissions." On the basis of the actual facts the MIPI report adduces here—and rational and reasonable extrapolations from those facts—one would have to conclude that the therapeutic performance of physicians generally must be pretty acceptable.

Actually, the majority of the data, if not practically all of it which we have available, have been developed by studies in a hospital, either total hospital population studies like the Philadelphia study or studies on medical floors of hospitals such as the Cluff and other similar type studies represent. Still it is true that in the time frame involved from the 50s through the 60s to the present, it would be most unlikely that a very large number of seriously ill patients—made ill by serious adverse reactions to drugs which they were prescribed or even took on their own—would not finally have found their way into hospitals where, it seems again quite unlikely, the majority of such cases would not have been properly related to the cause, namely, overdose or peculiar idiosyncrasies to specific drug products. Those would all seem reasonable and rational inferences on the basis of the total medical scene during the time frame involved. Of course, there could be those who would say that the therapeutic competence of physicians manning hospitals would not be adequate to detect the relationship between such serious signs and symptoms as the patient presented and the drug which he had taken. To some degree this may be true, one must admit, but it would be certainly a tremendous indictment of the practice of hospital medicine, largely medical school hospital medicine, to say that the majority of physicians manning such hospitals are that incompentent in the diagnosis of disease from whatever cause. Furthermore, when the MIPI report indicates that the more accurate figures for hospital admissions due to adverse drug reactions of a serious nature are as limited as noted above, again, one would have to conclude that the general level of therapeutic practice of physicians outside hospitals must be quite good overall—and this has to include the local medical doctor within reasonable transportation distances from such hospital centers.

It is true that Doctor Irey's carefully documented summarized studies, extrapolating an accuracy figure of less than 50% for the clinical diagnosis of serious adverse drug reactions, also bears on this matter. This would suggest that the clinical diagnostic data on specific drug products responsible for serious adverse drug reactions are really over reported. This could be interpreted to support the inference that less than 50% of those the MIPI report projects, within the realms of reasonable accuracy, are actually due to the drug products to which they are clinically ascribed. In short, as we look at all the facts available, even admitting that they leave something to be desired, the appropriate, reasonably documentable inferences and extrapolations are in the opposite direction from those which have been made and widely publicized, namely, that the practice of therapy in our country during and since the drug explosion has, overall, apparently been in the patient's best interest with a relatively minimal amount of serious potential or actual damage demonstrable in patients due to the drug products which those patients received, particularly if and when the physician's directions were followed. When one further realizes that there are patients who have peculiar idiosyncrasies to specific drug products which are not detectable before exposure to those products, one again begins to wonder if the total numbers of validated, severe, adverse drug reactions that one can extrapolate as accurately as possible from the total available literature are not approaching the lowest likely levels that could be reasonably expected. That would imply that near-perfect therapeutic activity is carried out by the whole medical profession—obviously far from a true statement in some validatable instances. Nevertheless, the total real picture which emerges here is not the picture of the incompetent therapeutic medical graduate whose prescribing arm is solely activated by the detail man on behalf of the pharmaceutical industry and at the expense of the patient.

HOSPITAL DEATHS DUE TO ADVERSE DRUG REACTIONS

Other statements or implications made in the Rather-Schorr report refer to "large numbers" of deaths in hospitals due to adverse drug reactions. Here the numbers validatable in the MIPI report certainly are far and away below the numbers one had heard stated or implied in a variety of places elsewhere and reiterated in the Rather-Schorr report. Actually, the numbers which the MIPI report suggests are validatable by the total published data and appropriate extrapolation thereof—and would seem to be further validated by the total experience of the Registry of Tissue Reactions to Drugs of the Armed Forces Institute of Pathology [3], under the leadership of Doctor Nelson Irey—are more in line with the total data dealing with hospital admissions because of or due to serious adverse drug reactions. It is also in reasonably good consonance with the data the MIPI report projects so far as the development of serious adverse drug reactions in hospital—particularly in the medical wards of hospitals—are concerned. It also points out that in many cases the listing of a fatal reaction as due to a drug product involves patients in the late stages of terminal diseases who were given very toxic drug products as the only thing that could be offered them to militate against the early fatal outcome of this disease. This again relates to Doctor Irey's findings of only about a 50% validatable clinical adverse reaction from a drug product in the cases reported to his registry. The MIPI report states, "In summary the prevalence of fatal adverse drug reactions in hospitalized medical service patients has varied from 0 to 0.56% in those reports which have presented sufficient data for analysis."

NEEDLESS ADVERSE DRUG REACTIONS

Then one must refer to the Rather-Schorr comment as to the needlessness of such great numbers (80%) of severe adverse drug reactions. One certainly wonders how anyone could come to this conclusion on the basis of the actual data published in the literature so far. The MIPI report considers this matter and comes to the conclusion that there are no data available permitting any statement that any specific percent really could be prevented. The MIPI report states further "the available data do not document the incidence of preventable adverse drug reactions."

SUMMARY

If we put it all together and attempt to come up with rational information as to the serious toxic effects of drug products, considering primarily those prescribed by physicians and taken according to the directions the physician supplied, one would have to say, generally, that the adverse drug reaction problem is not nearly the massive problem which has been presented to the public and even to the profession.

One must keep in mind that practically all the available information in the literature is information derived from rather carefully conducted studies of whole hospital populations, but most commonly of the populations of medical areas of the hospital where one expects to find very ill people and people who are taking a variety of drug products. Many of them may have been taking such products for long periods before coming to the hospital and are either continued on those products or deprived of them. Depending upon the state of their chronic illness, many are admitted to adjust doses under the supervision of the physician. Again, many are probably placed on continuing additional therapy of one sort or another. They are the chronically ill to a large degree. This is admittedly a high risk population and one would expect to find a substantially larger number of adverse drug reactions of all sorts in such a population than one would in the whole hospital population or in the total population of our country. A cardiac patient being adjusted to varying doses of digitalis products or a diabetic being stabilized on insulin are examples of chronically ill patients hospitalized for dose adjustments of potent drug products. Actually a review of the total published data involved validates such rational and reasonable inferences as have been noted. One certainly ought to use different kinds of thinking in relationship to the therapeutic management of admittedly very ill people on medical wards as compared with the therapeutic management of ambulatory patients—or of the population as a whole.

It would not be surprising to find such hospital populations demonstrating large numbers of minor adverse reactions to drugs depending upon one's definition thereof and even major reactions involved in, or associated with, severe morbidity and mortality in such ill populations. On the other hand, it would seem sensible and reasonable for those who did such studies to put their results in proper perspective related more to the particular population which they were studying and the likelihood that such a population would show significant numbers and degrees of adverse drug reactions compared with a total hospital population or to the total population of our country. It seems apparent that many such people, however, blinded to some degree by what they saw, perhaps used language a bit loosely in referring to the potential for adverse drug reactions of the drug products in common use in therapy in or out of hospital. One hesitates to level such a charge, but actually, it can scarcely be avoided. From the foregoing it would seem clearly evident that there has been a lack of common sense and good judgment on the part of professional and nonprofessional alike in dealing with the actual facts available relative to serious adverse drug reactions in our country for a good many years.

Since the majority of reported adverse drug reactions are relatively minor functional disturbances, many of which can be elicited in the absence of any drug of any sort and in the absence of any disease of any clinically observable sort, as stated above, to consider these reactions as drug produced or drug induced in all cases is certain playing fast and loose with what we know. So far as the severe adverse drug reactions are concerned, those unquestionably associated with morbidity and mortality, these have been tremendously exaggerated by loose statements on the part of professional and nonprofessional alike. It may well be that many such statements were well designed or well intended to point up a problem which, to the individual involved, appeared to be a tremendous problem, about which information had to be made available to the public with sufficient shock value to have that public take cognizance of it. However, it would appear that this has been massively overdone, and that as a result of excessive exaggeration since the early 50s, we have seen a picture of drug hazard develop that is out of line with reality. A medico-legal malpractice situation that is counter-productive to the best therapeutic care of our people has been created. It has been made to appear as though our prime therapeutists, our physicians, are uncaring, unknowing, and are contributing massively to the problem when, in fact, the total picture available would seem to indicate they are doing rather well, all things considered, and that they have done this all these years!

So far as the pharmaceutical industry relationship is concerned, the usual story has been to throw it all off on their detail men as having mislead and brainwashed the physician. The way the picture looks now, if it is indeed the detail man who teaches the physician, then, by and large, over this whole period one must infer he has done a mighty fine job when compared with what has been contributed by the medical undergraduate and post graduate therapeutic teaching to which young medical students and house officers are exposed in academia! We would prefer to think however, that the physician's overall acceptable therapeutic performance is a function of their intelligence, common sense, and ability to learn by experience.

WHAT KINDS OF DRUGS ARE MOST ASSOCIATED WITH ADVERSE DRUG REACTIONS?

Another clear cut finding stated in the MIPI report has interesting ramifications worthy of careful consideration. For many years this finding has been apparent to all who would consult the literature. That is, it is not the newer, the more modern, the more sophisticated, the more potentially hazardous, the patented, the more difficult to use drug products that are mainly associated with the severe morbidity and mortality that the MIPI report clearly related to drug products [3]. On the contrary, it is the multi-source drug products in broad and deep use for over 25 years, the aspirins, the diphenylhydantoins, the digoxins and other cardiac drug products, that are the major ones clearly responsible and reliably shown to be related to adverse drug reactions of the more severe types. The Harlem Hospital Study is a documented, published case in point here.

By implication, from the foregoing, the medical profession as a whole, dealing with the therapy of patients, can be concluded to have managed quite well to use effectively and safely the newer agents still under patent or just off patent. At least that conclusion would be accurate when compared with their ability, on record, to use the older, multi-source drug products on the market.

To put it another way, we can conclude that physicians have more trouble safely using insulin, aspirin, and all the cardiac glycosides than they do in using the new antibiotics, the new anti-gout agents, and any of the other newer agents which have come on the market in the 60s and 70s. (And remember, the numbers of new products marketed since 1962 is relatively small!)

Why is this? It certainly does not seem reasonable to us that their therapeutic competence in using the older drugs should be any less than in using the newer drugs. (The corollary here might be that the pharmaceutical industry, if it be true that they are the sources of drug information to the medical profession on the newer drugs, have done a fine job of educating the physician in the therapeutic handling of such agents, as noted above and as is worth repeating.)

The one fact that stands out clearly is that all these older drugs in common use, in relatively large amounts overall, are the ones which are obtained from many sources. In short, it is these agents which are the multi-source drug products produced by many producers but containing the same generic chemical. These are the "generic" drugs, using that word loosely.

Relative to the price of drugs, again, it is the older drugs in common use where the lowest prices for drug products exist. Furthermore, since they are made by many producers, in some instances, at least, there is probably more price competition in the multi-source drug products than in the newer patented ones. In addition to that, since more producers produce them, there is more likelihood of variations in the formulation of these and in the substances other than the generic chemical which they contain as well as in the mechanical processes of formulating and producing them. In short, they are not likely to be precisely interchangeable in their therapeutic use.

Yet, on the other hand, we have lived for many years now—even before the drug explosion—with the concept before us at all times of the generic equivalency of drug products containing the same generically named chemical. This has surfaced most recently in the stated concept of generic drug product interchangeability which was implied before but never stated. A diamond and a chunk of coal are generically (chemically) as equivalent as many marketed generic drug products of different manufacture!

If it is these older "generic," multi-source drug products which are the ones where one can shop on a price basis, assuming equivalence otherwise, and if the hospital formularies do such shopping—as they congratulate themselves on doing—and if it is from among the academic hospitals that our total information relative to adverse drug reactions has recently been codified, analyzed, and summarized, as it has, and if the decision as to therapeutic equivalence of such selected products is based arbitrarily on the opinion of pharmacist or physician members of the therapeutic committee without adequate substantiation by the appropriate clinical and scientific studies, then conceivably (a) the money saved by all hospital formulary committees, (b) the convenience of the pharmacist's stock problems, and (c) the pressures to have staff physicians conform to the formulary in their therapeutic activities—all these things which equate with progress in the academic mind, may well not be progress. These may well have been purchased at a risk in morbidity and mortality in the patients there hospitalized, as suggested by the Harlem Hospital Study, let alone the MIPI report findings. In short, with cardiac deaths alone in hospital—and many occur in hospitals—what percentage of these are absolutely due to the rigors of the disease and what percentage of them are due to therapeutic malpractice, to use a very blunt term, engendered by the wrong concepts of price related to quality of the drug products imposed interchangeably on patients in the hospital by the Hospital Formulary Committee?

Now we find similar pressures—and even yielding to such pressures—to have the government impose a statewide formulary committee on the physicians and patients in their respective states. We have in the Weinberger Maximum Allowable Cost (MAC) program a similar attempt on the part of the federal government.

If we refer to the mass of published data available, it is absolutely clear that there is but minimal evidence of available valid medical and scientific studies demonstrating clearly therapeutic equivalence and therefore therapeutic interchangeability of any of the multi-source generically (chemically) similar drug products available for the physician to prescribe and for the patient to use.

We also have the unequivocal military experience [4] as to what happened in the way of life-threatening complaints when they embarked on a "cheapest drug" procurement; that is, a generic drug procurement policy in the late 50s. Their total experience over a good many years is unequivocal—when they paid too much attention to price they bought cheap drug products at the expense of severe morbidity and mortality type reactions. When they adequately insisted upon quality drug products being used in their establishment—and such insistence on quality cost them money—they had a much better record of many fewer serious side effects and, as well, the medical officers were much more satisfied with the effect of the drug products against their diagnosis of disease.

With the foregoing—and this comprises all of the really valid information available in this area—one might well ask himself or herself why any further legislation is needed. Particularly, one should question the utility, the safety, and, in the long run, the actual cost saving of any kind of formulary. One might also simply raise the question as to how medico-legally liable are the members of the Hospital Formulary

Committee who approved a drug product which, by bio-availability tests not yet run, proves to be an inferior product, to say nothing of its being not therapeutically interchangeable by any available published—or other—evidence, and what might be the liability of the state which mandates the use by the physicians of such agents?

Legislating in an area as difficult as this is tricky at best. Legislation which has been in effect for many years delegates therapeutic responsibility to the physician—as it properly should, since he or she is the most trained therapeutician available. It makes him or her medico-legally liable for any shortcoming he or she has in this area.

To legislate in such a fashion that the control of an arm of the state decides what the physician must prescribe and what the pharmacist must or may dispense for what patients under what circumstances gets the state into the practice of medicine, an area in which they have no competence whatsoever. Furthermore, they are going into this area, not on the basis of proven lack of therapeutic competence by the mass of physicians in the state, but apparently to legislate away the incompetences of the few—manifestly a totally impossible task. They are also going into this in a way which directly or indirectly puts pharmacists, who have no competence in the therapeutic field whatsoever, in a position of making what, in the last analysis, are therapeutic decisions—that is the decision of selecting which drug product the patient will get regardless of what the physician desires based on his actual examination of that patient and knowledge of the patient's history and, in many instances, total health background for many years—together with his total therapeutic experience with the disease.

One of the major reasons given for legislating therapeutics is the large numbers of serious drug side effects and the physicians' supposed incompetence therapeutically without which such would not occur! The total picture reported above negates this.

Altogether, if one takes all the foregoing into consideration, it would seem that this is an area where the total record shows that the use of drugs in patients for the most part has been done safely and effectively. In those instances where this is not true—mainly derived from information on patients in the great academic centers—it is true that drugs of potentially different therapeutic qualities are being used clinically and interchangeably, largely on the assumption that, because they contain the same chemical substance in the same amount, they are sure to give the same therapeutic performance. This last statement is challenged time after time after time in the total literature available and there is no substantial segment of the literature—only opinions—which can be brought to bear in support of that concept; in fact quite the reverse is true.

Under all these circumstances and after consideration of all these facts, opinions, inferences, and what have you, certainly the picture is not clear enough so that any legislative body could honestly recommend taking any activity in the way of producing a law which would in any way interfere with the physician's control of the therapy of his patient since there are no guidelines available that one can use to override the physician's proven competence as a therapeutician, overall. In fact, to do so in the light of all the foregoing data on adverse drug reactions in humans is flying in the face of the facts. To insist on doing so is almost certain to lead to an enhancement of adverse drug reactions in the future since all such legislation mandates, permits, or promotes the increasing use of the multi-source generic drug products—those shown to be most associated with the greater numbers of more severe adverse drug reactions.

So it is then, that this whole picture of the side effects of drugs has been distorted into one that is absolutely unrecognizable as it relates to the real facts developed and published. Much needless legislation relative to therapy has been proposed, considered, and some of it passed!

An interesting phenomenon here also is the degree to which pharmacy has felt it necessary to join the anvil chorus of denigrating the physician's therapeutic competence and freely asserting a competence in that area which they, in fact, do not have nor can they even obtain under present circumstances.

However, willing legislators have listened to the simplistic, self-serving arguments, backed up by a few rather unusual and seemingly incontrovertible supporting facts, to the degree that they consistently overlook the whole picture and willingly go along with pharmacists and consumers, also probably activated by such pharmacists, to press for third party interference, control, and meddling with the therapy which only the physician thoroughly understands to be needed by the patients whom he or she has diagnosed.

DRUG INTERACTIONS

It has only been more recently that the idea of drug interactions as a potential cause of adverse drug reactions of a severe nature has come into the picture. It is interesting that the MIPI report shows how inconsequential are supportable numbers of reported real adverse drug reactions on the basis of drug interactions. Actually, again, it is pharmacists (and physicians associated with them) who have added this potential source of adverse reactions to all the other sources to help arrive at the distorted figures and concepts that we have referred to above. Such overemphasis, unsupported by actual facts, cannot fail to have been counter-productive and lend itself to data distortion!

SUMMARY AND DISCUSSION

Clearly, all the foregoing is in no way to be considered as an attempt to say that there are no adverse reactions to drug products. Obviously there are, there have been, there always will be, and the physician will have to take cognizance of these in the practice of effective and safe therapy for his patients based on the real data available. However, what does come out in the foregoing—and designedly so—is the incontrovertible picture based on all the published data available that (a) the majority of physicians are reasonably accomplished therapeuticians for the majority of the patients with whom they deal; (b) there has been a gross distortion of the severe morbidity and mortality type of adverse drug reactions; (c) it is the older, multi-source drug products which are most responsible for most of the severest adverse drug reactions. This is probably true because of the teaching that generically equivalent drug products equate with their therapeutic equivalency, regardless of source, and therefore the concept that drug products with the same generic chemical content are interchangeable. This interchangeability has been pushed in hospital formularies; it has been pushed by government; it has been pushed by pharmacists individually; it has been pushed by some academic physicians; and, probably, it is this mistaken concept, absolutely unsupported for the most part by <u>any</u> published data, that is perhaps responsible for the fact that the majority of severe adverse drug reactions are due to the older, multi-source, so-called generic products where the physician, the pharmacist, the hospital administrator, and even the patient have been brought to believe that if the same kind of chemical is there the same kind of effect will occur. This is just not so on the basis of the total published data.

In short, then, taking a bird's-eye overall view of the whole picture, let's admit it—we have been seriously misinformed by a variety of individuals for a variety of reasons to believe what just isn't so, namely, that the physician is an incompetent therapeutician; that the pharmaceutical industry dictates to the physician what he will prescribe and in so doing, dictates that he prescribe drug products that are unsafe and unworkable; that regulatory and legislative activity is necessary to "force the physician" to prescribe more rationally so as to avoid these purported large numbers of serious adverse drug reactions and lighten the load on the patient's pocketbook.

The picture that seems to be supported by the evidence and that should superimpose itself on the foregoing is that the majority of physicians are thoroughly competent therapeuticians in the use of the drug products available in those situations which they treat most frequently.

It is clear that the pharmacists can be of some assistance to physicians in supplying information to them relative to drug products with which the individual physician has not had frequent personal experience.

It is equally apparent that the pharmacist is not a therapeutician in his own right in any way, shape, or form. It is equally obvious that those legislators, political pundits, and purveyors of news by the various types of media involved, themselves certainly incompetent therapeutists despite their insinuation of competence in being overtly critical of the medical profession in that particular area, have compounded the problem.

It would seem high time that we get back to a more rational consideration of the therapeutic aspects of medicine, leave it in the hands of those who are trained, knowledgeable, and, based on the total record available, quite competent in this area and stop meddling with them. The meddling done in the past has probably caused more adverse drug reactions and more mistaken and ineffective therapy through promoting the "defensive" therapy it has engendered, than any help it has been to a physician or to an ill patient.

In other words, the physician, as a practitioner of the therapeutic art and science has been much maligned over this whole period of time, primarily by nonprofessionals who know nothing of therapeutics and who are readily mislead by the distortions caused, perhaps, by a few well meaning professionals visualizing adverse drug reactions as a substantial problem—perhaps more substantial than would seem to be the case in the light of the total objective evidence now available and now objectively considered.

All toxicologists should know of these findings and it would be advisable for all of them to read the MIPI report to get themselves well oriented on the story of what the human toxicity picture is relative to drug products used in therapy. After all, it is toxicologists who should know these matters and who should be able to explain them to professional and nonprofessional alike if they are thoroughly conversant with the facts.

It is a little bit unsettling to us to find that, despite all the efforts made in the 60s to attempt to get this matter of adverse reactions to therapeutic agents put in some rational and reasonable perspective, it has persistently become more nonobjective, more irrational, and more derogatory of those therapeutists who are the best we have, namely the physicians who are charged with combating disease and with using drugs to the extent they can effectively and safely so do in their patient's best interests.

Altogether it would seem that this whole matter of a 25-year consideration of the development of the story of adverse drug reactions is not one for which the medical profession can take much credit or much pride in what has been allowed to develop in the way of misinformation with all the associated, undesirable fall-outs. It seems clearly to have abrogated its educational responsibility in this area.

Furthermore, it is clear that the communications media have never even bothered to attempt to evaluate the data available before they put out strongly biased and absolutely incorrect reports on the relationships of drugs effective against disease to the development of toxicity in human beings; in short, they have completely ignored the objectively demonstrable benefit-risk aspect of drug use.

Also, governmental agencies, particularly the FDA, can take little if any pride in their contribution in this area. If anything, their officials seem to have used this as a political ploy to help them get additional appropriations and to help further the governmental careers of some of their leaders rather than to attempt to deal with the problem on an objective basis for the best interest of the people of our country. Cursory reading of the package insert (or any other of their publications), which they absolutely control, makes clear the fact that they overplay risk and underplay benefit.

Similarly, one can fault legislators who have fished in these troubled waters without taking the time or the trouble to get the real facts before making pronouncements based on what were obviously not facts.

There is much blame available to be applied to and shared by all involved.

Perhaps now, with the MIPI report available, it is going to be possible to pin the tail on the donkeys who brayed loudest and most blatantly relative to the physician's incompetence as therapeutists, the tremendous hazards of modern drug products promoted by the pharmaceutical industry to the physician, and so on, and the virtues of generics. If this occurs some progress will finally have been made.

REFERENCES*

[1] H. S. Reidenburg, Registry of Adverse Drug Reactions, Report of the Drug Reaction Registry Subcommittee of the Greater Philadelphia Committee for Medical-Pharmaceutical Sciences, JAMA, 203, 31 (1968).

[2] J. K. Weston, The present status of adverse drug reaction reporting, JAMA, 203, 35 (1968).

[3] Medicine in the Public Interest, Adverse Drug Reactions in the United States, 600 New Hampshire Ave., N.W., Suite 720, Washington, D.C., 20037 (1975).

[4] Allegations of Conspiracy Between the Department of Defense and Large Drug Manufacturers, Investigation of the Office of Special Investigation, U.S. Air Force, Department of the Air Force, Office of Special Investigations, HQ D 58-7145, July 5, 1974.

*Since all the major bibliographic sources are listed in Ref. 3, above, no further references will be listed.

ADDENDUM

Note must be taken that the foregoing was written and submitted in the fall of 1975, well over a year ago. The following summarized statements are an abridgment of what has developed of significance in the Adverse Drug Reaction Area in the interim, at least in the judgment and opinion of the authors:

1. The MIPI report was deemed of sufficient interest that it was revised, shortened, updated, and published by Karch and La Sagna in JAMA in late 1975 [1] so that the analysis of the factual published data would be readily and widely available to physicians, especially. There is now no excuse for anyone further disseminating misinformation on human adverse drug reactions.
2. The Tufts Drug Surveillance Program has been continuingly productive.
3. The AFIP Registry on Tissue Reactions to Drugs has been continuingly productive.
4. A sensible editorial appeared in the New England Journal of Medicine [2]. NB. All the foregoing have been in substantial support of much of the data, inferences, surmises, opinions, and conclusions advanced in the instant report.
5. As a result, perhaps, of the foregoing, the cutting edge of the Adverse Reaction alarmists seems to have been somewhat blunted over the past year or so—or perhaps only redirected into the environmental pollutant area in the broad sense, where one notes considerable similar "viewing with alarm."
6. That there are still oncoming, active, vocal, and altogether generically similar adverse reactionists of the Rather-Schorr vintage can be unequivocally demonstrated by the relatively recent appearance of one, Joe Graedon, for instance, who apparently ignores the valid, published data now widely available in favor of laying about him lustily and extrapolating a bumper crop of similar misinformational and outmoded cliches related to the adverse reaction field [3].
7. A somewhat intermediate type of consideration of certain aspects of the adverse drug reaction field has recently appeared from Britain [4]. Hopefully, for the future, more and more of those interested who

become involved in the adverse drug reaction area will thoughtfully consider and reflect upon the valid data and information now becoming increasingly available in this field, will produce more of the same and will also challenge, as stridently and as often as necessary, any and all counterproductive, misinformational efforts of any type from any source.

REFERENCES

[1] F. E. Karch and L. La Sagna, Adverse drug reactions—a critical review, JAMA, 234, 12 (1975).
[2] F. Ingelfinger, Counting adverse drug reactions that count, New Engl. J. Med., 294, 18 (1976).
[3] J. Graedon, Killing combos, Esquire (May, 1976).
[4] J. P. Griffin and P. F. D'Arcy, A Manual of Adverse Drug Interactions, John Wright & Sons, Ltd., Bristol, 1975.

Poisoning with Tricyclic Antidepressant Drugs

ANTHONY S. MANOGUERRA, Pharm. D.

Assistant Professor
College of Pharmacy
University of Minnesota

and

Supervisor, Poison Control Center
Department of Emergency Medicine
Hennepin County Medical Center
Minneapolis, Minnesota

LAWRENCE C. WEAVER, Ph.D.

Professor and Dean
College of Pharmacy
University of Minnesota
Minneapolis, Minnesota

One of the most serious types of poisoning that appears to be increasing in frequency in both adults and children is that due to ingestion of excess amounts of the tricyclic antidepressant drugs. These drugs were introduced into psychiatric practice in the early 1960s for the treatment of severe forms of depressive disorders. They are now widely prescribed for this purpose. This has resulted in easy availability of these drugs to individuals who wish to commit suicide or perform a suicidal gesture. Recently, these drugs were approved by the Food and Drug Administration for use as an adjunct in the treatment of nocturnal enuresis in children. This latter use has placed these drugs into homes where they are now more available for accidental ingestion by young children.

During the one-year period from October 1973 to September 1974, American physicians prescribed these drugs, either alone or in combination with other drugs, more than 24 million times. Amitriptyline ranks 29th, imipramine 92nd, and doxepin 100th, in order of prescription frequency in the United States [1].

Imipramine and amitriptyline were the first tricyclic antidepressants to be marketed in the United States. Since their introduction, chemical alterations of the basic three-ringed molecule have led to the marketing of numerous similar drugs. The chemical structures of these drugs are illustrated in Fig. 1. Table 1 lists the 11 commercial drug products that are available on the United States market and that contain a tricyclic antidepressant either alone or in combination with another psychoactive drug [2]. Doxepin, which is promoted as a unique drug having both antianxiety and antidepressant activity, is pharmaologically and toxicologically a tricyclic antidepressant and is included in this discussion.

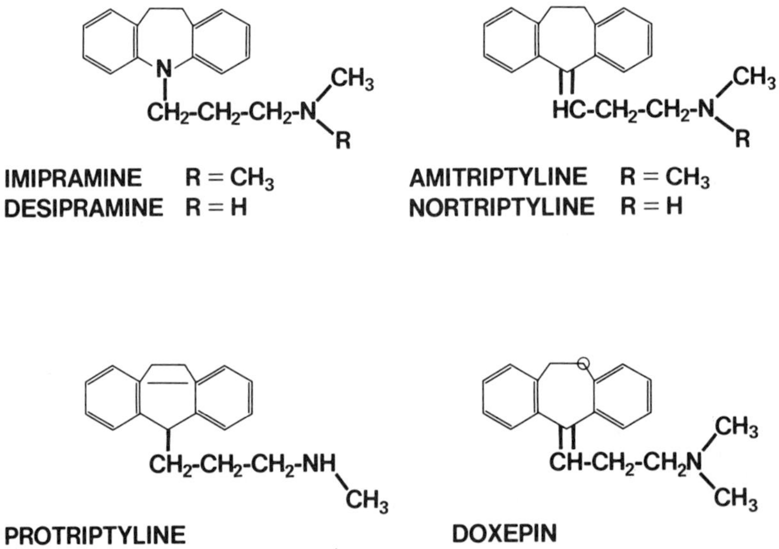

FIG. 1. Chemical structures of tricyclic antidepressants.

TABLE 1[a]

Generic name	Brand name—manufacturer
Amitriptyline	Elavil—Merck Sharp & Dohme
Amitriptyline and perphenazine (in combination)	Triavil—MSD Etrafon—Schering
Desipramine	Norpramin—Lakeside Pertofrane—USV
Doxepin	Adapin—Pennwalt Sinequan—Pfizer
Imipramine	Tofranil—Geigy Presamine—USV
Nortriptyline	Aventyl—Lilly
Propriptyline	Vivactil—USV

[a]Source: 1975 Physicians Desk Reference.

ACUTE TOXICITY

It is very difficult to predict the severity of an acute intoxication with the tricyclic antidepressants based on the amount of drug ingested. For example, with amitriptyline, fatalities have occurred in children with as little as 375-500 mg of the drug, whereas survival has occurred after ingestion of 1750 mg. The data in adults show fatalities from ingestion of 500 mg of amitriptyline and survival after ingestion of as much as 3925 mg [3]. With this wide range of toxic dosages and considering that this class of drugs may produce irregularities in cardiac rhythm when given in therapeutic doses [4], it would be prudent to consider the ingestion of any quantity of these drugs as potentially lethal and to treat and observe the patient accordingly.

The symptoms from poisoning with these drugs may become apparent from less than 1 hr to as long as 12 hr after ingestion. The most dangerous period seems to be during the first 12 to 24 hr, with recovery of consciousness usually occurring about 24 hr after ingestion. However, prolonged coma has been reported and deaths from cardiac arrhythmias have occurred as long as five days after ingestion [5].

Patients poisoned with these drugs are usually unconscious, after going through a brief phase of excitement, often with visual and auditory hallucinations. While awake the patient may complain of blurred vision, photophobia, and difficulty with speech. The patient may progress from a state of being alert and lucid to unconsciousness in a very short period of time. The patient's pupils will usually be dilated and unresponsive or minimally responsive to light. Mucous membranes may be dry, bowel sounds diminished or absent, and the patient may have urinary retention. Hyperreflexia with involuntary twitching is common and may progress to seizures, particularly when the patient is externally stimulated as during endotracheal intubation or during the usual procedure of determining the depth of coma by eliciting a pain response. Respirations are usually not markedly depressed in rate but may be very shallow in depth. Severe poisoning will result in apnea. Hyperpyrexia is a common finding. Sinus tachycardia is an expected finding with a variety of arrhythmias occurring frequently, often associated with hypotension.

The above symptoms are primarily the result of the potent anticholinergic activity of the tricyclic antidepressants. These symptoms are not unlike those seen in poisoning with other anticholinergic drugs. It has recently been demonstrated that the hyperreflexia, twitching, and seizure activity are also most likely the result of the anticholinergic properties with a reduction of central nervous system activity of acetylcholine leading to an excess dopamine influence [6].

The arrhythmias seen are probably the result of a combination of the anticholinergic-induced tachycardia, a direct effect of the tricyclic antidepressant on the myocardium, and the acidosis and hypokalemia that has been reported [7-9]. The direct effect is postulated to be an inhibition of the adenosine triphosphate (ATP)-phosphohydralase enzyme, which is considered to be the enzyme involved in the maintenance of sodium and potassium balance across the myocardial cell membrane [10, 11].

The toxicity of the tricyclic antidepressants may be increased by factors that influence their binding to serum proteins. Acidosis has been shown to increase the amount of tricyclic antidepressant unbound to serum proteins. As it is the unbound fraction of the drug that is pharmacologically active, acidosis will worsen the toxicity [9]. In addition, acidosis imposed the added hazard of depression of myocardial contractility.

PHARMACOKINETICS

Tricyclic antidepressants are rapidly absorbed from the gastrointestinal tract, and because of their high lipid solubility, rapidly distribute to body tissue sites leaving only small amounts of the drug in the blood. Of the drug remaining in the blood, 90% is bound to plasma proteins. Elimination of these drugs occurs via hepatic metabolism to active metabolites which undergo enterohepatic recycling followed by further metabolic degradation to inactive forms which are renally excreted. In the first 24 hr after ingestion only 3% of a given dose can be recovered in the urine in active or inactive forms. The half-life for elimination of these drugs is greater than 24 to 48 hr [12] with significant patient variability. Gard et al. [13] showed that significant amounts of amitriptyline and its metabolites, as much as 20% of a given dose, appear in gastric secretions in the first 24 hr after ingestion. This amount, coupled with the drug excreted through the biliary system, can account for as much as 30% of a given dose during the first day after ingestion. Most of this secreted drug is reabsorbed as it has been shown that very small amounts appear in the feces [14].

TREATMENT

In poisoning with tricyclic antidepressants, as in all other poisoning situations, good, intensive supportive care is of the utmost importance. Initial therapy should be aimed at maintenance of a patent airway and support of respiratory and cardiovascular function. The patient should be placed on a cardiac monitor as soon as respiratory maintenance is accomplished and should remain on the monitor for at least 48 hr. Laboratory studies for electrolytes should be done as well as a blood gas determination to judge the degree of existing acidosis. The bladder should be catheterized because of the urinary retention that will most likely occur.

If the patient is alert and appears to be in no immediate danger of losing consciousness, vomiting can be induced with syrup of ipecac. If the patient is unconscious, lavage should be carried out using a large bore tube, after the airway has been secured by placement of a cuffed endotracheal tube. Because of the rapid absorption of these drugs, the effectiveness of emesis or lavage is decreased. Gard et al. found that at $2\frac{1}{2}$ and 3 hr after ingestion, 5.4 and 9.6%, respectively, of the ingested drug was removed by gastric lavage in two different patients [13]. Obviously, the lavage technique used will greatly influence the effectiveness of the procedure. In any case, lavage may only remove a small portion of the ingested quantity of drug.

Following either induced emesis or lavage, a slurry of activated charcoal should be instilled into the stomach. In vitro studies have shown that 1 gm of charcoal will adsorb 250 mg of imipramine in gastric juice [15]. Gard also postulates [13], based on data from his in vitro work, that 100 gm of charcoal is capable of binding 4 gm of amitriptyline. He then suggests that because of the large component of gastric and biliary excretion, charcoal, administered every 4 to 6 hr after ingestion, should speed the elimination of these drugs from the body. We are currently testing this hypothesis in an animal model in our laboratory. Concurrently, we are studying, in overdosed patients, the effect of repeated administration of charcoal on the kinetics of elimination of tricyclic antidepressants and their active metabolites. If this work proves the effectiveness of this regimen, this procedure will be valuable in reducing the critical time period during which the patient is at greatest risk. Even with the current information, the routine administration of activated charcoal following emesis or lavage is strongly suggested.

Following the administration of the charcoal, the patient should be given a saline cathartic to stimulate movement of the charcoal and adsorbed drug through the gastrointestinal tract. For this purpose sodium or magnesium sulfate or magnesium citrate can be used.

A procedure that has been utilized by some clinicians is continuous gastric lavage or continuous gastric suction. Theoretically, this procedure should remove that amount of drug that is secreted into the gastric juices. Penny [10] utilized this procedure in a $3\frac{1}{2}$-year-old child who had ingested imipramine and removed 2.78 mg/liter of lavage fluid.

The seizure activity induced by the antidepressants may be controlled by the intravenous injection of diazepam. However, a more pharmacologically rational approach to this problem is to use physostigmine. Physostigmine is a reversible acetycholinesterase inhibitor that, unlike neostigmine or pyridostigmine, is capable of crossing the blood-brain barrier thus affecting the central cholinergic blockade induced by the antidepressant. Physostigmine has been shown effective in rapidly reversing the choreathetosis and myocolonus that is commonly seen [2]. Because physostigmine is centrally active, it is also effective in reversing the coma that results from poisoning with tricyclics and other anticholinergic drugs [6, 16-19]. Other authors [20] have suggested that physostigmine be given to patients to make them alert enough for vomiting to be induced with syrup of ipecac. This is a dangerous procedure, as the duration of activity of physostigmine, is 30 to 45 min and the patient may lose consciousness before or while vomiting is occurring. The use of physostigmine to treat the patient who is comatose but otherwise stable is a subject of controversy. Newton [17] states that "in the routine management of tricyclic antidepressant poisoning in patients free of complications, physostigmine should not be used because of its potentially dangerous effects." He supports this statement by referring to the experience at the Edinburgh Regional Poisoning Center where 609 cases of tricyclic antidepressant overdose have been treated with supportive care alone with no fatalities. The dangerous effects that Newton refers to are related to the excess cholinergic effects that can result following physostigmine administration. These effects are severe bradycardia, excessive salivation leading to respiratory difficulties, and grand mal seizures. Also, spontaneous emesis, urination, and defecation can occur. To reverse these excessive cholinergic effects, atropine can be administered in a dose of 0.5 mg for every 1 mg of physostigmine that has been given. The possibility of seizures can be minimized by administering the physostigmine over a 2- to 5-min period.

TABLE 2. Dosage of Physostigmine Salicylate (Antilirium) in Anticholinergic Poisoning [21]

Pediatric dose:	0.5 mg i.v., injected over 2 to 5 min. Repeat every 5 min until toxic effects are relieved or cholinergic effects develop. Repeat the effective dose as needed.
Adult dose:	2 mg i.v., injected over 2 to 5 min. Repeat every 20 min until reversal of toxic effects occurs or cholinergic symptoms are produced. Repeat the effective dose as needed.

Atropine in a dose of 0.5 mg for every 1 mg of physostigmine administered should be available to reverse excess cholinergic symptoms if they develop.

The dosage schedule of physostigmine that was developed by Rumack [21] and that is most commonly employed is outlined in Table 2.

The experience in the Emergency Department at Hennepin County Medical Center with physostigmine has led to recommending its use in anticholinergic poisoning only in situations where the patient has one of the following complications:

1. seizures
2. hallucinations or delirium, where the patient cannot be easily restrained and where the patient may injure himself or others
3. severe tachycardia or arrhythmia
4. coma with respiratory depression and/or hypotension.

Patients who are comatose and without the above listed complications are treated supportively.

Physostigmine [19], neostigmine [22], and pyridostigmine [23] have been said to be effective in reversing the arrhythmias seen in tricyclic antidepressant poisoning. However, the evidence of this effectiveness does not appear conclusive and warrants further study. Physostigmine should be effective in reversing those arrhythmias that are the result of vagal blockade, while those arrhythmias developing from the direct effect of the antidepressant on the myocardium would most likely not be affected. For these latter arrhythmias, measures such as the infusion of potassium [7, 10, 19], and bicarbonate [9, 19] or the administration of lidocaine [24, 25] or propranolol [24, 26] have been suggested.

Hypotension should be treated with the administration of intravenous fluids. Vasopressors should be reserved because of the possibility of further sensitizing the myocardium and inducing or worsening arrhythmias. If necessary, a vassopressor such as phenylephrine, that can increase blood pressure without increasing the heart rate, should be used. Other vasopressors, such as levarterenol, epinephrine, metaraminol, and similar sympathomimetics should be used only with extreme caution, if at all. When the vagal influence on the heart is blocked, as it is by the tricyclic antidepressants, these sympathomimetic drugs will produce a dramatic increase in heart rate and may precipitate arrhythmias [27].

Because of the high tissue and serum protein affinity of the tricyclic antidepressants, forced diuresis and dialysis are of no usefulness in the treatment of these poisonings. Bailey [28] showed that forced diuresis yielded only 43 mg of imipramine in 23,370 ml of urine in a patient that ingested "a large quantity" of the drug. Hemodialysis [29] and peritoneal dialysis [30] have also been shown to remove very small quantities of these drugs.

CONCLUSION AND SUMMARY

The tricyclic antidepressant drugs produce a serious and complex poisoning in patients who either accidently or intentionally ingest them. Fatality rates, even with intensive care, may be exceedingly high. As these drugs are very useful in the treatment of severe depression, it is unlikely that prescriptions for them will decrease. Prescribing physicians should, therefore, be thoroughly familiar with the toxicity of these drugs and the methods of treatment. When the drugs are prescribed for patients in households with small children or when the drugs are used for childhood nocturnal enuresis, parents should be made aware of the dangers of these drugs so that they can take the necessary precautions. In all cases, the minimum quantity possible should be prescribed and dispensed in an attempt to minimize the severity of any poisonings that may occur.

Editor's Comment: Clinically it has been noticed that digitalization may reverse the cardiotoxicity of tricyclic antidepressants.

REFERENCES

[1] National Disease and Therapeutic Index, IMS America, Ambler, Pennsylvania.
[2] Physicians Desk Reference, Medical Economics, Inc., Oradell, N. J., 1975.
[3] Merck, Sharpe and Dohme product information for Elavil.
[4] L. Meyler and A. Herxheimer, Side Effects of Drugs, Volume VI, Excerpta Medica Foundation, Amsterdam, 1968.

[5] A. B. Masters, Delayed death in imipramine poisoning, Brit. Med. J., 1967-3, 866.
[6] J. S. Burks, J. E. Walker, B. H. Rumack, and J. E. Ott, Tricyclic antidepressant poisoning, reversal of coma, choreoathetosis and myoclonus by physostigmine, JAMA, 230, 1405 (1974).
[7] S. Fargharson, Poisoning by tricyclic drugs, Brit. Med. J., 1972-1, 378 (1972) (Letter).
[8] J. C. Fouron and R. Chuoine, ECG changes in fatal imipramine (Tofranil) intoxication, Pediatrics, 48, 777 (1971)
[9] T. C. Brown, G. A. Barker, M. E. Dunlop, and P. M. Loughman, The use of sodium bicarbonate in the treatment of tricyclic antidepressant induced arrhythmias, Anesth. Intensive Care, 1(3), 203 (1973).
[10] R. Penny, Imipramine hydrochloride poisoning in childhood, Am. J. Diseases Child., 116, 181 (1968).
[11] V. Tane and M. Brechtlone, Effect of imipramine and ouabain on the sodium and potassium activating ATPase from brain microsomes and cooperating interaction with the enzyme, J. Neurochem., 14,
[12] B. Alexanderson, Prediction of steady state plasma levels of nortriptyline from single oral dose kinetics, Europ. J. Clin. Pharmacol., 5, 181 (1973).
[13] H. Gard, D. Knapp, T. Walle, and I. Havenson, Qualitative and quantitative studies on the disposition of amitriptyline and other tricyclic antidepressants in man as it relates to the management of the overdosed patient, Clin. Toxicol., 6, 571 (1973).
[14] E. Von Eschenof and J. Rieder, Untersvchungen uber das schicksal des antidepressivums amitriptylin im organismus der ratte und des menschen, Arz. Forsch., 19, 957 (1969).
[15] J. Crammer and B. Davies, Activated charcoal in tricyclic drug overdose, Brit. Med. J., 1962-1, 527.
[16] A. S. Manoguerra and E. Ruiz, Physostigmine treatment of anticholinergic poisoning, J. Am. Coll. Emergency Physicians, 5, 125 (1976).
[17] R. W. Newton, Physostigmine salicylate in the treatment of tricyclic antidepressant overdosage, JAMA, 231, 941 (1975).
[18] B. D. Snyder, L. Blonde, and W. R. McWherter, Reversal of amitriptyline intoxication by physostigmine, JAMA, 230, 1433 (1974).
[19] T. L. Slovis, J. E. Ott, D. T. Teitelbaum, and W. Lipscomb, Physostigmine therapy in acute tricyclic antidepressant poisoning, Clin. Toxicol., 4, 451 (1971).
[20] Z. E. Brashere and W. R. Conley, Physostigmine in drug overdose, J. Am. Coll. Emergency Physicians, 5, 46 (1975).
[21] B. H. Rumack, Anticholinergic poisoning; treatment with physostigmine, Pediatrics, 52, 449 (1973).
[22] A. I. Aruff and E, A. Friedman, Coma following non-narcotic

drug overdosage: management of 208 adult patients, Am. J. Med. Sci., 266, 405 (1973).
[23] J. Rasmussen, Amitriptyline and imipramine poisoning, Lancet, 1965-2, 850.
[24] J. A. Young and W. H. Galloway, Treatment of severe imipramine poisoning, Arch. Diseases Child., 46, 353 (1971).
[25] C. M. Steel, J. O'Duffey, and S. Brown, Clinical effects and treatment of imipramine and amitriptyline poisoning in children, Brit. Med. J., 1967-3, 633.
[26] J. W. Freeman and M. G. Loughhead, Beta blockage in the treatment of tricyclic antidepressant overdosage, Med. J. Australia, 1(25), 1233 (1973).
[27] L. S. Goodman and A. Gilman, The Pharmacological Basis of Therapeutics, 4th ed., Macmillan, New York, 1970.
[28] R. R. Barly, J. R. Sharman, J. O'Rourke, and A. L. Buttemore, Hemodialysis and forced diuresis for tricyclic anti-depressant poisoning, Brit. Med. J., 1974-4, 231.
[29] J. W. Hawthorne, A. M. Marcus, and M. Kaye, Management of massive imipramine overdosage with mannitol and artificial dialysis, New Engl. J. Med., 268, 33 (1963).
[30] P. Sunshine and S. J. Jaffe, Amitriptyline poisoning, clinical and pathological findings in a fatal case, Am. J. Diseases Child., 106, 501 (1963).

Drugs and Children: Methods for Therapeutic Monitoring

KEITH B. HAMMOND, M.S., F.I.M.L.S.

Pediatric Microchemistry Laboratories
University of Colorado Medical Center
Denver, Colorado

INTRODUCTION

The value of monitoring blood concentrations of drugs to assess therapeutic efficacy and prevent toxicity is well established [1, 2]. Hospital laboratories are experiencing an increasing number of requests for this type of assay, and it might be expected that this trend will continue as new analytical methods are made available. However, while many clinical laboratories perform assays for a variety of therapeutic agents used for adult patients, the particular needs of pediatric patients are seldom met. The factors which affect optimal dosage requirements are often exaggerated in younger patients, particularly in the newborn period when there is rapid alteration of rates of metabolism and elimination as both liver and renal function mature. Since protein-binding and the integrity of the blood-brain barrier may be altered in early infancy, drug therapy in this age group should not be undertaken lightly. While the development of micro-analytical techniques has done much to enhance the availability of clinical chemistry assays in pediatrics [3], many procedures in current use for the determination of drug levels require amounts of blood which are difficult to obtain from very young children. The purpose of this chapter is to describe a variety of analytical procedures which have particular value in monitoring drug therapy in children.

METHODS OF ANALYSIS

Colorimetry

Most colorimetric assays in use today for the measurement of drug concentrations in biologic fluids have their origins in the old literature. The success of a colorimetric method depends on the production of a colored complex of sufficient absorptivity that the levels of drug ordinarily encountered during therapy are accurately measured without significant interference from inactive metabolic products, or from other endogenous or exogenous constituents of blood. It is well documented that this ideal situation is seldom achieved and for this reason colorimetric procedures have in general been replaced by other, more specific methods of analysis.

Spectrophotometry

Since many drugs contain chromophoric groups as a component of their chemical structure (e.g., unsaturated carbon-carbon linkages, carbonyl and thiocarbonyl groups, etc.) they can be quantitated by measurement of their absorptivity in the ultraviolet region of the spectrum. As with colorimetric analyses the specificity of spectrophotometric assays is sometimes questionable [4-6].

Gas-Liquid Chromatography

The rapidity and ease with which structurally similar compounds can be simultaneously differentiated and quantitated has led to the wide acceptance of gas-liquid chromatography as a technique for measuring drug levels in biologic fluids. The precision of gas-chromatographic determinations of drugs has been greatly enhanced by the commercial availability of internal standards that are chemically similar to the drugs to be measured. However, a number of published gas chromatographic procedures are of uncertain specificity since the authors do not report a comprehensive listing of drugs and other substances that have been shown not to interfere. The analyst should constantly bear in mind the danger of ascribing a definite identity to a peak appearing on a chart recorder on the basis of a single relative retention time obtained on one column under a single set of conditions. The hydrogen-flame detector recognizes nothing more than the presence of a molecule containing carbon atoms. It is therefore important to establish to one's own satisfaction the lack of interference from other compounds or to apply a confirmatory method such as derivatizing and re-chromatographing each sample. The recent application of the organic nitrogen-selective detector in measuring plasma drug concentrations represents a real advancement toward the elimination of interferences from such compounds as lipids and plasticizers. However this detector is somewhat more troublesome in operation than the more robust and simple hydrogen flame detector [7].

Immunoassay

There has been considerable growth in the application of this technique to the measurement of a variety of substances of interest in the clinical laboratory. This range of substances has recently been extended to include drugs such as diphenylhydantoin, phenobarbital, carbamazapine, primidone, and gentamicin for which reagents are commercially available in kit form. Immunoassay procedures applied to drug determinations include radioimmunoassay, spin-labeled immunoassay, and enzyme-labeled immunoassay. The extent of cross reactivity from closely related compounds should be established for any antibody preparation used. In some published procedures there is an indication that this technique could give quite erroneous results if a variety of therapeutic agents are being given simultaneously. Assuming that a specific antibody is available, this technique would seem to lend itself particularly to the large batch processing of large numbers of samples. Of particular interest in pediatrics is the extraordinary sensitivity of the method permitting the use of finger-stick or heel-stick samples. In common with all other immunoassay procedures, however, there is a need for meticulous technical skill in the performance of these assays without which results of adequate precision cannot be obtained. For laboratories with sufficiently large workloads, a variety of automated or semi-automated systems are available which can reduce the overall error of the methods considerably.

STANDARDIZATION AND QUALITY CONTROL

The increasing frequency of requests for blood levels of drugs has resulted in the transfer of responsibility for the performance of these tests from the research laboratory to the clinical laboratory. Most larger hospital and commercial clinical laboratories now perform a variety of drug determinations. It has become apparent that the stanard of performance achieved by many of these laboratories is less than adequate, and these impressions have been recently confirmed by a number of quality control surveys both in the United States and in Europe [8-10]. The accuracy of drug determinations could be greatly improved if suitable standard materials of high purity were made readily available. At the present time the National Bureau of Standards is involved in an investigation concerning the preparation and evaluation of drug reference materials for use in the monitoring of anti-convulsant blood levels [11].

Quality control is a vital component in the performance of any clinical laboratory procedure and drug assays are no exception. Each laboratory involved in such determinations should be aware of the day-to-day error of the methods used, and the only way to monitor this parameter is to perform an assay on a control material of known composition with each batch of patient samples. For many drugs there are no commerically available control preparations, and consequently they should be prepared in the laboratory by adding suitable quantities of drugs to either pooled plasma or to a solution of bovine serum albumin. Such materials may then be aliquoted in suitable small quantities and stored frozen until needed. Although there appears to be no consensus on what constitutes an acceptable degree of precision in drug assays it might reasonably be inferred that a result deviating no more than ±10% from the "true" value is adequate in most instances.

ESTABLISHING THERAPEUTIC AND TOXIC RANGES

The value of monitoring blood drug concentrations is totally dependent on there being some correlation among the blood level, achievement of therapeutic effect, and onset of toxicity. The desired blood concentration, therefore, is one which can be maintained above the level at which the desired response can be achieved but below the level at which toxicity results. Blood level information is particularly useful for those drugs which have a low therapeutic index (low ratio between the median toxic dose and median effective dose). For ease of interpretation, the plasma half-life of the drug should be sufficiently long for minor differences in timing in the collection of specimens to have only an insignificant impact on the value obtained. Subsequent sections deal with specific drugs and indicate to the reader that the therapeutic and toxic ranges for many drugs are not at all well defined. A complicating factor in interpreting previously published data is the variety of methodologies used, and the recent finding of substantial interlaboratory variability in the values obtained. Since interpretation of blood drug values are clearly subjective at best, clinicians are well advised to establish therapeutic ranges and toxic levels to their own satisfaction using the facilities of a laboratory of proven competence.

CHLORAMPHENICOL

Clinical Commentary

In the newborn, treatment with chloramphenicol is accompanied by the risk of shock and death ("gray baby syndrome") unless the blood levels of unconjugated drug are carefully monitored. Dosage should be controlled so that blood levels are not allowed to exceed 25 μg/ml. Beyond the neonatal period it is important to monitor blood levels to guard against bone marrow suppression. Blood for chloramphenicol determination can be drawn at any time since there is relatively little variation in the blood level after the first 24 hr of therapy.

Technical Commentary

Chloramphenicol (D (-) threo-1-p-nitrophenyl-2-dichloroacetamido-1,3-propanediol) is converted in the body both to its glucuronic acid conjugate and to a basic hydrolysis product (D (-) threo-1-p-nitrophenyl-2-amino-1,3-propanediol) [12]. Only free chloramphenicol is metabolically active and of importance in the evaluation of both its therapeutic and toxic effects. Dosage forms of chloramphenicol include the succinate and palmitate esters, which are hydrolyzed in the body, liberating free chloramphenicol. Following parenteral administration of these compounds, there are significant quantities of unhydrolyzed esters in the bloodstream. Consequently, in order to be of value in monitoring free chloramphenicol concentrations, any method used should not be susceptible to interference from either the unhydrolyzed esters or the inactive metabolites. Although the microbiologic assay is specific for free chloramphenicol, it is of limited value when the patient is receiving multiple antibiotics. Several chemical procedures have been described [13, 14] that depend on the reduction of the nitro group on the aromatic nucleus to an amino group which is then diazotized and coupled to N-1-naphthyl ethylenediamine to give a compound that absorbs at 550 nm. Since these methods also measure the metabolic products of chloramphenicol and other aryl amino compounds such as the sulfonamides and procaine penicillin [14, 15], they have been replaced by the method of Kakemi et al. [16, 17], which is described below. This procedure has been shown to be specific for the biologically active form of the drug. Occasionally falsely high values have been experienced in the author's laboratory in extremely icteric sera. This problem can be overcome by running an appropriate blank determination when indicated by the appearance of the isoamyl acetate extract.

Reagents

1. Saponin, 1.0%. Make up with water.
2. Isoamyl acetate.
3. Isonicotinic acid hydrazide, 3% in water.
4. Sodium hydroxide, 1.5 N. Use deionized water to dissolve 6 gm NaOH; and then bring the solution up to 100 ml using deionized water.
5. Phosphate buffer, pH 7.0, 0.1 M. Use deionized water to dissolve 2.21 gm $NaH_2PO_4 \cdot H_2O$ and 7.61 gm $Na_2HPO_4 \cdot 7H_2O$; dilute to 1 liter with deionized water.
6. Stock standard, 100 μg/ml. Use deionized water to dissolve 10 mg water-soluble chloramphenicol; dilute to 100 ml with deionized water.

Procedure

1. Pipet 0.5 ml saponin solution into a 12 × 75 mm stoppered test tube. Wash in 0.5 ml of heparinized whole blood or serum.
2. Pipet 1.0 ml standard solution or 1 ml water for blank into separate tubes.
3. Add 2.0 ml phosphate buffer and 3.0 ml isoamyl acetate.
4. Stopper and mechanically shake the tubes for 10 min. Centrifuge.
5. Transfer 2 ml upper layer to clean tubes. (If there is any yellow color due to bilirubin apparent at this stage, a second sample should be prepared as in steps 1 through 5 above for use as a test blank).
6. Pipet into the test, standard, and blank tubes 0.5 ml each of 3% isonicotinic acid hydrazide and 1.5 N sodium hydroxide.
7. If a test blank has been prepared, add 0.5 ml of water and 0.5 ml of 1.5 N sodium hydrazide.
8. Stopper, mix thoroughly, and incubate at 30°C for 45 min, shaking at frequent intervals.
9. Remove aqueous under-layer and read in a spectrophotometer at 430 nm in a cell of 10-mm light path with a path width of 4 mm (0.9 ml solution required).

Calculation

After subtracting the blank reading, plot the standards on a graph and read the concentration of the tests minus the blank (and test blank) readings from this graph, and multiply by 2.

GENTAMICIN

Clinical Commentary

Gentamicin is an aminoglycoside closely related chemically and biologically to streptomycin and kanamycin. It is used primarily in the treatment of urinary tract infections. However, its application in pediatrics is quite recent with a pediatric formulation available only since 1972. Since then there have been several published reports describing the clinical pharmacology of gentamicin in newborn infants and children 2 months to 2 years of age [18, 19]. Because the drug is eliminated by glomerular filtration, its elimination rate in the newborn period is probably prolonged, permitting potentially toxic blood levels to accumulate. Desirable therapeutic serum concentrations have been reported to be in the range of 2.5-7.5 μg/ml [20]. Sustained blood levels greater than 10-12 μg/ml may result in ototoxicity while levels below 2 μg/ml will not achieve full therapeutic effect.

Technical Commentary

A microbiologic assay using agar diffusion has been used for quantitating gentamicin in serum [21]. A result can be available in 3-5 hr by this method, but a knowledge of other antibiotics given simultaneously must be available so that the appropriate steps may be taken to inactivate them. More recently an enzymatic method has been developed which measures gentamicin by the formation of [^{14}C]-adenylated-gentamicin using [^{14}C]-adenosine triphosphate (ATP) in the presence of a specific adenylation enzyme derived from a gentamicin-resistant *E. coli* strain [22]. A further development was an acetylation method, in which gentamicin is labeled with a [^{14}C]-acetyl group from [^{14}C]-acetyl coenzyme A in the presence of an acetyltransferase enzyme, also obtained from *E. coli* [23]. Broughall and Reeves reported a comparison of assay procedures for gentamicin and concluded that the acetyltransferase method is the most satisfactory [24]. The assay can be performed on 20 μl of serum, and the results can be available in under two hours, readily enabling an eight hourly regime of gentamicin to be adequately monitored.

SULFONAMIDES

Clinical Commentary

Weinstein and Samet [25] have shown that there is wide variability between any given blood concentration of sulfonamide and antimicrobial activity. Therefore there is only occasional value in performing blood sulfonamide determinations, primarily to assure the physician that the drug is indeed present or that potentially harmful concentrations are not present. Toxicity to sulfonamides includes reactions involving the hematopoietic system, kidney, liver, skin, and peripheral nerves. While possessing no antibacterial activity, the acetylated metabolites of sulfonamides may be responsible for many of the toxic reactions [26]. The finding of a low blood level of free drug does not necessarily indicate the need to increase the dosage. Should the low level of free drug be the result of an increased rate of acetylation, increasing the dosage may result in the manifestation of severe toxic effects. Determination of total sulfonamide (free plus acetylated) may be of value in these circumstances.

Technical Commentary

The standard method for the determination of sulfonamides in biologic materials is that of Bratton and Marshall [27] and Annino [28]. The principle of the method is the formation of a diazonium salt of sulfonamide by the action of nitrous acid. The excess nitrous acid is destroyed by the addition of ammonium sulfamate. The diazonium salt is then coupled with N-(1-naphthyl) ethylene-diamine to give a red color. In order to measure total sulfonamide it is necessary to hydrolyze the acetylated metabolite by boiling the protein-free filtrate of plasma for 30 min with hydrochloric acid prior to formation of the diazo salt. The standard should be identical to the sulfonamide being determined since conversion factors cannot be computed on the basis of molecular weight relation [29]. The majority of sulfonamides in current use can be determined by this procedure. One notable exception is Mafenide (α-amino-p-toluene sulfonamide) which is used topically in the prevention of infections in burns. This compound soes not possess the p-amino group necessary for formation of the colored diazo complex.

Reagents

1. Trichloroacetic acid, 10%.
2. Sodium nitrite, 0.1%. Prepare fresh each day.
3. Ammonium sulfamate, 0.5%.
4. Standard, 10 mg/100 ml. Dissolve 100 ml of the sulfonamide to be determined in about 200 ml of water containing 1 ml of 10% sodium hydroxide. When dissolved, add 1 ml concentrated hydrochloric acid, and dilute to 1 liter.
5. N-(1-Naphthyl) ethylene diamine, dihydrochloride, 0.1%. Make up in water. Reagents should be kept in refrigerator.

Procedure

1. Pipet 1.0 ml water into a small stoppered tube.
2. Wash in 0.1 ml plasma, serum, whole blood, CSF, urine diluted to 1:10 or more, or standard. For blank, use 1.1 ml water. (Whole blood should now be allowed to hemolyze.)
3. Add 2.0 ml 10% TCA to all tubes, mix, allow to stand for 5 min, and then centrifuge.
4. Free sulfonamide. Pipet 1 ml supernatant fluid into a 5-ml stoppered tube.
5. Total sulfonamide. Pipet 1 ml supernatant fluid into another tube and add 0.1 ml 6 N HCl. Heat in oil or water bath at 100°C for 30 min, then cool.
6. Add 0.2 ml 0.1% sodium nitrite to all tubes. Mix and let stand 3 min.
7. Add 0.2 ml ammonium sulfamate and shake well. Let stand for 2 min.
8. Add 0.6 ml N-(1-naphthyl) ethylene diamine. Let stand for 5 min.
9. Read at 545 nm in a spectrophotometer using 50 × 4.3 × 10 mm cells.

Calculation

$$\frac{A_{test} - A_{blank}}{A_{standard} - A_{blank}} \times 10 = \text{sulfonamide/100 ml.}$$

THEOPHYLLINE

Clinical Commentary

Theophylline plays an important role in the management of bronchial asthma and bronchospasm associated with chronic obstructive lung disease. In seriously ill patients the most commonly used preparation of this drug is intravenous aminophylline (theophylline ethylenediamine). Optimum therapeutic serum concentrations range from 10-20 μg/ml [30-33]. Values greater than 20 μg/ml are often associated with signs of toxicity, which is manifested by gastrointestinal symptoms, including nausea, vomiting, and occasional diarrhea. Severe headaches are also common. Seizures, which are often intractable and potentially lethal, occur generally with serum concentrations over 40 μg/ml, although toxic symptoms are not universal even at this level [34].

A loading dose of theophylline is usually given in order to achieve rapid relief of symptoms [35]. If the patient has previously been receiving theophylline, it is important to obtain a baseline blood level before administering the loading dose. This requires the availability of a method that is both rapid and available at all times [36]. Further blood levels should be obtained at 30 min to 1 hr after the loading dose to assess the need for administering further smaller loading doses. For patients receiving continuous infusions of theophylline, blood levels should be monitored at 2-4 hr intervals to prevent the occurrence of toxic concentrations. When oral preparations are used, the most appropriate time for collection of blood samples is dependent on the dosage form used. For products either already in solution or theophylline tablets or capsules that undergo rapid disintegration and dissolution, 2 hr is a reasonable approximation for a peak level once the drug has been taken regularly for at least three days without missed doses.

It has been shown that salivary theophylline concentrations correlate closely to those in the plasma [37, 38]. Possibly there is some justification for assaying saliva in preference to blood samples, particularly in children who would undoubtedly prefer not to have to submit to frequent venipunctures.

Technical Commentary

Methods described for the determination of theophylline (1,3 dimethylxanthine) in blood have utilized spectrophotometry [39-41], gas-liquid chromatography [42-44], and high-pressure liquid chromatography [36, 45]. Spectrophotometric procedures have the disadvantage of being both time-consuming and subject to interference from a variety of other medications or dietary xanthines. Attempts to eliminate the problem of interferences have involved the use of sample blanks [41] or differential spectrophotometry [40]. Gas-liquid chromatographic procedures require an extraction of the serum into an organic solvent, followed by evaporation of the solvent, derivatization, and injection onto the column. While being much more specific than spectrophotometric procedures, these methods are still too time-consuming for emergency use. Gas chromatographic procedures are well suited for routine monitoring of blood and saliva theophylline, particularly in out-patient population for whom reliable dietary information may not be available. Such estimations can be performed on instruments that are readily available in most well-equipped clinical laboratories. The method of Weinberger and Chidsey [36] utilizing high-pressure liquid chromatography is extremely rapid, specific, and simple to perform. It requires only 0.1 ml of serum which from pediatric patients may be conveniently obtained by finger-stick. An assay can be completed within 30 min of receipt of the sample in the laboratory, making the procedure particularly well suited for emergency situations. The reader is referred to the original paper for precise details of this technique, which due to the nature of the instrumentation does not allow for meaningful abstraction here [36].

PHENOBARBITAL

Clinical Commentary

Phenobarbital has enjoyed much popularity as an anticonvulsant since its introduction into clinical medicine in 1912. While a wide variety of anticonvulsant drugs are now available to the physician, phenobarbital is usually the first medication prescribed for grand mal and focal seizures. In children with febrile convulsions, phenobarbital has been used successfully for prophylactic control of seizures [46] while such seizures may prove refractory to treatment with diphenylhydantoin [47]. Good correlation between serum phenobarbital levels and seizure control was demonstrated in a well-controlled study involving 60 children less than 3 years old with febrile convulsions [48]. The required serum phenobarbital concentration for control of these seizures has been reported to be over 1.5 mg/100 ml [49]. The necessity for ensuring regular medication in children with febrile convulsions has been well documented [50]. Should the phenobarbital level be allowed to fall below 1.5 mg/100 ml and convulsions ensue, they might not be alleviated by the administration of diazepam. In addition the risk of respiratory arrest following diazepam is much greater when phenobarbital has previously been given [51].

Tolerance to the depressant action of phenobarbital is acquired rapidly, and drowsiness due to the drug abates rapidly during the first few days of therapy [52]. Toxic symptoms due to overdosage with phenobarbital do not in general occur until serum levels exceed 3.0 mg/100 ml. It is not uncommon, however, to encounter serum phenobarbital levels as high as 6.0 mg/100 ml in patients with no signs of toxicity. Hypersensitivity reactions requiring withdrawal of therapy occur rarely and are not related to the blood level.

Technical Commentary

Published methods for the determination of phenobarbital levels in serum have included spectrophotometric [53, 54], gas-liquid chromatographic [55-58], and, more recently, immunoassay techniques. Gas-chromatographic procedures are currently enjoying wide popularity. They are free of the interferences from other drugs that plagued users of spectrophotometric techniques, and many are used to measure other anticonvulsant drugs simultaneously. The propensity of published procedures, however, provides some indication that the best method for any particular laboratory depends on its users' particular requirements. Baylis et al. have described a micro-technique applicable to the simultaneous determination of phenobarbital and diphenylhydantoin using only 200 μl of serum [55]. This quantity of serum is easily obtainably from a finger-stick collection of blood. Because of the necessity to operate the gas chromatograph at a high-sensitivity setting when such small sample volumes are used, it is not possible to utilize a solvent-injection technique. Interference, which would be created by the tailing solvent peak, is eliminated by the use of a solid-sample injector. However, this accessory is not readily available to most users of gas chromatographs in clinical laboratories. A solvent-injection technique using an extract obtained from only 100 μl of serum has been described by Kållberg et al. [56]. This method also would appear to be susceptible to interference from the tailing solvent peak because of the high sensitivity setting required. Most other published procedures for the gas-chromatographic determination of phenobarbital utilize 1.0-2.0 ml of serum [57, 58].

A frequently encountered problem in the gas-chromatographic analysis of phenobarbital (and other similar compounds) is tailing and reduction in size of the peak due to absorption of the drug onto the column support material. This makes accurate quantitation by peak height measurements impossible. One commonly utilized technique to minimize tailing is to reduce the polarity of the barbiturate nucleus by methylation which forms the 1,3-dimethyl barbituric acid derivitive [59]. A disadvantage of applying this technique to the determination of serum phenobarbital is that both mephobarbital (N-methyl-phenobarbital) and phenobarbital are converted to 1,3-dimethyl phenobarbital and are not differentiated from each other. Accurate quantitation of underivitized phenobarbital can be achieved if the column is saturated by injecting a relatively large quantity of phenobarbital (10 μg) onto the column prior to performance of the assay [60]. This technique has been used successfully in my own laboratory in the method described below.

Reagents

1. Sodium acetate, 1 M. Prepare by dissolving 82.04 gm of $C_2H_3O_2Na$ in distilled water and dilute to 1 liter
2. Acetic acid, 1 M. Dilute 60.06 gm of glacial acetic acid to 1 liter with distilled water.
3. Acetate buffer, 1 M, pH 4.8. Add 566 ml of Reagent #1 to 434 ml of Reagent #2 and mix.
4. Chloroform.

5. Internal standard. Dissolve 25 mg of hexabarbital in and dilute to 100 ml with ethanol.

6. Stock phenobarbital standard. Using ethanol, dissolve 100 mg of phenobarbital and then dilute to 100 ml.

7. Working standard (5 mg/100 ml). Dilute 5 ml of stock phenobarbital standard to 100 ml with distilled water.

8. Control serum (3.5 mg/100 ml). Dilute 3.5 ml of stock phenobarbital standard to 100 ml with 5% bovine serum albumin. Freeze in 1.5 ml aliquots.

Procedure

1. Pipet 1 ml of serum (working standard or control serum) into a 15-ml glass-stoppered conical centrifuge tube.

2. Add 1 ml of acetate buffer to each tube.

3. Using a 200 μl Lang-Levy pipet, add 200 μl of internal standard to each tube.

4. Add 7.5 ml of chloroform to each tube.

5. Shake each tube for 60 sec and centrifuge.

6. Aspirate off the top aqueous layer with a Pasteur pipet, and transfer 5 ml of the clear chloroform to a clean conical test tube.

7. Evaporate the chloroform extract to dryness under a stream of nitrogen in a fume hood. This can be aided by placing the tubes in a water bath maintained at 60°C.

8. Redissolve the residue in 25 μl of chloroform and inject 3-4 μl onto a gas-chromatographic column (6 ft × 0.08 in i.d.) packed with 3% OV-17 on 100-120 mesh Gas Chrom. Q. The column temperature is maintained at 190°C, and the injector and detector manifold temperatures are both 300°C. Prior to injection of the standard, control, and test samples, the column should be saturated by the injection of 10 μg of phenobarbital dissolved in 10 μl of ethanol (stock phenobarbital standard).

9. The peaks for the hexobarbital internal standard and phenobarbital are identified and the peak heights measured to the nearest millimeter.

Calculation:

$$\frac{\text{Phenobarbital peak height}}{\text{Hexobarbital peak height}} = \text{R}$$

then

$$\frac{\text{R (test)}}{\text{R (standard)}} = \times 5 = \text{mg/100 ml.}$$

DIPHENYLHYDANTOIN

Clinical Commentary

Diphenylhydantoin (Dilantin) is the drug most frequently adopted after an adequate trial with phenobarbital has failed to alleviate convulsions in patients with grand mal, focal motor, sensory, and psychomotor seizures. It has been shown to be of no value in the treatment of febrile convulsions in children under three years of age [47] or in the treatment of petit mal seizures [61]. Blood levels of the drug correlate poorly with the dosage given, particularly in children [62]. This is not surprising when one considers the numerous factors affecting the rate of diphenylhydantoin metabolism. These factors include genetic variability in hydroxylation capacity [63], liver function, and the concommitant ingestion of other drugs. Therapeutic agents which have been shown to decrease the rate at which diphenylhydantoin is metabolized include sulthiame [64, 65], chloramphenicol [67], dicoumarol [68], antituberculous drugs [69], disulfiram and phenyramidol [70]. Modifications to the extent of protein binding (which is normally approximately 90%) have been reported to occur in uremic patients changing the proportion of free or metabolically active drug [71]. Fortunately, with the exception of the latter situation, serum levels of total diphenylhydantoin correlate well with the control of seizures. The therapeutic range is usually accepted as being 1.0-2.0 mg/100 ml [72], although a narrower range of 1.0-1.5 mg/100 ml has been suggested [73].

The appearance of toxic symptoms correlates less well with the blood level of diphenylhydantoin than does the control of seizures. This is important to pediatricians since the onset of toxicity may be more difficult to ascertain in children than in adults [74, 75]. The frequency of toxicity, however, does seem to be less in children than in adults and the toxic manifestations vary with age [47, 72]. Toxic symptoms due to chronic overdosage with diphenylhydantoin include nystagmus on far lateral gaze, ataxia, dizziness, and occasionally an increased frequency of seizures [76]. Evidence of toxicity is usually associated with blood levels above 2.0 mg/100 ml [63, 77], although mild toxic symptoms can occasionally be seen with levels as low as 1.5 mg/100 ml [73].

Blood levels may be drawn at any time of the day providing that a steady-state has been attained, which, unless a loading dose has been given, may take as long as 8 or 9 days [78]. The time taken to reach a new steady-state when dosage is increased or decreased should be considered when requesting repeat blood levels.

Technical Commentary

Diphenylhydantoin levels in blood have been measured by a number of techniques including colorimetry [79], spectrophotometry [80, 81], thin-layer chromatography [82], gas-liquid chromatography [83-89], and immunoassay. As with phenobarbital and most other anticonvulsant drugs the determination of diphenylhydantoin in serum is most commonly performed by gas chromatography. Techniques involving both underivatized [84, 87, 88, 90], methylated [83, 85, 89], and trimethylsilylated [86] extracts of plasma have been described. The formation of nonpolar derivatives prevents the tailing of the gas-chromatographic peaks experienced by some workers and also permits the use of lower column temperatures. The method described below is used in the author's own laboratory for the simultaneous determination of diphenylhydantoin, primidone, and carbamazepine.

Reagents

1. Saturated borate buffer, pH 8.3. Prepare approximately one liter of saturated sodium borate. Adjust the pH to 8.3 by the addition of solid boric acid and decant the saturated solution into a suitable container.
2. Chloroform.
3. Internal standard. Dissolve 30 mg of 5(p-methyl-phenyl)-5-phenylhydantoin in 100 ml of ethanol.
4. Stock mixed diphenylhydantoin, primidone, carbamazepine standard. Dissolve 100 ml of diphenylhydantoin, 100 mg of primidone, and 100 ml of carbamazepine in 100 ml of ethanol.
5. Working mixed standard (2 mg/100 ml). Dilute 2 ml of the stock standard to 100 ml with distilled water.
6. Control serum. Prepare by diluting 2 ml of a 1 mg/ml ethanolic solution of diphenylhydantoin together with 1 ml of a 1 mg/ml solution of both primidone and carbamazepine to 100 ml with 5% bovine serum albumin. Freeze in 2.5-ml aliquots.

Procedure

1. Pipet 2 ml of serum (working standard or control serum) into a 15-ml glass-stoppered conical centrifuge tube.
2. Add 0.5 ml of saturated borate buffer to each tube.
3. Using a 200-μl Lang-Levy pipet, add 200 μl of internal standard to each tube.

4. Add 7.5 ml of chloroform to each tube.

5. Shake each tube for 60 sec and centrifuge.

6. Aspirate off the top aqueous layer with a Pasteur pipet and transfer 5 ml of the clear chloroform to a clean conical test tube.

7. Evaporate the chloroform extract to dryness under a stream of nitrogen in a fume hood. This can be aided by placing the tubes in a water bath maintained at 60°C.

8. Redissolve the residue in 25 μl of chloroform and inject 3-4 μl onto a gas-chromatograph column (6 ft × 0.08 in i.d.) packed with 3% OV-17 on 100-200 mesh Gas Chrom. Q. The column temperature is maintained at 240°C and the injector and detector manifold temperatures are both 300°C. The column temperature should be adjusted so that adequate resolution of the three anticonvulsants is achieved. The retention times of the three anticonvulsants relative to the internal standard are 0.66 (diphenylhydantoin), 0.58 (carbamazepine), and 0.54 (primidone).

9. The peaks for the internal standard and the anticonvulsants are identified and the peak heights measured to the nearest millimeter.

Calculation

$$\frac{\text{Anticonvulsant peak height}}{\text{Internal standard peak height}} = R$$

then

$$\frac{R\text{ (test)}}{R\text{ (standard)}} \times 2 = \text{mg/100 ml.}$$

PRIMIDONE

Clinical Commentary

Primidone (Mysoline) is an anticonvulsant that is usually applied when attempts at therapy with phenobarbital and diphenylhydantoin alone have failed. It is metabolized by the liver to form phenobarbital and phenylethylmalonamide (PEMA), both of which are present in the blood in addition to unchanged primidone. Due to the frequent presence of other anticonvulsant drugs in addition to the two active metabolites of primidone, there is very little information showing the correlation of primidone levels in the serum with seizure control. Because phenobarbital has a longer half-life than primidone, patients receiving the drug tend to accumulate phenobarbital until the serum phenobarbital levels approximate those found in patients given phenobarbital alone.

In one study described in the literature [91], phenobarbital was substituted for primidone in 19 chronically institutionalized subjects with uncontrolled seizures, all of whom were deceiving a variety of anticonvulsant drugs. Although the number of patients involved was too small for meaningful statistical interpretation of the data, more patients showed deterioration of seizure control on phenobarbital alone than showed improvement, suggesting that primidone itself may exert some anticonvulsant activity.

The mean blood level of primidone in one survey of patients receiving the drug in addition to other anticonvulsants was found to be 0.8 mg/100 ml [92]. There was no difference between the mean blood level of patients with controlled versus uncontrolled seizures. It seems clear therefore that the routine monitoring of serum primidone levels has little or no value in maintaining therapeutic control of seizures. The primary usefulness of serum primidone assays would appear to be in the early detection of toxicity due to the drug. Undesirable side-effects of primidone treatment include sedation, vertigo, nausea, ataxia, diplopia, and nystagmus. There is some evidence indicating that the appearance of toxicity correlates with increasing serum primidone levels. In view of this some clinicians attempt to maintain serum primidone levels below 1.0 mg/100 ml [93]. Because of the shorter half-life of primidone compared with diphenylhydantoin and phenobarbital it may be more important to relate the time of collection of the blood sample to the time of dosage. The average time to reach peak levels has been reported to average 3.1 ± 1.0 hr (mean $\pm$ S.E.M.) [92].

Technical Commentary

A spectrophotometric assay for primidone in serum has been described by Bush and Helman [94]. This procedure relies on the chemical oxidation of primidone to phenobarbital. This is accomplished following a determination of any phenobarbital that is originally present in the sample and which is then subtracted from the value obtained after chemical oxidation. Most recently published procedures for the determination of serum primidone levels utilize gas-chromatographic techniques [85, 90], although an immunoassay procedure has also been described.

CARBAMAZEPINE

Clinical Commentary

Carbamazepine (Tegretol) has become a useful adjunct to phenobarbital and diphenylhydantoin in the treatment of epilepsy. Its introduction into pediatrics is relatively recent, and its use appears to be increasing. Unfortunately there appears to be even less information regarding alleviation of symptoms and corresponding blood levels than there is for primidone. In one published study of blood levels found in 144 patients who has been receiving 200 mg of the drug t.i.d. for periods of time ranging from a few days to 5 years, a range of 0.1-0.9 mg/100 ml was found [95]. At the University of Colorado Medical Center the mean blood level of carbamazepine in 50 patients (adults and children) receiving the drug in combination with a variety of other anticonvulsants was 0.4 mg/100 ml (range 0.1-1.2 mg/100 ml). There is somewhat more information correlating blood levels with symptoms of toxicity (including nausea, drowsiness, disturbances of vision, and ataxia). At blood levels of 0.8-1.0 mg/100 ml, 50% of all subjects have been found to suffer from such undesirable side effects [95]. In light of these admittedly limited observations, it is probably unwise to ascribe a safe therapeutic range of plasma concentrations, and the practical value of monitoring carbamazepine levels seems in doubt.

Technical Commentary

Because of the relatively recent introduction of this drug into clinical practice, methods for its accurate measurement in plasma have only recently begun to appear in the literature. These have mostly involved gas-liquid chromatography [95-98], although an immunoassay procedure has also been described. Since the therapeutic blood levels are much lower than those encountered for other anticonvulsants such as phenobarbital and diphenylhydantoin, the analytical demands placed upon the assay procedure are somewhat greater. The method of Roger et al. [99] involving on-column methylation appear to achieve a coefficient of variation of 2%. The limit of detectability by this method is claimed by the authors to be 0.05 mg/100 ml.

SUMMARY

In this era of polypharmacy, the incidence of adverse reactions due to drug therapy has increased alarmingly since the precise effects on the metabolism of a drug given in combination with other drugs can never be predicted with certainty. Inadequate therapy due to insufficient medication or to factors which diminish absorption or enhance metabolism may be equally undesirable. The consequences to patients in terms of increased morbidity and financial cost of prolonged hospitalization may be considerable. For pediatric patients, particularly in the newborn period, these hazards may be much more dangerous.

There is a need for more investigation into the validity of procedures in current use for the determination of drug levels in biologic fluids and into the interpretation of the values they produce. In addition clinical chemists and clinical pharmacologists are faced with the challenge of defining those drugs for which blood level information would be advantageous and developing rapid, sensitive, and accurate assays which can be performed by the routine clinical laboratory. The day may be not too far away when a major proportion of the workload of the clinical laboratory consists of assays primarily designed as an aid to therapy rather than diagnosis.

REFERENCES

[1] V. Marks, W. E. Lindup, and E. M. Baylis, "Measurement of Therapeutic Agents in Blood," in Advances in Clinical Chemistry (O. Bodansky and A. L. Latner, eds.), Vol. 16, Academic, New York, 1974, pp. 47-109

[2] E. S. Vesell and G. T. Passananti, Utility of clinical chemical determination of drug concentrations in biological fluids: A review, Clin. Chem., 17, 851 (1971).

[3] D. O'Brien, F. A. Ibbott, and D. O. Rodgerson, Laboratory Manual of Pediatric Microbiochemical Techniques, 4th ed., Harper and Row, New York, 1968.

[4] S. Tompsett, Interferences from the presence of other substances in detecting and determining barbiturates in biological material, J. Clin. Pathol., 22, 291 (1969).

[5] R. Cooper, M. Greaves, and G. Owen, Diphenylhydantoin interferences with spectrophotometric barbiturate estimation, Clin. Chem., 19, 422 (1973).

[6] R. Gupta and P. Keane, Diphenylhydantoin interferences with spectrophotometric barbiturate estimations, Clin. Chem., 19, 1318 (1973).

[7] P. A. Toseland, M. Albani, and F. D. Ganchel, Organic nitrogen-selective detector used in gas-chromatographic determination of some anticonvulsants and barbiturate drugs in plasma and tissues, Clin. Chem., 21, 144 (1975).

[8] A. Richens, "Results of a Phenytoin Quality Control Scheme," in Clinical Pharmacology of Antiepileptic Drugs (H. Schneider, ed.), Springer-Verlag, Berlin, 1975, pp. 293-303.

[9] C. E. Pippenger, J. K. Perry, B. G. White, D. D. Daly, and R. Buddington, Interlaboratory variability in determination of antiepileptic drugs, Arch. Neurol., 33, 351 (1976).

[10] D. S. Reeves, Accuracy of gentamicin assays, Postgrad. Med. J., 50, Suppl. 7, 20 (1974).

[11] H. J. Kupferberg and J. K. Perry, "The Development of Matrix Reference Standard for Anticonvulsant Analysis," in Clinical Pharmacology of Anti-epileptic Drugs, Springer-Verlag, Berlin, in press.
[12] A. J. Glazko, W. A. Dill, and M. C. Rebstock, Biochemical studies on chloramphenicol (chloromycetin). III. Isolation and identification of metabolic products in urine, J. Biol. Chem., 183, 679 (1950).
[13] J. Levine and H. Fischbach, The chemical determination of chloramphenicol in biological materials, Antibiot. Chemotherap. (Basel), 1, 59 (1951).
[14] A. J. Glazko, Colorimetric Procedure for the Determination of Chloramphenicol and Related Nitro Compounds, Parke Davis Research Laboratories, Ann Arbor, Michigan.
[15] D. W. O'G. Hughes and L. K. Diamond, Chloramphenicol in blood: Simple chemical estimations in patients receiving multiple antibiotics, Science, 144, 296 (1964).
[16] K. Kakemi, T. Arita, and S. Ohashi, Absorption and excretion of drugs. IV. Determination of chloramphenicol in blood, J. Pharm. Soc. Japan, 82, 342 (1962).
[17] K. Kakemi, T. Arita, and S. Ohashi, Absorption and excretion of drugs. V. Determination of chloramphenicol in urine and its metabolic rate, J. Pharm. Soc. Japan, 82, 345 (1962).
[18] J. B. Andersen, N. Rosdahl, and R. Vejlsgaard, Aspects of pharmacology of gentamicin in newborn infants, Acta Pediat. Scand., 61, 343 (1972).
[19] G. H. McCracken, Clinical pharmacology of gentamicin in infants 2-24 months of age, Am. J. Diseases Child., 124, 884 (1972).
[20] G. H. McCracken and L. G. Jones, Gentamicin in the neonatal period, Am. J. Diseases Child., 120, 524 (1970).
[21] R. E. Winters, K. D. Litwack, and W. L. Hewitt, Relation between dose and levels of gentamicin in blood, J. Infect. Diseases, 124 (Suppl.), 590 (1971).
[22] D. H. Smith, B. Van Otto, and A. L. Smith, A rapid chemical assay for gentamicin, New Engl. J. Med., 286, 583 (1972).
[23] M. J. Haas and J. Davies, Enzymatic acetylation as a means of determining serum aminoglycoside concentrations. Antimicrob. Agents Chemotherap., 4, 497 (1973).
[24] J. M. Broughall and D. S. Reeves, The acetyl transferase enzyme method for the assay of serum gentamicin concentrations and a comparison with other methods, J. Clin. Pathol., 28, 140 (1975).
[25] L. Weinstein and C. A. Samet, Sulfonamide blood levels and serum antibacterial activity, Arch. Intl. Med., 110, 794 (1962).
[26] L. Weinstein, "The Sulfonamides," in The Pharmacological Basis of Therapeutics, (L. S. Goodman and A. Gilman, eds.), MacMillan, New York, 1970, p. 1184.

[27] A. D. Bratton and E. K. Marshall, A new coupling reagent for sulfanilamide determination, J. Biol. Chem., 128, 537 (1939).

[28] J. S. Annino, "Sulfonamides," in Standard Methods of Clinical Chemistry, Vol. 3 (D. Seligson, ed.), Academic, New York, 1961, p. 200.

[29] D. O'Brien, F. A. Ibbott, and D. O. Rodgerson, "Determination of Sulfonamides in Biological Fluids," Laboratory Manual of Pediatric Micro-Biochemical Techniques, 4th ed., Harper and Row, New York, 1968, p. 306.

[30] M. Turner-Warwich, Study of theophylline plasma levels after oral administration of new theophylline compounds, Brit. Med. J., 1957-ii, 67.

[31] J. W. Jenne, E. Wyze, F. S. Rood, and F. M. MacDonald, The pharmacokinetics of theophylline: application to adjustment of the clinical dose of aminophylline, Clin. Pharmacol. Therap., 13, 349 (1972).

[32] P. A. Mitenko and R. I. Ogilvie, Rational intravenous doses of theophylline, New Engl. J. Med., 289, 600 (1973).

[33] M. M. Weinberger and E. A. Bronsky, Evaluation of bronchodilator therapy in asthmatic children, J. Pediat., 84, 421 (1974).

[34] C. W. Zwiech, F. D. Sutton, T. A. Neff, W. M. Cohn, R. A. Matthay, and M. M. Weinberger, Theophylline-induced seizures in adults: Correlation with serum concentrations, Ann. Int. Med., 82, 784 (1975).

[35] K. M. Piapky and R. I. Ogilvie, Dosage of theophylline in asthmatic children, New Engl. J. Med., 292, 1218 (1975).

[36] M. Weinberger and C. Chidsey, Rapid analysis of theophylline in serum by use of high-pressure cation-exchange chromatography, Clin. Chem., 21, 834 (1975).

[37] R. Koysooko, E. F. Ellis, and G. Levy, Relationship between theophylline concentration in plasma and saliva of man, Clin. Pharmacol. Therap., 15, 454 (1973).

[38] G. Levy, E. F. Ellis, and R. Koysook, Indirect plasma theophylline monitoring in asthmatic children by determination of theophylline concentrations in saliva, Pediatrics, 53, 873 (1974).

[39] J. A. Shack and S. H. Waxler, An ultraviolet spectrophotometric method for the determination of theophylline and theobromine in blood and tissues, J. Pharmacol. Exptl. Therap., 97, 283 (1949).

[40] R. D. Gupta and G. D. Lundberg, Quantitative determination of theophylline in blood by differential spectrophotometry, Anal. Chem., 45, 2403 (1973).

[41] E. Ellis, J. Cordell, D. Clemente, and K. Hammond, Determination of theophylline in biological fluids, submitted for publication.

[42] V. P. Shah and S. Riegelman, Gas-liquid chromatographic determination of theophylline in biological fluids, J. Pharm. Sci., 63, 1283 (1974).

[43] G. F. Johnson, W. A. Dechtiaruk, and H. M. Solomon, Gas-chromatographic determination of theophylline in human serum and saliva, Clin. Chem., 21, 144 (1975).
[44] W. Dechtiaruk, G. F. Johnson, and H. M. Solomon, Faster gas-chromatographic procedure for theophylline, Clin. Chem., 21, 1038 (1975) (Letter).
[45] R. D. Thompson, H. T. Nagasawa, and J. W. Jenne, Determination of theophylline and its metabolites in human urine and serum by high-pressure liquid chromatography, J. Lab. Clin. Med., 84, 584 (1974).
[46] O. Faerø, K. W. Dastrup, J. C. Melchior, and I. Thom, Phenobarbital as prophylaxis for febrile convulsions: A preliminary report, Epilepsia, 12, 109 (1971).
[47] J. C. Melchior, F. Buchthal, and M. Lennox-Buchthal, The ineffectiveness of diphenylhydantoin in preventing febrile convulsions in the age of greatest risk under three years, Epilepsia, 12, 55 (1971).
[48] O. Faerø, K. W. Kastrup, E. Lykkegaard Nielsen, J. C. Melchior, and I. Thom, Successful prophylaxis of febrile convulsions with phenobarbital, Epilepsia, 13, 279 (1972).
[49] F. Buchthal, O. Svensmark, and H. Simonsen, Relation of EEG and seizures to phenobarbital in serum, Arch. Neurol. (Chicago), 19, 567 (1968).
[50] M. A. Lennox-Buchthal, Febrile convulsions: a reappraisal, Electroenceph. Clin. Neurophysiol., Suppl. 32, 1973.
[51] S. McMorris and P. K. A. McWilliams, Status epilepticus in infants and young children treated with parenteral diazepam, Arch. Diseases Child., 44, 604 (1969).
[52] O. Svensmark and F. Buchthal, Accumulation of phenobarbital in man, Epilepsia, 4, 199 (1963).
[53] L. R. Goldbaum, Analytical determination of barbiturates, Anal. Chem., 24, 1604 (1952).
[54] P. M. G. Broughton, Ultraviolet method for the determination and identification of barbiturates in biological material, Biochem. J., 63, 207 (1956).
[55] E. M. Baylis, D. E. Fry, and V. Marks, Micro-determination of serum phenobarbitone and diphenylhydantoin by gas-liquid chromatography, Clin. Chim. Acta, 30, 93 (1970).
[56] N. Kållberg, S. Agurell, B. Jalling, and L. O. Boreus, Rapid gas chromatographic determination of phenobarbital in small plasma samples, Europ. J. Clin. Pharmacol., 3, 185 (1971).
[57] H. J. Kupferberg, Quantitative estimation of diphenylhydantoin, primidone and phenobarbital in plasma by gas-liquid chromatography, Clin. Chim. Acta, 29, 283 (1970).
[58] J. W. A. Meijer, Simultaneous quantitative determination of antiepileptic drugs including carbamazepine in body fluids, Epilepsia, 12, 341 (1971).

[59] E. Brochmann-Hannessen and T. Olawuji-Oke, Gas chromatography of barbiturates, phenolic ankaloids, and xanthine bases: Glask heater methylation by means of trimethylanilinium hydroxide, J. Pharm. Sci., 58, 370 (1969).
[60] M. W. Anders, Rapid Micro-method for gas-chromatographic determination of blood barbiturates, Anal. Chem., 38, 1945 (1966).
[61] W. G. Lennox, The petit mal epilepsies; their treatment with Tridione, JAMA, 129, 1069 (1945).
[62] O. Svensmark and F. Buchthal, Diphenylhydantoin and phenobarbital. Serum levels in children, Am. J. Diseases Child., 108, 82 (1964).
[63] H. Kutt, W. Winters, R. Kokenge, and F. McDowell, Diphenylhydantoin metabolism, blood levels and toxicity, Arch. Neurol., 11, 642 (1964).
[64] J. M. Hansen, M. Kristensen, and L. Skovsted, Sulthiame (Ospolot) as inhibitor of diphenylhydantoin metabolism, Epilepsia, 9, 17 (1968).
[65] O. V. Olesen, Determination of sulthiame (Ospolot) in serum and urine by thin-layer chromatography: serum levels and urinary output in patients under long-term treatment, Acta Pharmacol. Toxicol., 26, 22 (1968).
[66] J. W. Huisman, H. W. VanHeycep Tentham, and C. H. W. Van Zyl, Influence of ethylphenacemide on serum levels of other anti-epileptic drugs, Epilepsia, 11, 207 (1970).
[67] L. K. Christensen and L. Skovsted, Inhibition of drug metabolism by chloramphenicol, Lancet, 1969-ii, 1397.
[68] J. M. Hansen, M. Kristensen, L. Skovsted, and L. K. Christensen, Dicoumarol-induced diphenylhydantoin intoxication, Lancet, 1966-ii, 265.
[69] H. Kutt, W. Winters, and F. McDowell, Depression of p-hydroxylation of diphenylhydantoin by antituberculous chemotherapy, Neurology, 16, 594 (1966).
[70] H. M. Solomon and J. J. Schrogie, The effect of phenyramidol on the metabolism of diphenylhydantoin, Clin. Pharmacol. Therap., 8, 554 (1967).
[71] M. M. Reidenberg, I. Odar-Cederlof, C. Von Bahr, O. Borga, and F. Sjoquist, Protein-binding of diphenylhydantoin and desmethylimipramine in plasma from patients with poor renal function, New Engl. J. Med., 285, 264 (1971).
[72] F. Buchthal, O. Svensmark, and P. J. Schiller, Clinical and electroencephalographic correlations with serum levels of diphenylhydantoin, A.M.A. Arch. Neurol., 2, 624 (1960).
[73] H. Kutt and F. McDowell, Management of epilepsy with diphenylhydantoin sodium, JAMA, 203, 969 (1968).
[74] W. J. Logan and J. M. Freeman, Psuedodegenerative disease due to diphenylhydantoin intoxication, Arch. Neurol., 21, 631 (1969).

[75] H. Patel and J. V. Chrichton, The neurologic hazards of diphenylhydantoin in childhood, J. Pediat., 73, 676 (1968).
[76] E. Roseman, Dilantin toxicity: A clinical and electroencephalographic study, Neurology (Minneapolis), 11, 912 (1961).
[77] H. Kutt, W. Winters, R. Scherman, and F. McDowell, Diphenylhydantoin and phenobarbital toxicity, Arch. Neurol., 11, 649 (1964).
[78] R. A. Buchanan, A. W. Kinkel, J. R. Goulet, and T. C. Smith, The metabolism of diphenylhydantoin (Dilantin) following once-daily administration, Neurology, 22, 126 (1972).
[79] W. A. Dill, J. Bankema, T. Chang, and A. J. Glazko, Colorimetric assay of 5,5-diphenylhydantoin (Dilantin) and 5-(-p-hydroxyphenol)-5-phenylhydantoin, Proc. Soc. Exptl. Biol. Med., 137, 674 (1974).
[80] G. L. Place and C. H. Hine, A method for the simultaneous determination of phenobarbital and diphenylhydantoin in blood, J. Lab. Clin. Med., 47, 649 (1956).
[81] O. Svensmark and P. Kristensen, Determination of diphenylhydantoin and phenobarbital in small amounts of serum, J. Lab. Clin. Med., 61, 501 (1963).
[82] G. E. Simon, P. I. Jatlow, H. T. Seligson, and D. Seligson, Measurement of 5,5-diphenylhydantoin in blood using thin-layer chromatography, Am. J. Clin. Pathol., 55, 145 (1971).
[83] D. H. Sandberg, G. L. Resnick, and C. Z. Bacallao, Measurement of serum diphenylhydantoin by gas-liquid chromatography, Anal. Chem., 40, 736 (1968).
[84] C. E. Pippenger and H. W. Gillen, Gas chromatographic analysis for anticonvulsant drugs in biological fluids, Clin. Chem., 15, 582 (1969).
[85] H. J. Kupferberg, Quantitative estimation of diphenylhydantoin, primidone, and phenobarbital in plasma by gas-liquid chromatography, Clin. Chim. Acta, 29, 283 (1970).
[86] T. Chang and A. J. Glazko, Quantitative assay of 5,5-phenylhydantoin by gas-liquid chromatography, J. Lab. Clin. Med., 75, 145 (1970).
[87] D. Sampson, I. Harasymit, and W. J. Hensley, Gas-chromatographic assay of underivatized 5,5-diphenylhydantoin (Dilantin) in plasma extracts, Clin. Chem., 17, 382 (1971).
[88] C. Gardner-Thorpe, M. J. Parsonage, P. F. Smethurst, and C. Toothill, A comprehensive gas chromatographic scheme for the estimation of antiepileptic drugs, Clin. Chim. Acta, 36, 223 (1972).
[89] E. B. Solow and J. B. Green, The simultaneous determination of multiple anticonvulsant drug levels by gas-liquid chromatography, Neurology, 22, 540 (1972).

[90] M. A. Evenson, P. Jones, and B. Darcey, Simultaneous measurement of diphenylhydantoin and primidone in serum by gas-liquid chromatography, Clin. Chem., 16, 107 (1970).
[91] O. V. Olesen and M. Dam, The metabolic conversion of primidone (Mysoline) to phenobarbital in patients under long-term treatment, Acta Neurol. Scand., 43, 348 (1967).
[92] H. E. Booker, K. Hozokown, R. D. Burdette, and B. Darcey, A clinical study of serum primidone levels, Epilepsia, 11, 395 (1970).
[93] H. E. Booker, "Primidone: Toxicity" in Antiepileptic Drugs (D. M. Woodbury, J. Kiffen Penny, and R. P. Schmidt, eds.), Raven Press, New York, 1972, p. 380.
[94] M. T. Bush and E. Helman, Quantitative determination of primidone, Life Sci., 4, 1403 (1965).
[95] H. Meinardi, "Carbamazepine" in Antiepileptic Drugs, (D. M. Woodbury, J. Kiffen-Penny, and R. P. Schmidt, eds.), Raven Press, New York, 1972, p. 487.
[96] J. W. A. Meijer, Simultaneous quantitative determination of anti-epileptic drugs, including carbamazepine, in body fluids, Epilepsia, 12, 341 (1971).
[97] H. J. Kupferberg, Gas-liquid chromatographic determination of carbamazepine in plasma, J. Pharm. Sci., 61, 284 (1972).
[98] P. Friel and J. R. Green, Quantitative assay for carbamazepine serum levels by gas-liquid chromatography, Clin. Chim. Acta, 43, 69 (1973).
[99] J. C. Roger, G. Rodgers, and A. Soo, Simultaneous determinations of carbamazepine ("Tegretol") and other anticonvulsants in human plasma by gas-liquid chromatography, Clin. Chem., 19, 590 (1973).

Private Forensic Toxicology: The Adversary System

LAWRENCE C. KIER

Kier Laboratories, Inc.
6740 East Hampden Avenue
Denver, Colorado

"Adversaries in law strive mightily but eat and drink as friends."

—Shakespeare

The author has largely drawn on his personal experience in over 25,000 private forensic cases, and hundreds of court appearances. He has testified in most of the county and district courts in the state of Colorado, and he is mentioned by name as qualified by the Colorado State Supreme Court. He has also testified in county and district courts in the states of Wyoming, Nebraska, and Washington; county court in Ohio; United States District courts in Denver, Colorado; Cheyenne, Wyoming; and Twin Falls, Idaho, as an expert witness in forensic toxicology.

The cases were from both sides of the criminal adversary system, for the prosecution and for the defense and for the plaintiff and the defendent in civil cases, and sometimes for both sides in the same case. Although most of the cases cited are factual, the names and places have been changed.

Most of the cases were those in which he had personally conducted the scientific measurements. Thus, he could testify both as a "fact witness" as to the results of the scientific measurement and also as an expert witness about the effects of such a measurement. These were conducted for local law enforcement agencies, the state patrol, and sheriff's offices on living subjects and for coroner's offices, medical examiners' offices, FAA, and FBI on deceased persons.

Forensic toxicology is the study of the harmful actions of chemicals and the presentation thereof in a court of law. The adversary system is the system of law where one side contends with, or opposes, the other; in criminal cases the people (prosecution) vs. the defendant, or in civil cases the plaintiff vs. the defendant. The application of forensic toxicology may be expressing an expert opinion in response to a hypothetical question based on facts in evidence and/or on the results of analytical toxicologic determinations either personally performed or performed by others. This is not intended to be a treatise on law with pertinent citations, although practical examples will be given.

Some of the facts in a given case are based on scientific evidence which is usually based on actual scientific measurement. The facts may be the actual concentration (weight/volume) of ethyl alcohol in a given blood sample or other biologic fluid at a particular time, or other quantitative measurements.

FORENSIC TOXICOLOGY APPLIED TO LIVING SUBJECTS

The subject is usually contacted because of an alleged violation of the law. The majority of cases involve driving while under the influence of either alcohol or drugs. Usually erratic driving or other violations are involved (such as an accident, speeding, etc.) which draws attention to the alcohol or drug content of the person; or the subject may be charged with being intoxicated (alcohol or drug usage) in a public place. The consumption of alcohol or drugs should be considered in cases of homicide (defendant). The victim of homicide or suicide will be discussed under "deceased subjects."

We utilize symptom charts (Figs. 1 and 2) in training law enforcement officers, district attorneys, etc., as to the various symptoms caused by various chemicals [1, 2]. Law enforcement agents, of course, are used to using the standardized visual sobriety questionnaire. Alcohol is the number one drug of abuse or recreational drug. In 1974, the per capita adult consumption was 3.11 gallons. Ethanol, of course, should be the first drug tested for. We also point out in the effects of ethanol (Fig. 2) that the frontal lobe areas affected by the lower levels, of course, are affected first. We designate these effects as invisible effects, i.e., effects not observable (by a measurement of the alcohol concentration) as distinct from the visible effects which most people are familiar with. We have been able to demonstrate in hundreds of subjects the various effects of alcohol. The invisible effects include those that low blood ethanol levels

KIER LABORATORIES
6740 East Hampden Ave.
Denver, Colorado 80222

SYMPTOMS

DRUG	MENTAL										SPEECH				COORDINATION							EYE				AP.				SAMPLES
	Drowsy	Excited	Belligerence	Anxiety	Euphoria	Depression	Hallucinations	Panic	Irrational Behavior	Confusion	Talkativeness	Rambling Speech	Slurred Speech	Laughter	Tremor	Staggering	Impaired Coordination	Dizziness	Hyperactive Reflexes	Depressed Reflexes	Increased Sweating	Constricted Pupils	Dilated Pupils	Bright Shiny Eyes	Inflamed Eyes	Decreased Appetite	Increased Appetite	Insomia	Space & Time Distort.	Available Tests Preferred Samples
*CNS Depressants	X		X		X	X			X				X			X	X			X					X		X			
Alcohol	X	X	X	X	X	X	X		X	X	X		X	X	X	X	X			X	X				X		X		X	Bl,Ur,Br*
Barbiturates	X		X		X	X			X	X			X	X		X	X			X	X	X								Blood
Codeine	X			X	X								X				X			X		X				X				Urine
Dilaudid	X			X	X								X				X			X		X				X				Urine
Heroin	X			X	X								X				X			X		X				X				Urine
Methadone	X			X	X								X				X			X		X				X				Urine
Morphine	X			X	X		X						X				X			X		X				X				Urine
Phencyclidine(PCP)	X			X				X		X				X			X	X												Urine
Demerol	X			X	X		X						X				X			X		X				X				Urine
*Marijuana	X	X		X	X	X	X	X			X			X			X								X		X		X	Swabs
*CNS Stimulants		X		X	X		X				X				X				X				X							
Amphetamines		X		X	X		X	X			X				X			X	X		X		X	X		X		X		Urine
Cocaine		X		X	X		X				X				X				X				X			X		X		Urine
DMA		X		X	X	X	X		X			X									X		X			X			X	Urine
DMT		X		X	X	X	X		X			X									X		X						X	Urine
LSD		X		X	X	X	X	X	X			X			X						X		X						X	Urine
Methamphetamines		X		X	X		X											X			X		X	X		X				Urine
Peyote		X		X								X											X							Urine
Psilocybin		X		X	X	X	X		X			X									X		X						X	Urine
STP					X	X	X		X	X		X			X														X	Urine

*Bl - Blood
Ur - Urine
Br - Breath

FIGURE 1.

(0.100% or less) have on vision (actual change in curvature of the cornea) and delayed recovery of night vision (around 0.050% ethanol). This is consistent with the findings of James Olds of the California Institute of Technology that different parts of the brain develop at different times and that reactions in different parts of the brain to various stimuli were correlated with changes in behavior [3].

"Changes appeared first in the hypothalmus (the part of the brain that controls temperature, hunger, and thirst) before any effect on the rat's behavior was evident. The reticular formation, a network of small nerve cells that control sensory and motor activities,

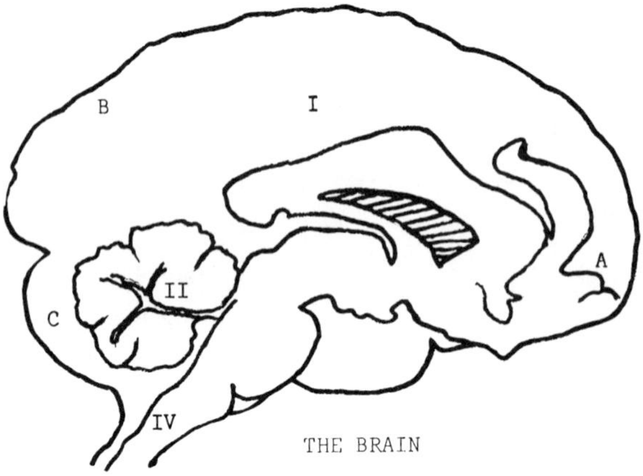

FIGURE 2

I. Cerebrum: Principle portion of brain including all parts within skull except medula, pons, and cerebellum

A. Frontal Lobe: .001-0.100% blood alcohol

Reaction is colored by the individuals personality	Increased confidence
Removal of inhibitions	Expansiveness
Less self control	Generosity
Weakening of will power	Altered judgment
Development of euphoria	Increased good fellowship
Feeling of well being	Loquaciousness (talkative)
Exaltation	Dulling of attention

B. Parietal Lobe:

1. Psychomotor area 0.10%-0.20% blood alcohol

Ataxia (loss of the power of muscular coordination)	Tremors
Apraxia (disorder of voluntary movement)	Slurred speech
Agraphia (loss of the power of writing)	Loss of skill

2. Somestheto-psychic area 0.10%-0.30% blood alcohol
   Dulled or distorted sensibilities

C. Occipital Lobe:

1. Visual - Psychic areas 0.20%-0.30% blood alcohol
   Disturbance of: Color perception, Form, Dimensions, Motion, Distance, and Diplopia.

responded as the rat began to look toward source of sound. The extrapyramidal motor system, which directs movement, showed changes while the rat learned to move toward the food. The sensory cortex which perceives sensory impulses responded as the rat's movements became smooth and fast.

"Only after the rat's movements were perfected did changes appear in the frontal cortex which may be important in higher intellectual activities."

The areas of the brain that developed first (primitive and essential to life) are affected adversely by high alcohol levels. The first area affected by the lowest blood alcohol level is the frontal lobe (invisible effects). Then as the alcohol level rises the more vital centers (more central) are affected until the most primitive center, the medulla, is affected by the highest level and death ensues. In summary, increasing alcohol levels affect areas of the brain in the inverse order of functional development of these areas.

The law enforcement agent may make a determination (breath testing) of the subject's alcohol content and feel that the results are inconsistent (negative or too low) with the visual observations. The observable effects may be due to a combination of alcohol and other drugs, either "uppers" or "downers." Law enforcement officers have been trained so that when they find tablets, powders, pills, etc., they send them along with the biologic specimens. These are a tremendous aid in the "unknown" biologic drug determination.

The odor of the breath (alcoholic beverage) is, of course, only a qualitative indication that some alcohol has been consumed. The recre-

---

FIG. 2. (continued)

II. Cerebellum: 0.15%-0.35% blood alcohol
Disturbance of equilibrium

III. Diencephalon: (inter brain, between brain) 0.25%-0.40% blood alcohol

Apathy	Sweating
Dilation of surface capillaries	Inertia
Tremors	Stupor
Cessation of automatic movements	Coma

IV. Medulla: 0.40%-0.50% blood alcohol
Depression of respiration
Peripheral collapse
Subnormal temperature
Death

ational drug user who is "hep" may consume only small quantities of beer to "flavor" his breath. When contacted he may exhibit some of the visual effects of ethanol. He has first choice as to the type of specimen to be used, i.e., blood. If he refuses to take a blood test, the officer has his choice of breath or urine in Colorado if blood is not used. The result of a blood test will only be available some days after his contact, and by the time the results are obtained any other drug used will have been metabolized. Even though he may have been kept in custody, at this point another drug test would not be valid for the time of the incident.

We point out that with most of the hallucinogenic drugs the effect is on the occipital lobe rather than on the cerebellum which controls equilibrium. The subject is "spaced out." Two classical cases are good examples of this. (a) A subject was contacted because he ran off the road and was found in a snow bank beside Berthoud Pass, elevation around 12,000 feet. He said he couldn't understand why the Colorado State Patrol had contacted him when he was in Ohio (some 1000 miles away). The subject was determined to be under the influence of peyote. (b) In another case the subject had rear-ended a police car stopped at the stop light. His response to why it happened: "A coyote ran across his path on Parker Road." Parker Road is a street 25 miles from the scene of the accident, and coyotes probably haven't been in that area for at least ten years. When he was asked when this happened, his response was, "Oh, last week." He was determined to be under the influence of Mepergan.

In these cases, although the visual psychic areas were disturbed there wasn't any disturbance in equilibrium, i.e., staggering, slurred speech, the visible signs of ethanol intoxication.

The important thing to stress in training is the subtle differences in observable signs. The subject who has an identical symptom picture to ethanol but no alcoholic beverage odor is a good candidate for being under the influence of barbiturates.

Most states have set a level of ethanol considered to constitute driving under the influence. This level is considered prima facia evidence. In some states the level may be divided as 0.050%-0.099% BAC being impaired and 0.100% and above as driving under the influence. This charge does require some symptom evidence as to the effect of ethanol.

In the case of drugs, the legal prima facia levels are not delineated even if the drug has been shown to be present by tests. The best way to demonstrate impairment is by the officer's testimony, giving his observations of the subject's behavior plus the scientific measurement of the chemical agent.

Some states have enacted legislation concerning driving under the influence per se. The charge is not rebuttable, i.e., only a measurement of the alcohol level is required.

Once a law enforcement officer has decided, based upon his training and experience, that someone is affected by any drug (under the influence), including alcohol, he then collects scientific evidence to substantiate the charge.

EVIDENCE COLLECTION AND PRESERVATION OF CHAIN ON LIVING SUBJECTS

The "kit" for the collection of evidence should be supplied by the individual who is going to do the testing, or it should at least be quality assured by the tester that the "kit" he is using doesn't contain anything that will interfere with the toxicology procedures, thus raising questions as to the validity of the final result (see Fig. 3).

One of the newer types of sealing materials is 3M Scotch Evidence Tape #566 which is better than the red sealing wax with impressed signet symbol. First class mail is adequate protection for the chain of scientific evidence. It may also be sent certified or registered with restricted delivery, i.e., only the person to whom it is addressed may receive it and sign for it; a return receipt may also be signed so that it will be returned to the sender for his records (the kit should have a quality control number). The outside mailing carton should be preserved and returned with the results as part of the chain to prove that a sample was exchanged. It should be identified with a number to relate it to the request form and the results.

In order for the scientific evidence to be accepted, it must be related to the subject by a "chain of evidence." The protection of the "chain of evidence" is challenged because of speculation that there might have been tempering with the evidence in a particular case. In a Colorado Supreme Court decision [4] (as published in Colorado Lawyer, Sept., 1973, pp. 119-120) "when it is only speculation that there was tampering, it is proper to admit the evidence and let the jury determine its weight. People v. Riser, 47 Cal. 2d 566, 305 P. 2d 1. See also, United States v. Von Roeder, 435 F. 2d 1004 (10th Cir. 1971); United States v. Freeman, 412 F.2d 1181 (10th Cir. 1969); State v. Riley, 24 Conn. Supp 234, 189 A.2d 518; State v. Cook, 17 Dan. 392; Commonwealth v. Mazarella, 279 Pa. 465 124 A.163; 2 Wharton Criminal Evidence R 665 (12th ed. R. Anderson 1955). In our view, under the circumstances present here, it would be pure speculation that the tube was tampered with prior to the placing of the blood sample into it. The prosecution was not required to negate every conceivable possibility of tampering, but only to establish with a reasonable degree of certainty that no such occurrence took place. The court did not err in admitting into evidence the result of the blood alcohol test. The weight to be given to it, taking into consideration the possibility of tampering, was for the jury."

It is extremely frustrating to spend a great deal of time and energy on a particular case and then find that the results of your scientific investigation are not admissible because the "chain has been broken," i.e., not adequately protected.

A written record of the chain of evidence should be included inside

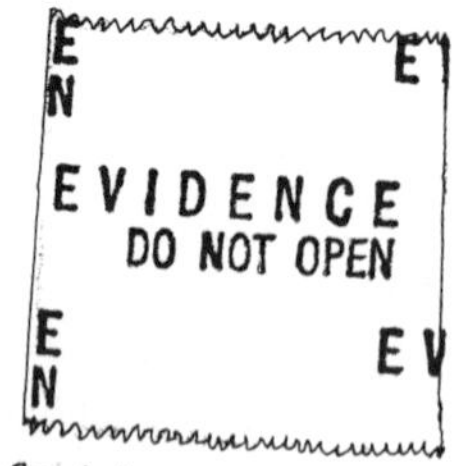

Scotch Evidence Tape No. 566

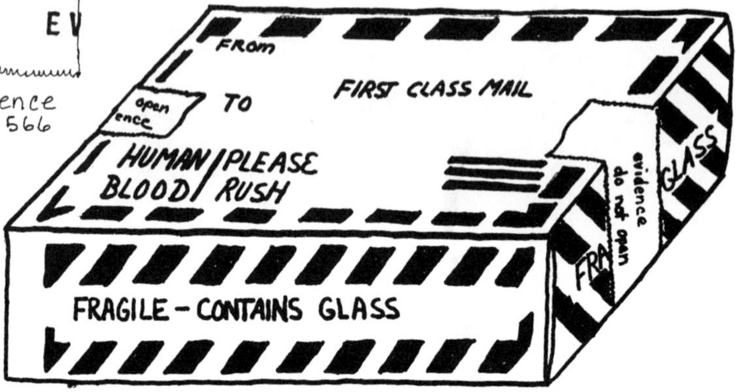

Polyfoam Packers Mailing Sleeve No. 340

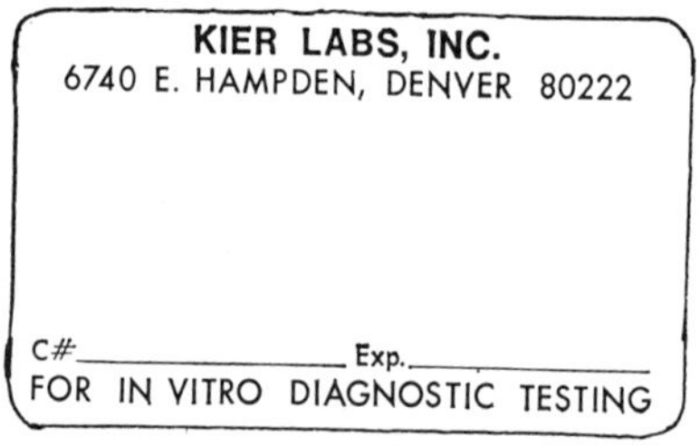

Paper Seal

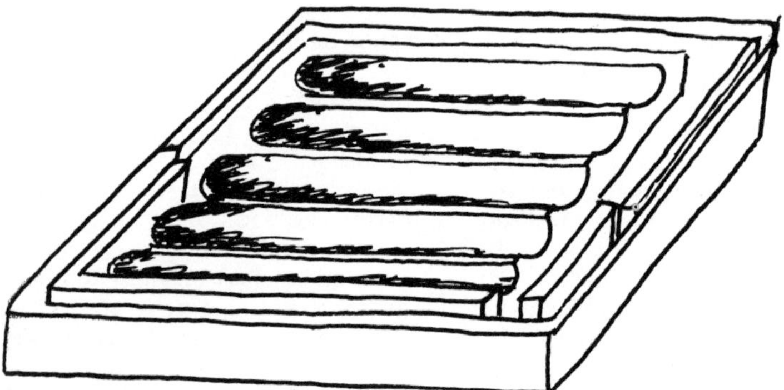

Polyfoam Packers Blood Mailer No. 339

FIGURE 3

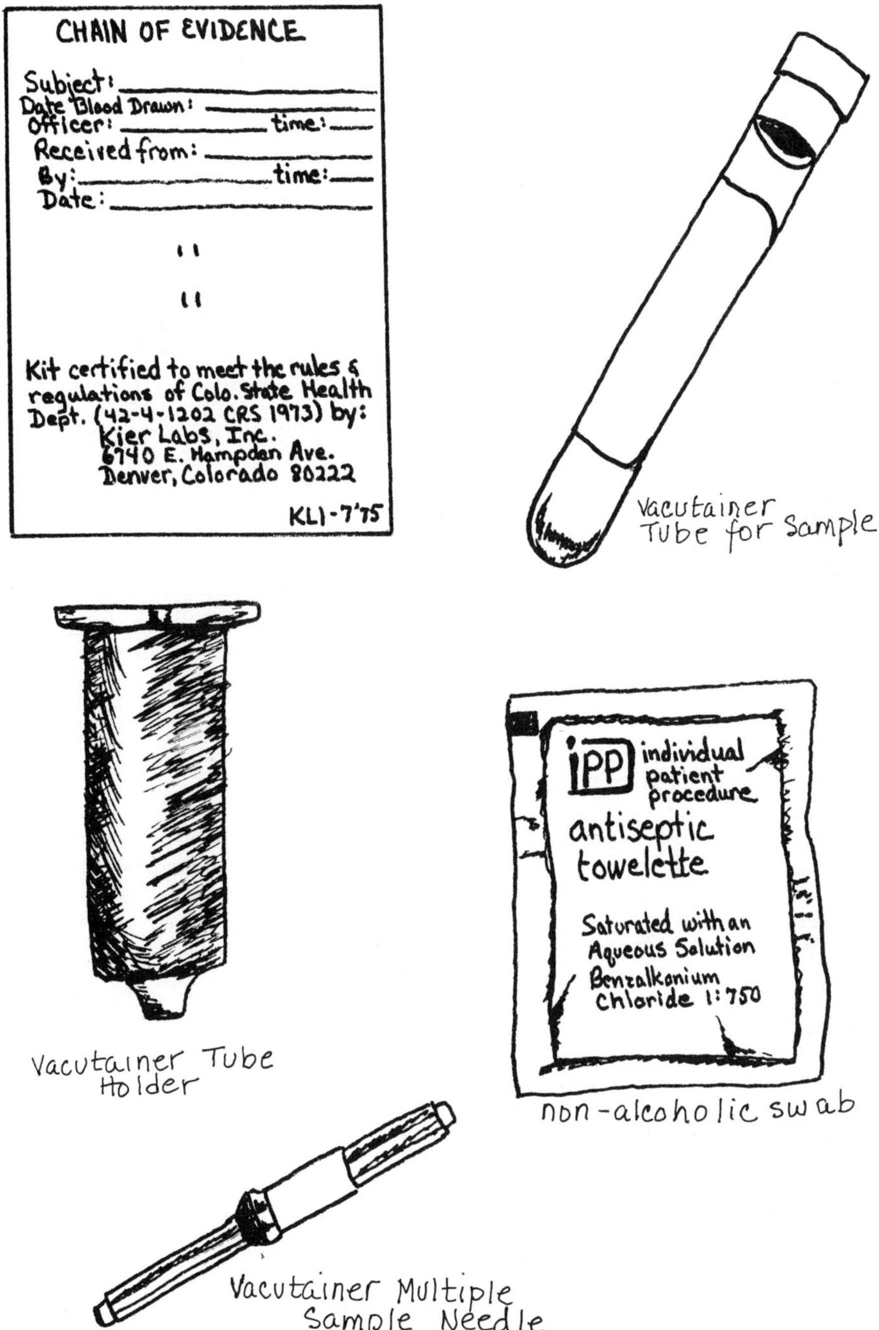

FIG. 3. (continued)

the kit. It should be filled out by each individual as he becomes part of the chain. Identification by a number for quality control is helpful. The inner Styrofoam carton protects samples in transit, is light weight, and meets U.S. postal regulations.

Inside the Styrofoam container are the materials for sample collection: nonalcoholic swab for sterilizing the venipuncture site (1:750 of aqueous Zephiran), sterile syringe and needle or evacuated tube and holder, and tubes to protect the chemical and physical integrity of the sample.

Results of our experience and experiments indicate that in living subjects utilizing "sterile technique," 0.2% fluoride and evacuated tube (Vacutainer v3200 PS) is adequate for blood or urine samples for tox-analysis. Filling the tubes full via vacuum also appears to limit the effect of alcohol oxidase (lowering of ethanol level). We have also checked tubes containing: (a) 20 mg potassium oxalate and 25 mg sodium fluoride (10 ml capacity) (BD#4726); (b) 100 mg NaF (10 ml capacity, sterilized) (BD#3200 XF 525); (c) 10 mg EDTA(Na_2) and 20 mg NaF (10 ml capacity), (BD#3200 XF 357); (d) 5 mg thymol and 50 mg NaF (7 ml capacity), (BD#4756). All of these appear adequate in maintaining ethanol (results to be published) and drugs. The BD 3200 PS (20 mg NaF and 25 mg potassium oxalate tube has been checked up to five years after sample collection without any significant change in either alcohol or drug levels. No increase in ethanol concentration after storage was found in any of the cases (1200). Results were presented in Paris, 1972, International Meeting of Accident and Traffic Medicine on fatal cases [5].

The Report Form (Fig. 4)

(1) or (2) with a check indicating the address where the sample was received. A C# (for certified mail) or R# (for registered mail) or PERS. DEL. (for personal delivery by an individual) may be marked next to the address if applicable. (3) The requesting agent's signature is authorization for testing and creates a financial obligation by the (5) requesting agency. (4) The requesting agency then may charge it to a particular division as part of their cost accounting. (6) "For Lab Use Only" is where the number is assigned to the particular request to identify the specimen (it should be chronological and may be prefixed by the year '77) and is used as a file number and log number. (7) The county establishes the legal jurisdiction. (8) This is the date of the offense. (9) The legal name of the subject is taken from a driver's license or other official document. (10) This is the ticket number or other law enforcement identification. (11) Location is the place (hospital, emergency room) where the blood is drawn. (12) The date when the sample was drawn is important in relationship to the date of the offense (it may be after midnight and thus not the same date as the of-

P. O. Box 22313 (1)
Wellshire Station
Denver, Colorado 80222

Science / Truth / Justice

KIER LABORATORIES, INC.

6740 E. Hampden Ave. (2)
Denver, Colorado 80222
(303) 759-4981

(3) Requesting Agent (Officer) ______________________ Division No. (4)

(5) Requesting Agency (PD) ______________________ (6) For Lab Use Only

(7) County ____________ Date (8) ______________________

(9) Name (Suspect) ______________________ Cr # (10) ________

PERMISSION FOR ALCOHOL AND/OR DRUG DETERMINATION

Location (11) ______________________ Date (12) ______________________

I, X (13) ______________________, give my consent to have a specimen
(Signature of suspect)

drawn for an alcohol and/or drug test. Witness (14) ______________________

****

Specimen drawn at (15) : ____ __A.M. __P.M. by (16) ______ (1) ______ (2) ______ (3)
(Signature of Doctor, Nurse or Technician)

Specimen drawn in my presence, after breaking seal, (17) and tube placed in small mailing carton(s) and sealed with Seal No. (18) ______, Seal No. (19) ______

by (20) ______________________ (Requesting Agent or Officer)

(21) Determination Requested: [A] Alcohol; [B] Drugs (Urine preferred); [C] Marijuana (Via Swabs Only)

(22) Specimen Submitted: [A] Blood; [B] Urine; [C] Breath; [D] Swabs [E] Fatal Victim

****

REPORT OF ALCOHOL AND/OR DRUG DETERMINATION

This is to certify that the undersigned removed, by breaking Seal No. (23) ______ the specimen described on this sheet and analyzed it for alcohol and/or drugs, that during the analysis the specimen was constantly under observation by the undersigned, and that the results of the analysis are as follows:

(24) The specimen contained not less than

(25) ____ mg. ethyl alcohol per 100 ml. of blood, or

(26) ____ mg. ethyl alcohol per 1 ml. of blood, or

(27) ____ % ethyl alcohol and/or a drug level of

(28) ______________________

(30) ______________________

(29) ______________________
(Signature of Toxicologist)

(31) ______________________
(Signature of Technician)

Date (32) ______________________

KLI 7/1/74
NO CARBON PAPER REQUIRED

FIGURE 4

fense). (13) The signature may be compared with the control signature (driver's license or other legal document) to demonstrate a "drug effect." It also provides legal protection (civil) for the individual drawing the sample, although in Colorado it is not necessary in felony cases or if the individual is deceased. (14) Witness should be the requesting officer for chain purposes, indicating that the individual that signed the form is the same individual named in 9. (15) Time of sample drawing in relation to the time of incident is important. This coupled with the questioning of the subject about when he stopped taking the drug (alcohol) can be extremely valuable in forming an opinion on what the level might have been at the time of the incident. (16) This is a person who by training and experience includes drawing blood in their normal duties, preferably a physician. This may also include a person with a state license, or an intern or resident if under supervision of a state licensed physician, or nurses in those states where their normal duties include drawing blood. Technician-technologist by state definition is one whose normal duties include drawing of blood. Legal requirements of qualification may be spelled out. (17) The seal that is applied by the laboratory that manufactured the kit (preferably the same laboratory that is doing the analysis in order to ensure that it was not tampered with from the time of manufacture and quality control until used. (18) and (19) May be "destruct" paper seal with same number as on outside of box (relates the outer mailing cover, or numbered metal box car seal, of type used to protect integrity of the sample. Box car seals in interstate transport once sealed can only be opened by cutting. Paper seals with the same number are used to seal tubes after specimen is placed in them to prevent tampering. Colorado State Health Dept. requires two samples to be drawn, one intact for future testing (by the defendant's expert) and stored under refrigeration (less than 4°C) for one year [6]. Some identifying mark should be placed on the tube by the person conducting the analysis, such as his initials and the date. (20) This should be the same as (3). (21) Determination requested (based on symptoms) (a) an alcohol should always be done. (b) In a driving situation drugs may or may not be done. The officer may want the drugs tested anyway because the suspect may have indicated that his problems are related to drugs and not alcohol. Drugs are screened by a comprehensive thin-layer chromatography system. Fortox positive results are confirmed by gas-liquid chromatography, or another thin-layer system. The same result by two different systems is preferred. (c) Marijuana method reported at the VI International Meeting of Accident and Traffic Medicine in Toronto [7] involves using isopropyl-soaked wooden-handled cotton applicator sticks. The area of the lips and particularly under the nose is the best place for sample collection to demonstrate the use of marijuana. (22) Specimen submitted is self-explanatory although if urine is submitted for alcohol (according to Colorado Health Dept. regulations), the subject should void, then the first sample should be taken and the second sample 20 min after the first sample to indicate if the ethanol level is rising. We automatically subtract 33% from urine to give an approximate equivalent blood alcohol level (this is based on 300 fatalities reported in AAFS February, 1970 [9]). (d) In a fatal motor vehicle accident, alcohol, drugs, and carbon monoxide tests are required where death occurs within 4 hr of the accident. (23) The number of either the self-destruct paper seal or the metal box car seal should relate to (18) or (19) with an indication of which second sample was saved for one year. (24) This indicates that three standard deviations of accuracy have been subtracted, because the law does not take this into account. (25) The BA (blood alcohol) level expressed as most physicians and medical personnel relate to it. (26) The concentration as many law enforcement agents relate to it. (27) The % ethyl alcohol (weight/volume) as expressed legally in most statutes. (28) The drug level found. (29) Signature of toxicologist if he personally performs the test; he may then testify as to the validity of the scientific measurement, and then express an expert opinion about the effect of such a level. (30) Confirming drug level or results of tablet or pill powder analysis. (31) Signature of the fact witness as to validity of the scientific measurement, which usually requires testimony of (29) as to the effect of such a level, which may or may not be consistent with (28). (32) Date on which the analysis is completed. A three-copy form is used.

After receipt of the sample, the specimen is logged into a toxicology laboratory record (see Fig. 5). This is a version modified from one suggested by Finkle [8]. It is $15 \times 8\frac{1}{2}$ in. and filed in a two-post cover.

FORENSIC TOXICOLOGY APPLIED TO DECEASED INDIVIDUAL

If the subject isn't found dead at the scene or dead on arrival (DOA) at an emergency treatment center, the subjective information as to symptoms (see Fig. 1 and presenting symptoms Fig. 6) are of much help in selection of tests. The rest of the information is critical to differentiate drug (chemical) levels that were present on arrival from those administered in treatment in an attempt at life-saving procedures. This information is critical in the final evaluation of the toxicology findings.

In the case of individuals who are found deceased and who don't have a previous medical history of disease or an attending physician willing to sign a death certificate, the death may have been caused by an accident, suicide, or homicide, or by unknown means.

The Forensic Toxicology Request (Fatal) is then used in those cases where the subject was found dead at the scene or DOA (see

1 Lab No.	2 Seal No.	3 Place Received	4 Received By	5 Date Sample Drawn	6 Type of Test	7 Subject	
Number assigned consecutively to identify the request form and is used to file all data connected with the case including TLC plates, GLC curves, etc.	Seal number taken from request form with an indication of the specimen saved.	Place received as indicated on request form	Person who received sample	Date sample was drawn as taken from request form. Helpful in location of request when requesting agent in DA's office inquires about result. To minimize the number of calls the original copy of the request form is returned to the requesting agency, the yellow copy is sent to the DA's office, and the pink one is kept on file.	Lists the types of test requested.	The individual which the test is being run on.	

8 Requesting Agency	9 Agency (Agent) ID#	10 Assign to	11 Requesting Agent	12 Date Completed	Completion Data			
					Tests Results	W T	Sent to	Billed Date
The requesting agency creating a financial obligation. (Who is to be charged)	Used to identify the fiscal agency.	Individual to who the test is assigned to. The chain is simplified if #4 and #10 are the same individual.	Requesting agent required by some agencies to create financial responsibility.	Date appearing in (32) of report (request) form.	Test results as indicated from request form.	W-written report sent T- date and time and to whom a telephonic report has been given(data may be placed on back of log sheet)	The individual or agencies to whom reports are sent.	The billing date is important for a private laboratory and should be completed only after the report has been sent out.

FIGURE 5

KIER LABORATORIES
6740 EAST HAMPDEN AVENUE / DENVER, COLORADO 80222 / (303) 759-4981

INFORMATION
IF SUBJECT NOT DEAD AT SCENE OR D.O.A. BUT EXPIRES LATER

Presenting Symptoms

System

Brain & Nervous
(1) Depression (a)Coma (b)Stupor (c)Drowsiness (d)Confusion (e)________
(2) Stimulation (a)Nervousness (b)Irritability (c)Anxiety (d)Fear (e)______
(3) Psychoses (a)Manic (b)Depressive (c)Dementia (d)________
(4) Reflex Excitability (a)Increased, decreased (b)Convulsive, clonic or tonic (c)Twitching (d)Tremor (e)________
(5) Temperature________

Visual
(1) General Appearance (a)Watery (b)Bloodshot (c)Pupils dilated, contracted (d)mobility (e)________

Auditory Effect________

Respiratory
(1) Respiration (a)Number____Type____ (b)Breath Odor________
(c)Cough (d)Pulmonary congestion or edema (e)________

Gastrointestinal Tract
(1) Appearance of tongue, lips or mouth________ (b)Constipation or Diarrhea (c)Urinary output______ (d) Urine Appearance________

Circulatory
(1) Heart rate______ (b)Blood Pressure______ (c)Shock Syncope
(d)________

SUSPECTED AGENT INGESTED
(accidental, suicidal or homicidal)

Information By
(1) History________
(2) Prescription Number(s) and where obtained________
(3) Pills or materials saved for analysis________
RESULT________

EMERGENCY TREATMENT

(1) Emesis, induced or spontaneous. Time______Material saved for analysis
RESULT________
(2) Lavage. Time______Material saved for analysis________
RESULT________
(3) Blood drawn for analysis of suspected agent. Time________
RESULT________
(4) Urine saved for analysis. Time______ RESULT________
(5) Medications given________Time________
Time______ Time______ Time______ Time______

FIGURE 6

Science

Truth Justice

KIER LABORATORIES

6740 EAST HAMPDEN AVENUE / DENVER, COLORADO 80222 / (303) 759-4981

FORENSIC TOXICOLOGY REQUEST (Fatal)

Requesting Agency__________________________By:_______________________________

Address:____________________________________Telephone:_______________________

City State Zip (Signature of Requesting Agent)

Subject Information

Name________________________Age____Sex____Wt.____Ht._______Date_____________

Time_____________Place_______________________Identification No._____________

Blood Type________

Suspected Cause of Death:____

Pertinent Autopsy Findings:____

Pertinent History:____

Chemicals or drugs implicated (Prescription # or Actual Samples)___________

Test Requested & Sample Required (Minimum) Results

Blood ___ 10cc____

Urine ___ 10cc*____

Gastric___ 10cc____

Vitreous___ 7cc (all)____

Bile ___ 10cc____

Tissues___ 4 oz.**____

Liver ___ Kidney ___ Lung ___ Brain (center if cyanide suspected)______

*If no urine is available send second 10cc tube of pericardial fluid with no anticoagulant (red stopper) for enzymes and other tests.

**Preserved separately and frozen for later analysis if required.

FIGURE 7

Fig. 7). Its purpose is to obtain the best materials for analysis and maintenance of the chain of evidence.

METHODS OF ANALYSIS

The best method of analysis is that which the tester uses and has successfully defended in court. They may be simple inexpensive thin layer or GLC testing of appropriate biologic specimens [Fortox]. Separations from the biologic specimen may be done by various liquid extraction procedures, column chromatography, ion exchange, etc. There are many fine volume of methodology. The most critical area is the standardization of the procedure and the validity of the standard. If you are a certified laboratory, state and/or federal, etc. (see Ref. [9], you are able to obtain standards. There are even standards available without a license requirement. The individual should assure himself that the certified standard supplied is a valid one by testing it himself. The use of melting point determination of organic chemicals (most drugs) is an excellent means of testing purity and specificity of the compound.

Most cases of analytical toxicology relate the unknown to the standard by comparative means. Instrumental, ultraviolet, visible, infrared spectrometry, gas liquid, thin layer, or high pressure chromatography and combinations such as separation by TLC then GLC, followed by mass spectrometry, work well on pure or relatively pure samples.

The most difficult analysis, of course, is application to biologic samples because of the wide variety of chemicals (some not identified even today) that normally occur in the specimen. This is further complicated as a result of metabolism, depending on the sample selected.

The choice of sample in living individuals is usually straight forward and a matter of law. This may, however, vary from jurisdiction to jurisdiction; one should be familiar with the legal requirements of the type of sample, how collected, preserved, and analyzed in his own particular jurisdiction. One should keep current with the new changes in this area.

The case of the deceased individual is one in which no set rules are readily available. The "unknown cause of death" is one of the most difficult and challenging problems a forensic toxicologist may face.

The types of sample required are based on scientific validity, although some regard this as undependable, having been told that "such and such" a test could not be run on "such and such" a sample. In light of his experience he might not be able to run the test, but this doesn't preclude someone else from making a satisfactory analysis.

Our personal choices and reasons in the forensic toxicology of deceased persons are the result of experience and use of scientific intuition.

Gastric

Physical examinations, including microscopic, are of a tremendous help in the unknown cases in establishing the time of death. The circumstances may be related to a meal shared by the victim with the suspect in homicide and witnessed by others. The presence of large amounts of tablet residue (type and color) is a clue as to what type of chemical (drug) was ingested. The pH is also of help in elucidating the type of chemical which might have been involved (as is a description of the gastric mucosa, which should be indicated on the report form by the examiner). One must keep in mind that the material here doesn't necessarily relate to the cause of death, because death may have ensued due to another agent ingested earlier and already absorbed. The latter material may not have been significantly absorbed.

The material in the stomach has probably not undergone metabolism and the pH of the gastric fluid may actually preserve the chemical integrity. It is usually in high concentration and relatively pure, making it an ideal sample for qualitative screening tests. The quantitative concentrations, i.e., the excess above that absorbed, may be important in differentiation between accidental and suicidal death. A great excess of drug (with even a large number of essentially intact tablets) is consistent with suicide. The particular tests applied to gastric content first would, of course, relate to evidence found at the scene, i.e., tablets, "pills," powders, prescription labels, glasses, cups, bottles, and the solutions contained therein.

The results of this preliminary information then serve as a guide to further testing on the biologic specimen. Optimum methods for quantitation of the specific agent may then be undertaken.

Urine

This is the form from which the most information may be obtained. The newer specific methods utilizing a small drop of urine are extremely important, i.e., hemagglutination, EMIT, and fluorescence. One has to be aware that the body metabolizes many drugs to more polar compounds (to make them more soluble in urine). The metabolites may actually be the agent detected; in the case of cocaine, it is the metabolite benzoyl ecgonine that is detected. The use of dip stick testing is also important in the evaluation of the health of an individual and is the first test performed.

Vitreous

This may be the fluid of choice in cases of trauma or extensive burns as it is well isolated from contamination. It does reflect the brain level better than other fluids. It is the fluid of choice for evaluation of the "state of health" of the deceased. Urea nitrogen (renal function) and sugar levels (carbohydrate metabolism) should be routinely done. The interpretation of quantitative analysis on other fluids will be influenced by the health status of the subject. For example, if there is evidence of renal failure (high vitreous urea nitrogen), low levels of a drug or chemical would be much more significant than if we assumed normal urinary excretion. This, of course, would effect the blood level of those drugs that are excreted in the urine.

Blood

This is the last of the biologic fluids to be tested. When one has some idea of which drug or chemical is involved, he will then be in a position to decide whether digestion with acid or alkali is required to release the compound; otherwise extremely low or negative values will be obtained.

Bile

This is an important source for some compounds that are metabolized or excreted via the liver through the bile. Keep in mind that IM or IV injection may show up in the gastric fluid by mucosal secretion of the drug (mucosal secretion may also be affected by the pH of the blood).

Pericardial fluid

An analysis of the pericardial fluid shows extremely elevated levels of drugs and further investigation is warranted as we reported at the AAFS meeting in Chicago, 1970 [10].

Tissue

Tissue analysis is called upon if one is unable to demonstrate adequate levels in biologic fluids. The brain may have increased levels of a drug compared with normal blood levels because of the effect of alcohol. (We have demonstrated that altered blood-brain barrier results from the combination of ethanol and drugs.) It may be a direct central nervous system effect or physiological alteration. Most drugs are organic and so are more soluble in alcohol than gastric juices, and the alcohol aids in the absorption of the drug. Liver-blood ratios of drugs may also be of value in interpretations.

The final interpretation of the analytical toxicology must consider the levels found in the different fluids and tissues and whether a combination of compounds are involved. When, for example, one of the compounds has a central nervous system depressant effect and the other has some central nervous system effect, and if they both act on the same center or place in the nervous pathway, the effect may be additive. If the drugs act on different centers, potentiation (effect greater than the simple additive) may occur. Trauma to the central nervous system must also be considered as potentiating or adding to a given drug level.

The forensic toxicologist must rely on the total picture, i.e., evidence at scene, including empty pill vials, the location and position of the decedent, etc. and then relate them to the pharmacologic picture based on drug level distribution. There may not be so much of a question as to what agent or agents caused the death as to whether accident, suicide, or homicide were involved. The answer to these questions may have a great economic impact on the outcome of insurance settlements—whether industrial or life.

The results of the forensic toxicology analysis may be accepted in the legal system by stipulation. This usually occurs when the forensic toxicologist has previously successfully defended his findings in court on many occasions.

THE PRIVATE FORENSIC TOXICOLOGIST AS AN EXPERT WITNESS

An article by Hauser and Erickson can be used as a guide for attorneys in selecting an expert, and it is particularly pertinent and serves as a guide to the "expert" [11].

"When the attorney needs the help of technical experts, his choice for assistance can be a crucial factor in the courtroom or at pretrial negotiations. Many attorneys lack sufficient information for selection of experts and may settle for the yellow pages or suggestions of associates. . .. In looking for an expert for court testimony, remember that you are hiring an expert, not buying him. As a professional he has a high ethical standard in the performance of his work. Here are some things you can reasonably expect from a well qualified technical expert":

> "1. He will interpret the technical facts to you and advise you of the validity of your client's position."

This may require a discovery motion as to what technical facts are available and the methodology used to determine them. If the scientific evidence is weak (revolves around the tester's personal knowledge of standardization), then the wise tactic may be to attack the validity of the available facts. You may want to test the evidence yourself; however, the results may work to the disadvantage of your client, by reinforcing the validity of the adversary's findings. In a case of receiving a split sample from the FBI at the request of a defendant, the author also received a supoena from the FBI for court appearance in the case even though the findings might not have been to the defendant's benefit.

> "2. He will probe beneath the obvious evidence to discover facts that may have a crucial bearing on the case."

The first area, of course, is to review the "chain of evidence" and the current regulations and laws applicable to the particular case. Having had to maintain the chain for the prosecution, he likewise would be able to point out "flaws" in the prosecution's chain. (See previous discussion of the chain of evidence.)

"3. He will honestly back your client's position, regardless of evidence which may be presented."

One should always be professional and unbiased in his presentation and answer the questions honestly, if it is possible to answer them. This doesn't preclude expanding on your opinion to your client's benefit. In response to a defense attorney (who had previously been a DA—haven't most of them!), "Dr., the answers to the questions propounded have changed." I replied, "The answers haven't changed, it's the questions."

This is where the adversary's advantage lies in questioning the expert. He is the one who is asking the questions. This may backfire on him if he hasn't done his homework, and doesn't know the answer. The best cross examination of an expert may be "no questions" in a large number of situations.

"4. He will communicate effectively with the judge and the jury."

The best way to do this is to look directly at the jury or judge when answering questions, no matter who asks them. The adversary isn't going to be convinced you know what you are talking about, nor admit it regardless of the answer. It is wise to "read" the jury. Are you boring them with detail? If so, cut it short and simplify your answers. If the adversary objects at some point in your testimony, look at the judge and wait for his ruling. Carefully listen to the objection, and try and meet the requirements in your further testimony. These moments may give you valuable time to reinforce something you may have forgotten to point out.

"5. He will remain calm under courtroom crossfire."

Remember, be cool. The initial time of losing one's cool will be long remembered even though it was 22 years ago. Being able to maintain one's cool usually makes the difference between successful and unsuccessful testimony. A personal satisfaction is achieved when, during the course of a trial, the judge suggests that a fifteen minute recess be called for the adversary (attorney) to regain his composure.

"When you have chosen the possible candidates, spend some time with each one. This will broaden your exposure to the technical community and give you a better basis for making a final choice. Ask penetrating questions. Ask embarrassing questions, if you wish, and note his reactions. Also note whether the expert asks penetrating questions of you. This is one of your best clues as to the expert's probing abilities. Be alert for both the snow job and the super-technical vocabulary of the expert. There is the possibility of over-sell by the expert—the broad-spectrum capability of an expert increases amazingly as he gets hungry. Does the candidate have access to suitable laboratory and technical facilities to provide adequate technical back-up for your case. Is this phase of the expert's services in keeping with the high ethical standards of a professional man? For example, does your expert intend to secure his laboratory data on his employer's equipment on a moonlighting basis? Will he use taxpayer-owned equipment? Will appropriation of taxpayer's equipment hurt your case? You may find it worthwhile to protect the credibility of testimony by avoiding such elements as moonlighting or use of taxpayer's equipment."

The private forensic toxicology laboratory that does testing and has qualified experts for testifying for both sides of the adversary system has the advantage of being at least impartial. The expert witness will be able to give a more valid testimony if he has personally done the testing, or at least if it has been done in his laboratory since then he will have established the statistical probability for the equipment and method used.

The private laboratory may be called upon to analyze a sample to reinforce the results that a governmental laboratory has obtained. It was taken as a compliment when the director of a regional laboratory commented, "Keep up the good work." The author inquired puzzledly, "What for?" In reply he said, "For keeping my boys on their toes."

The expert may reinforce a fact witness in a case by presenting his observation of the validity of a particular testing procedure and then the toxicologic effects of the level which is presented.

The chief disadvantage of a private forensic laboratory is the cost involved, either for testing or testimony. The cost from a business standpoint can only be reduced as the result of an increased volume of tests performed (greater efficiency). A private laboratory can offer good service. When a governmental agency is available, the testing can be done at little or no cost, although the work load may result in poor service (a long time interval in obtaining results). Nonroutine testing done by a technician is usually based on an hourly rate ($15-$30). The expert's time in testing, conference, and literature search is $50-$100 per hour (plus expenses) based on the complexity of the trial and expertise of the individual, with a minimum fee of $100 locally, or more if travel is involved.

There is a need for private forensic toxicology in the United States and their involvement in the adversary system. Governmentally supported facilities have a large work load and for professional reasons (political or economic reprisal) are unable to handle any private forensic cases.

In England, for example, there are seven district forensic science laboratories plus the central research establishment which are set up and paid for by the government [12]. They undertake work mainly for the police in their district. Since their inception, around 1935, they have regarded themselves as interested merely in ascertainment of the truth. They are equally available to the defense as they are to the prosecution; however one laboratory will not supply scientific help both to the prosecution and defense at the same time.

Such a system, as described by Curry, with either governmental financial support or private financial support, or both, would help solve the problem of the limited private forensic toxicology that is available.

REFERENCES

[1] Modified from Bureau of Narcotics and Dangerous Drugs, Terms and Symptoms of Drug Abuse, Washington, D.C. (chart).

[2] Modified from R. B. H. Gradwohl, Legal Medicine, Mosby, 1954, p. 760, fig. 195.

[3] The World Book Science Annual, Science Year, 1976, Field Enterprises Educational Corp., Chicago, pp. 332-334.

[4] Colorado Lawyer, September, 1973, pp. 119 and 120.

[5] "The Incidence of Alcohol & Drugs in Motor Vehicle Fatalities," IV International Conference of the Association for Accident and Traffic Medicine, Paris, 1972.

[6] Rules & Regulations of Colorado State Health Department (42-4-1202 CRS 1973).

[7] L. C. Kier, "A Simple Method for the Determination of the Smoking of Marijuana," VI International Conference on Alcohol Drugs & Traffic Safety, September, 1975. Proceedings, pp. 623-626. Toronto, Canada.

[8] B. S. Finkle (personal communication).

[9] News & Views, A Forum for Forensic Toxicologists, American Academy of Forensic Sciences, August, 1975.

[10] L. C. Kier and J. O. Kier, "Differential Distribution of Drugs in Tissues and Fluids," American Academy of Forensic Sciences, Toxicology section, Chicago, 1970.

[11] R. L. Hauser, Obtaining test & testimony in Colorado, Colorado Lawyer, May, 1974.

[12] A. S. Curry, Law Medicine, Science and Justice, Charles C Thomas, Springfield, Ill., 1964.

Drug Abuse Proficiency Testing

GORDON O. GUERRANT, Ph.D., and CHARLES T. HALL, Ph.D.

Proficiency Testing Branch
Licensure and Proficiency Testing Division
Center for Disease Control
Public Health Service
U.S. Department of Health, Education, and Welfare
Atlanta, Georgia

INTRODUCTION

An estimated 15 million urine specimens are tested each year in the United States for the presence of drugs of abuse [1]. These tests are performed by personnel with varying levels of skills using equipment and methods that differ in effectiveness. These variations impair the accuracy of laboratory results. In an effort to improve the performance of laboratories doing these tests, the Center for Disease Control (CDC) conducts an extensive proficiency testing program.

With a view toward laboratory improvement, CDC began its proficiency testing efforts in 1964. These efforts received added impetus with the passage of the Clinical Laboratories Improvement Act of 1967 (CLIA). The Act requires that laboratories processing human specimens which have crossed a state line meet standards promulgated under the Act in the areas of personnel, quality control, proficiency testing, records, equipment, and facilities. Laboratories testing interstate urine specimens for drugs of abuse came under the purview of the Act.

In 1972, CDC entered into an agreement with the Special Action Office for Drug Abuse Prevention (SAODAP), an organization within the Executive Office of the President. On July 1, 1975, SAODAP was, however, transferred to the National Institute on Drug Abuse (NIDA). All laboratories reimbursed for testing urine samples for drugs of abuse through federally funded methadone programs are currently required to participate in the CDC proficiency testing program in addition to the interstate laboratories. Under the methadone programs, drug addicts are given methadone as "substitute" therapy. In any drug addiction rehabilitation program, treatment centers have an addict's urine screened by a reliable laboratory service for the presence of drugs or their metabolites, or both. One cannot rely on an addict's word to determine what drugs have been taken. Present programs are directed toward the detection of abuse of morphine (heroin), methadone, barbiturates, amphetamine, and cocaine. For a certain time after a drug has been administered, the presence of each drug in the body can be monitored by detecting the drug or its metabolite, or both, in the urine.

GOALS

Through these proficiency testing surveys, we hope to encourage laboratories to improve the quality of services. In testing simulated urine specimens in surveys, laboratories will have to incorporate controls of known reactivity and reference samples into test procedures. This action encourages them to incorporate these controls and reference samples into their routine test procedures. Because methods, reagents, and laboratory skills are so varied, the laboratory worker must make sure that the methods in use are satisfactory and, further, that test protocol is strictly adhered to. Quality control checks confirm that the protocol is being properly followed, that all reagents are reactive, and that the methods are specific and capable of detecting minimum concentrations of interfering substances in urine samples.

It is difficult for an individual laboratory to evaluate its methodology, but it can make this easier by participation in a proficiency testing program. In such programs, urine samples simulating urine specimens of drug addicts are sent to participating laboratories as unknowns to be processed as patient specimens. The results of the proficiency tests are reported to the evaluating agency, which informs participants of the composition of the samples and summarizes the results.

DRUGS AND METABOLITES FOUND IN URINE

For morphine, methadone, and cocaine abuse, the drugs themselves and their primary metabolites are detected; for the barbiturates and amphetamines, only the parent drugs are detected.

Once in the body, heroin is metabolized to morphine and is eliminated in the urine as free morphine and as the conjugate morphine-3-glucuronide in a constant ratio of one part free morphine to five parts of the conjugate [2, 3]. Methadone is found as the free drug and as two metabolites: primary, 2-ethylidine-1,5-dimethyl-3,3-diphenylpyrrolidine, and secondary, 2-ethyl-5-methyl-3,3-diphenylpyrroline [4, 5]. Unlike morphine, where the ratio of parent compound to metabolite remains constant, the ratio of methadone to its metabolites [6] in urine decreases. Soon after methadone is ingested, only the parent compound can be detected in the urine sample; later, the parent compound can be found in diminishing concentrations, and its ratio to the primary metabolite decreases. In time, the parent compound diminishes to levels beyond the sensitivity of the test, and only the metabolite can be detected. The secondary methadone metabolite is present in low concentrations and is of significance in confirming the presence of methadone.

With barbiturates [7] and amphetamines [8], both the drug and its metabolites are present in the urine. Usually, only the primary drug is detected. Detecting cocaine is a special problem because cocaine is seldom found in the urine of addicts [9, 10]. Thus, laboratories must screen for the presence of benzoylecgonine, a metabolite of cocaine, rather than cocaine. Bastos et al. found benzoylecgonine in the urine of 259 of 3000 drug addicts [10].

THE PROFICIENCY TESTING SAMPLE

In the initial proficiency testing survey in January 1972, CDC mailed samples to 114 participant laboratories. These samples contained varying concentrations of morphine and methadone. Some were prepared in a water matrix to which caramel and urea were added to give the appearance and specific gravity of urine. Incorporating simulated urines in the early surveys was critical to the evaluation of methodologies. If the basic analytical procedures were to be evaluated, the samples had to be free of nonspecific interferences. The remainder of the samples were prepared in normal human urines diluted with water to one-half concentration. In these early samples, the concentration of morphine and methadone was so high that participating laboratories could detect the drug with any method they used. These samples were submitted to the participating laboratories to establish which methods in routine use were best for detecting drugs of abuse under ideal conditions. The plan was to then disseminate this information to the participants. However, the wide variety of methods and procedures and combinations thereof used were not described in sufficient detail for valid conclusions to be drawn on the performance and reliability of particular methods. After separating the drugs from the urine by solvent extraction or XAD-2 exchange resin, most laboratories used thin layer chromotography for drug detection. The percentage of participating laboratories that correctly identified all drugs in all proficiency testing samples ranged between 50 and 70% for the different laboratory specialty categories, with the exception of the hospital laboratories in which only 29% obtained correct results. A possible explanation for the poor performance of the latter was lack of experience in drug abuse monitoring of urine for morphine and methadone. Usually, of course, hospital laboratories monitor therapeutic drug levels and detect acute overdoses. Later results indicate that the performance of these laboratories improved, but as a group their performance is still somewhat below the overall average for participating laboratories.

In June 1972, the levels of morphine in samples were reduced to concentrations which, being just above the lower limits of sensitivity for methods in use, challenged the participants' capabilities. Morphine was submitted at concentrations of 2, 1, and 0.5 μg/ml. As might be expected, higher percentages of laboratories failed to detect lower concentrations of drugs. When the concentrations were reduced by one-half and one-fourth, the percentage of laboratories failing to detect morphine almost doubled, that is, it increased from 12 to 21% and from 21 to 40%. In this survey d-amphetamine was introduced at 10 and 5 μg/ml, and 8 and 15%of the laboratories, respectively, reported false negative results. Secobarbital was introduced at 5 and 2 μg/ml, and 12 and 19% of the laboratories reported false negatives.

In 1973, the practice of sending simulated urine specimens free of interfering substances was continued, and cocaine was put into the samples. The information derived from these samples was useful in comparing the sensitivity and specificity of methodologies. Responses from the participants were summarized by the methods used, and sensitivities were established for the most generally used methods. The minimum detectable concentrations that laboratories could reasonably be expected to identify routinely by any of the methods were: morphine, 0.2 μg/ml, and the other drugs, methadone, amphetamines, barbiturates, and cocaine, 1 μg/ml.

Beginning in 1974, the program was again modified by incorporating undiluted urine samples into the testing protocol so that the matrix of the sample would be similar to that of routine patient specimens. Thus, detection of the drugs was complicated by the presence of significant common interferences, such as metabolites of caffeine and nicotine.

In the 1974 surveys, morphine, methadone, d-amphetamine, and secobarbital were submitted in samples at the minimum detectable concentrations, and the respective true positive results laboratories reported were 53, 87, 74, and 84%. Based on the laboratories' poor response to 0.2 μg/ml of morphine, the minimum concentration was increased to 0.5 μg/ml. Late in 1974, the metabolites of cocaine, morphine, and methadone were added to the samples in concentrations that would be expected to be found with that concentration of parent drug. In 1975, laboratories were expected to detect cocaine and benzoylecognine at concentrations of 2 and 4 μg/ml or higher, respectively.

GENERAL INDICATION OF EFFECTIVENESS OF PROFICIENCY TESTING

It is difficult to measure the degree of improvement resulting directly from a proficiency testing effort. A pertinent question is: Has proficiency testing improved the ability of laboratories to screen urines for the presence or absence of drugs of abuse? Of course, a laboratory's improvement in its ability, under special circumstances, to perform a particular drug test is not necessarily reflected in routine drug screening. The CDC has long recognized that proficiency testing samples sometimes receive special treatment that is not given routine day-to-day patient specimens. Unfortunately, in some instances, the results of the proficiency testing survey may be submitted to the users of the service as evidence of the laboratory's ability to perform the drug screens. The proficiency testing agency provides only limited opportunities for evaluating participant laboratory performance because a small number of samples are offered infrequently; also these samples are expected to contain a large number of drugs. Thus, the samples are subjected to refined analyses which are ordinarily reserved for specimens which have first been implicated by screening procedures. Consequently, many drugs that might escape detection by the usual screen are detected in proficiency testing samples.

Despite the qualifications noted, proficiency testing has much to offer the participant and the testing agency. Specimens submitted from an external source constitute another approach to performance evaluation. Properly used, the samples offer the participant laboratory an opportunity to evaluate its day-to-day performance as opposed to the performance reflected by a report of the mean of numerous carefully controlled repeated tests of each proficiency testing sample. The testing agency obtains useful information on variability of results, and it can also identify certain methods with which laboratories have problems.

Proficiency testing results can alert laboratory directors to possible problems in the laboratory. If quality control is inadequate, proficiency testing may indicate problems with sensitivity and specificity. It is not, however, a substitute for quality control which would detect variations resulting from failure to follow the prescribed procedure, from failure to use reagents that do not have the required reactivity, or failure to use standards or calibrators that test the method near the minimum detectable level in the presence of likely interferences.

Over the years, the performance of laboratories in the CDC Proficiency Testing Program has improved. Participants are now more readily detecting the presence of drugs in minimal concentrations. In some surveys, they have detected the presence in samples containing concentrations approaching the limits of sensitivity of the method used. Laboratory performance has been directly influenced by advancements in methodology and improvement in reagents. Proficiency testing has contributed at least in part to this trend by permitting a laboratory to compare its performance with a given methodology to that of a peer population. Such comparisons have apparently caused some laboratories to reevaluate their methodologies, with the result that some procedures have been refined and some replaced.

Comparison of the incidence of failure to detect drugs in past and present surveys shows this improvement. Table 1 shows the average percent of false negative results reported by laboratories for the detection of morphine, methadone, cocaine, benzoylecgonine, and d-amphetamine by concentration and by year for 1972 through the first three quarters of 1975. The false negative responses shown for each year are average results of the surveys for each concentration and drug.

Improvement in the detection of morphine is shown by the decrease in frequency of false negative results. In 1972, at a concentration of 0.5 μg/ml of morphine, 30% of the laboratories failed to detect morphine, and in 1975, only 5%, or one-sixth as many, did not detect morphine. At the higher concentrations of 1 and 2 μg/ml, similar improvement is shown. The frequency of false negative results has decreased for methadone as well as for morphine. In 1972, the percentage of false negative results reported for a 2 μg/ml concentration of methadone was 22% and for 4 μg/ml and higher concentrations, 7%. In the first two surveys of 1975, the percentages of false negative results were 4 and 3% for methadone present at respective concentrations of 1 and 1.5 μg/ml. Thus, the percentage of false positive results was lower for methadone than for any other drug in the surveys.

Data on the ability of laboratories to detect cocaine or its primary metabolite, benzoylecgonine, in urine are insufficient to draw valid conclusions of true laboratory performance. Data in Table 1 indicate a slight improvement in the detection of free cocaine. In 1973, the percentage of false negative results reported for a 3 μg/ml concentration was 17%, whereas in 1975 the corresponding percentages for 2 and 2.5 μg/ml concentrations were 16 and 11%. For the determination of the metabolite benzoylecgonine, false negative results decreased from 89% in 1973 to 72% in 1974 for a 4 μg/ml concentration and from 62% in 1974 to 44% in 1975 for a 5 μg/ml concentration. Of the 322 laboratories participating in the November 1974 and April 1975 surveys, only 220 and 201 laboratories, respectively, indicated that they routinely screen for cocaine. Of those that do screen for cocaine, only 83 and 113 of the participant laboratories, respectively, detected the presence

TABLE 1. Drugs Undetected by Laboratories in Proficiency Testing Surveys Summarized by Concentration and Year

Drug	Concentration, μg/ml	Average percent of false negatives			
		1972	1973	1974	1975
Morphine	0.5	30	22	11[a]	5[a]
	1	22	9	6[a]	4[a]
	2	12	7	4	nd[b]
Methadone	1	nd	12	nd	4[a]
	1.5	nd	8	5	3[a]
	2	22	7	5	2.5[a]
	≥4	7	6	nd	nd
Cocaine	2	nd	nd	nd	16[c]
	2.5	nd	nd	nd	11[c]
	3	nd	17	nd	nd
Benzoylecgonine	4	nd	89	72	nd
	5	nd	nd	62	44
D-Amphetamine	1	nd	nd	20	nd
	1.5	nd	nd	15	11
	2	nd	nd	7	7
	3	nd	13	6	8

[a]Contained the primary metabolite.
[b]Not determined.
[c]Contained benzoylecgonine at twice the concentration of cocaine.

TABLE 2. Methamphetamine Undetected by Laboratories in 1975 Proficiency Testing Surveys Summarized by Concentration and Survey Number

Concentration	Average percent of false negatives		
μg/ml	I	II	III
1.5	nd[a]	34	28,29
2	48	nd	nd
3	nd	24	nd

[a]Not determined

of 5 μg/ml of benzoylecgonine, indicating that only one of every four drug laboratories in 1974 and one of every three drug laboratories in 1975 was proficient in detecting the abuse of cocaine at this relatively high concentration. The poor performance in detecting benzoylecgonine appears to be due to the laboratories' lack of experience and the unusual chemical properties of benzoylecgonine. A separate procedure is required for its detection.

The detection of low concentrations of amphetamine is a problem, as shown in Tables 1 and 2; only slight improvement has been demonstrated during this study. At a concentration of 3 μg/ml of d-amphetamine, false negative results were reported by 13, 6, and 8% of the laboratories in 1973, 1974, and 1975, respectively. The worst performance was that indicated by false negative responses of 20% for 1 μg/ml in 1974. Methamphetamine was first introduced into the surveys in 1975 at a concentration of 2 μg/ml, and 48% of the laboratories reported false negative results. A survey with concentrations of 1.5 and 3 μg/ml followed, and 34 and 24% of the laboratories, respectively, reported false negative results. In the third survey, a concentration of 1.5 μg/ml was submitted in duplicate, and 28 and 29% of the laboratories reported false positive results. These results indicate that approximately half (48%) of the laboratories were proficient in the determination of methamphetamine at the time of the first survey in 1975. However, after three surveys only 28 to 29% of the reporting laboratories were not proficient in detecting methamphetamine.

Results for the detection of barbiturates are presented in Table 3 as the percent of laboratories failing to detect various concentrations in the 1973, 1974, and 1975 surveys. In 1973, phenobarbital and secobarbital were submitted at 2 μg/ml or greater concentrations, and 10% of the laboratories reported false negative results. Only a slight improvement has been shown after the first three quarters of 1975 in which 6, 2, and 7% of the laboratories reported false negative results on phenobarbital and pentobarbital. At concentrations of 1 and 1.5

TABLE 3. Barbiturates Undetected by Laboratories in Proficiency Testing Surveys Summarized by Concentration, Specific Barbiturate, and Year

Barbiturate	Concentration, μg/ml	Average percent of false negatives		
		1973	1974	1975
Pheno-	1	nd[a]	20	nd
Seco-		nd	20	nd
Pheno-	1.5	nd	nd	14
Seco-		nd	10	nd
Pento-		nd	nd	6
Pheno-	2	10	9	6
Seco-		10	7	nd
Pento-		nd	nd	2
Pheno-	>2	10	6	7
Seco-		10	5	nd

[a]Not determined.

μg/ml, false negative results were reported by 10 to 20% of the laboratories for phenobarbital and secobarbital in 1974 and 1975. Thus, only a slight improvement in the detection of barbiturates has occurred over three years. Probable reasons for lack of improvement in detecting amphetamines and barbiturates are that more than one drug must be considered for each, closely related compounds may interfere with the test, and metabolites of the drugs are not used for confirmation.

Laboratories participating in the program are given a numerical percentage grade on performance. A score of 100 indicates accurate reporting of all drugs present in the survey and not reporting any drugs not present (false positives). A penalty is assessed for each false negative and false positive result, and the numerical value of the penalty is deducted from the score. The grades received are plotted in Fig. 1, where the grades for the surveys are paired and averaged over the $2\frac{1}{2}$-year period of 1973, 1974, and the first two surveys of 1975. A minimum grade of 80 points represents satisfactory performance. In surveys I and II of 1973, 41% of the laboratories made a perfect score and 63% received a passing grade of 80. Initially, the samples contained only morphine and methadone in high concentrations without interferences, and the high level of competency of a large number of good laboratories that were willing to join the program as

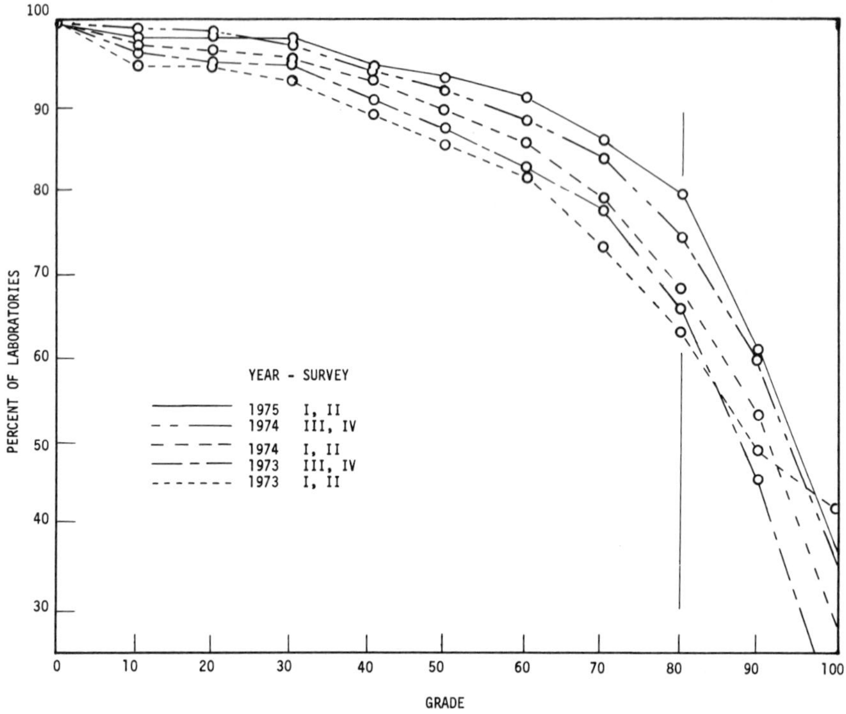

FIG. 1. Cumulative grade distribution for drug abuse proficiency testing.

part of their quality control program accounted for the large number of perfect scores. In later surveys, certain laboratories which had been unwilling to participate earlier were required to join the program as part of the basis for their funding. These laboratories were somewhat less proficient, and they reduced the percentage of laboratories receiving a perfect score. The percentage of laboratories with the established passing grade of 80 points has gradually increased to 78%. This percentage was reached after the first two 1975 surveys. Thus, the plot of the numerical grades the laboratories received, as shown in Fig. 1, indicates that the laboratories have improved in detecting drugs of abuse. The CDC Proficiency Testing Program has had an important role in this improvement.

SUMMARY

Concerning drugs in general, proficiency testing has undoubtedly been a major contributing factor to improved detection. Some of the improvement may be due to advances in technology, and this is possibly the case with improvement in the detection of morphine and methadone. The improvement in the determination of methamphetamine within three surveys over six months can clearly be attributed to proficiency testing. In drug screening for cocaine abuse, the poor results in proficiency testing for the detection of the primary metabolite, benzoylecgonine, has clearly demonstrated that laboratories are not proficient in this screening.

REFERENCES

[1] Drug Abuse Screening Market, USA, Market Potential Corporation, New York, 1972.

[2] E. B. Way and T. K. Adler, The biological disposition of morphine and its surrogates, Bull. World Health Org., 25, 227 (1961).

[3] F. W. Oberst, Free and bound morphine in the urine of morphine addicts, J. Pharmacol. Exptl. Therap., 69, 240 (1940).

[4] A. Pohland, H. E. Boaz, and H. R. Sullivan, Synthesis and identification of metabolites resulting from the biotransformation of dl-methadone in man and in the rat, J. Med. Chem., 14, 194 (1971).

[5] H. R. Sullivan and S. L. Due, Urinary metabolites of dl-methadone in maintenance subjects, J. Med. Chem., 16, 909 (1973).

[6] J. A. Mcintire, private communication.

[7] K. D. Parker, H. W. Elliott, J. A. Wright, N. Nomof, and C. H. Hine, Blood and urine concentrations of subjects receiving barbiturates, meprobamate, glutethimide or diphenylhydantoin, Clin. Toxicol., 3(1), 131 (1970).

[8] L. G. Dring, R. L. Smith, and R. T. Williams, The metabolic fate of amphetamine in man and other species, Biochem. J., 116, 425 (1970).

[9] F. Fish and W. D. C. Wilson, Excretion of cocaine and its metabolites in man, J. Pharm. Pharmacol., 21 Suppl., 135s (1969).

[10] M. S. Bastos, D. Jukofsky, and S. J. Mule, Routine identification of cocaine metabolites in human urine, J. Chromatogr., 89, 335 (1974).

Toxicology of Ipecac: A Review

BARBARA R. MANNO, Ph.D.

Associate Professor
Department of Pharmacology and Therapeutics
Louisiana State University Medical Center
School of Medicine in Shreveport
Shreveport, Louisiana

JOSEPH E. MANNO, Ph.D.

Associate Professor
and
Chief, Section of Toxicology
Department of Pharmacology and Therapeutics
Louisiana State University Medical Center
School of Medicine in Shreveport
Shreveport, Louisiana

INTRODUCTION

The effectiveness of syrup of Ipecac as an emetic has been well established [1-16]. Its long lived popularity is a tribute to its clinical effectiveness and relative safety. Although the fluid extract of Ipecac has not been available commercially for over ten years, a recent incident occurred with which the authors were associated whereby fluid extract of Ipecac was accidentally dispensed by a pharmacist for syrup of Ipecac. In reviewing the literature to determine the anticipated toxic actions of Ipecac, several reports regarding the ingestion of fluid extract of Ipecac were found, but very little investigative data regarding the pharmacology and toxicology of Ipecac were available in review format. The purpose of this review is to present a survey of the literature and to consolidate pertinent references which deal with the toxic actions of Ipecac extract and its component alkaloids, emetine and cephaeline, on the mammalian organism.

PREPARATION AND THERAPEUTIC USE OF IPECAC

Ipecac (Cephaelis ipecacuanha) has long been used by the natives of Brazil in the treatment of diarrhea. It was found in 1912 that the responsible chemical for its antiamebic activity was emetine [17, 18]. Ipecac also contains the alkaloids cephaeline and psychotrine [19]. Cephaeline produces more nausea and vomiting than does emetine, but emetine is more toxic to the heart and other organs. Psychotrine is considered to have low toxicity [19]. Several preparations of Ipecac are listed in the United States Pharmacopeia XVIII [20]. These include powdered Ipecac, i.e., Ipecac reduced to a fine powder and adjusted to contain not less than 1.9% and not more than 2.1% of the alkaloids of Ipecac (emetine and cephaeline). The other official preparation is Ipecac syrup. Ipecac syrup is prepared from powdered Ipecac. The concentration of alkaloid in the syrup is then 1/14 that of the powdered Ipecac. The only official use in the United States for Ipecac is as an emetic. The dose of Ipecac syrup for this purpose is 1 to 2 tablespoonfuls. It has been shown that syrup of Ipecac is as effective or more effective as other methods for termination of toxic exposure associated with the ingestion of poisonous substances [1-16]. Although Ipecac has been known for many years to be a very potent emetic, its common use as an antidotal agent in the treatment of accidental, oral ingestion of poisons or other intoxicants began in the 1960s when it was realized that this compound was an effective emetic, capable of removing large quantities of stomach contents rapidly and efficiently. Although the efficacy of gastric emptying has more recently been questioned [4, 6, 16], it is quite safe for use in children and adults in doses used per os. Prior to the issuance of the 1970 United States Pharmacopeia, the official method for preparation of syrup of Ipecac was by dilution of fluid extract of Ipecac. The Ipecac fluid extract is approximately 14 times more concentrated than the syrup. Unfortunately, fluid extract of Ipecac has been dispensed occasionally by mistake to unsuspecting mothers or physicians who in turn administered the concentrated product to a child with serious untoward effects. Several reports appeared in the literature during the 1960s regarding these accidental poisonings by fluid extract of Ipecac [21-23]. As a result of these accidental poisonings, the use of syrup of Ipecac was seriously questioned and was considered by the F.D.A. during the 1960s to place syrup of Ipecac under the dangerous drug regulations. However, because of the great value of syrup of Ipecac for the treatment and termination of accidental poisonings, it was deemed more suitable to remove the fluid extract of Ipecac from pharmacy shelves and thereby preclude accidental dispensing of the fluid extract. The removal of fluid extract of Ipecac was accomplished by a change in the United States Pharmacopeia. The 1970 U.S. P. did not list the fluid extract of Ipecac but rather powdered Ipecac and syrup of Ipecac, prepared from the powder.

SELECTED PHARMACOLOGY AND TOXICOLOGY OF IPECAC

Mechanism of Emesis

The Ipecac alkaloids, emetine and cephaeline, have been identified as the emetic-producing substances contained in syrup of Ipecac [19, 24-28]. Cephaeline was demonstrated to be twice as potent as emetine in producing vomiting [26, 28, 29]; however, cephaeline represents less than 50% of the combined total alkaloid content (emetine plus cephaeline) contained in the syrup of Ipecac [30].

Evidence supporting the centrally mediated emetic action of syrup or fluid extract of Ipecac include the work of Thumas [31], which showed that local application of emetine in the area of the medulla produced vomiting in dogs. Eggleston and Hatcher [27] administered emetine to dogs both orally and intravenously. Their findings are indicative of a central emetic action since the onset of vomiting was slower after oral administration than after intravenous dosing suggesting that time is necessary for absorption to occur. However, as discussed below, the local irritant effects of emetine could account in part for the production of the emesis after oral administration of syrup or fluid extract of Ipecac. Eggleston and Hatcher [27] further reported that emetine and cephaeline caused vomiting movements and symptoms of nausea in animals whose stomachs were completely removed. Recent reports of the use of syrup of Ipecac in cases of overdose or accidental ingestion of phenothiazines stated that emesis did not occur [23, 32]. Since phenothiazines are known to be antiemetic due to the suppression of the chemoreceptor trigger zone (CTZ) [33], these reports support earlier studies elucidating the central nervous system mediated vomiting produced by the administration of syrup or fluid extract of Ipecac.

Weaver and Griffith [34] distinguish between early and late phases of vomiting after administration of syrup of Ipecac. They have demonstrated that early vomiting (within 30 min) is due to the direct action of Ipecac on the gastrointestinal tract. Late vomiting or vomiting occurring at 30 min or more after ingestion of the drug is a result of centrally induced vomiting. Therefore, a secondary component of Ipecac-induced emesis which should not be discounted is local irritation of the gastric mucosa which produces a reflex vomiting.

Mechanism of Other Gastrointestinal Disorders Associated with Ipecac Alkaloids

Clinical reports have described a variety of disturbances of the gastrointestinal tract including stenosis of the lumen of the esophagus, bloody diarrhea, and protracted vomiting [21-23, 35-38]. Reports of the emetic action using syrup of Ipecac are summarized in Table 1. The data presented in Table 2 summarize the delayed onset of emesis and the protracted duration of vomiting occurring with fluid extract of Ipecac. Bloody diarrhea has been observed in animals administered syrup of Ipecac [5]. Although diarrhea has been a prominent toxic manifestation of fluid extract of Ipecac poisoning, no reports are available describing the precise mechanism of the diarrhea. Extrapolation of data from emetine toxicity studies provides us with a reasonable hypothesis that diarrhea encountered after fluid extract of Ipecac administration is a result of the presence of emetine. Emetine has been shown to produce increased intestinal peristalis [39, 40], hence the production of diarrhea.

Magendie and Pelletier as quoted by Pellini and Wallace [41] describe a definite inflammatory reaction along the mucous membrane of the alimentary tract after Ipecac is administered orally or parenterally. Cephaeline is more locally irritating than emetine [41].

TABLE 1. Summary of Onset of Emesis by Syrup of Ipecac in Humans

Number studied	Mean onset of vomiting	Dose and % responding	Ref.
214	18.7 min	20 ml syrup of Ipecac; 88% of children responded within 30 min	[16]
125	15 min or more	10-15 ml syrup of Ipecac; 55% responded	[14]
14	15 min	Syrup of Ipecac; patients responded within 5-40 min	[1, 3, 6]

TABLE 2. Summary of Onset and Duration of Emesis from Fluid Extract of Ipecac

Age	Sex	Ingested "poison"	Total dose fluid extract of Ipecac	Onset of emesis	Comments	Ref.
$2\frac{1}{2}$ yr	male	(6)-4 mg Chlor-trimeton	15 cc over 30 min	approx. 30 min	Violent for first 8 hr. Intermittent for $2\frac{1}{2}$ days.	[35]
4 yr	female	baby acetylsalicylic acid	10 cc over 15 min	1st emesis time not noted	Began vomiting second time in $7\frac{1}{2}$ hr. Vomiting occurred for 6 days; death ensued on 7th day.	[22]
34 mo	male	baby acetylsalicylic acid	5 cc	failed; lavaged	Intermittent vomiting for $2\frac{1}{2}$ days; intermittent vomiting began again 4th and 5th days.	[22]
4 yr	male	calcium carbonate antacid	30 cc; 30 cc repeated in 15 min	first dose failed within 15 min; vomiting occurred within 2 min of second dose.	Re-admitted to hospital approx. 12 hr after Ipecac fluid extract given; died within 8 hr of admission.	[21]

Pellini and Wallace [41] also state that rarely was the gastric mucosa affected when small doses of emetine was administered to animals where death was delayed for several days. Characteristic hemorrhagic changes occurred in the duodenum and jejunum but the lower part of the small intestine appeared normal. The cecum and large intesting assumed a hemorrhagic appearance. They described gastrointestinal tract changes with emetine similar to those observed with colchicine, diptheria toxin, and heavy metals. Large doses of emetine produced a highly injected, hemorrhagic mucosa covered with bile-stained secretions. Walters et al [28] demonstrated that irritant responses occurred when Ipecac alkaloid salts were placed in contact with the oral mucosa and conjunctiva. These irritative changes also occurred when application of the drug was by subcutaneous or intramuscular injection. Onset of irritant action was delayed for several hours. Chopra et al. [42] have reported emetine-induced irritation of the tongue with a marked increase in saliva flow. Others [29, 41] have also reported local irritant effects of emetine. Production of asthma in several men from the dust of Ipecac root has been reported as well as local irritation of the conjunctiva and nasal mucosa by Ipecac alkaloids [27, 28]. When exposed to dust of Ipecac root from which the alkaloids had been removed, the asthmatic condition returned. It was suggested that a plant protein was the causative agent for the asthma.

The mammalian body has been observed to dispose slowly of emetine with as much as 35% of the drug being retained after 35 days [43]. These same investigators concur that toxicity is the same whether exposure is due to relatively high doses of the drug or repeated small doses, e.g., 1/20 MLD (minimum lethal dose) of emetine. Tissue storage and subsequent slow excretion of emetine could explain the protracted vomiting and diarrhea which is reported with Ipecac fluid extract overdose. The following statements summarize the possible mechanism(s) explaining the gastrointestinal disorders associated with overdose of fluid extract of Ipecac. The diarrhea results from emetine-induced gastrointestinal peristalis. Bloody diarrhea is the result of local irritation of the mucosa of the alimentary tract. Allport [35] suggests that stenosis of the lumen of the esophagus is either due to local irritation by acidic gastric contents or regurgitation of emetine, which itself is irritating. The protracted diarrhea and vomiting results from the slow breakdown and excretion of emetine from the body.

Mechanism of the Emetine Cardiotoxicity

Cardiac toxicity has been reported in humans receiving emetine for the treatment of amebiasis [44-51], and after overdose with fluid extract of Ipecac (see Table 3). These untoward effects generally include a tachycardia which often precedes ECG irregularities. The

TABLE 3. Summary of Case Reports Involving Ipecac Intoxication

Age/Sex	Comment	Ref.
Adult Male	Ipecac extract, quantity ingested unknown. Violent uncontrolled vomiting within 1 hr. Rapid pulse; abdominal pain; death ensued after 2-3 hr. Necropsy revealed subacute congestion of stomach and first 2 ft of intestine.	[36]
$2\frac{1}{2}$ yr male	Ipecac fluid extract administered for chlorpheniramine maleate tablet ingestion. Course complicated by prolonged vomiting and diarrhea; leukopenia and neutropenia, etiology unknown—perhaps secondary to chlorpheneramine or ipecac; acute fluid and electrolytes disturbance leading to low sodium state and convulsions necessitating 5% NaCl administration; pneumonia and pleural effusion; phlebitis, secondary to 5% NaCl administration; ECG changes (ST and T-wave). Discharged from hospital on 17th day. However, did incur stenosis of the lumen of esophagus requiring bouginage in order to eat bulky foods.	[35]
4 yr male	Ipecac fluid extract administered for ingestion of antacid tablets containing precipitated calcium carbonate, magnesium carbonate, magnesium trisilicate, oil of peppermint, sugar. Symptoms: continuous vomiting; anorexia; anuria; diarrhea; fever; severe abdominal pain; bloody vomitus; irrational behavior; tachycardia; hypotension; coarse rhonchi in chest. Death ensued in approximately 24 hr after ingestion of drug. Necropsy findings: dehydration, moderate esophagitis, acute mucosal erosions of stomach and duodenum; acute moderate colitis with lymph-follicle hyperplasia; visceral congestion; hyaline-droplet degeneration of the renal tubules; fatty infiltration of the liver; focal interstitial proliferation in the myocardium.	[21]

(continued)

TABLE 3. (continued)

Age/Sex	Comment	Ref.
4 yr female	Ipecac fluid extract administered for ingestion of baby aspirin. Continuous vomiting began $7\frac{1}{2}$ hr after Ipecac. Listless twitching movements of extremities, admitted to hospital next morning. Symptoms on admission: fever; tachycardia; pale; no system abnormality. Lab findings: leukocytosis with atypical lymphocytes; second day—leukocytosis; proteinuria; stool, guaiac positive; protracted vomiting; 3rd hospital day—ECG abnormalities (depressed RS-T segment and inverted T-wave); 6th hospital day—drowsy, facial edema, fever; later semicomatose, no proteinuria but bloody urine. Death ensued on 7th day. Necropsy findings: heart and liver—normal; lungs—moderately congested and edematous; spleen—80 gm with moderate vascular congestion; GI tract including esophagus—no petechiae, ulcerations, congestion or inflammation; kidneys—moderately congested on cross section with no microscopic changes; bone marrow grossly pale and showed maturation arrest of granulocytic series; other organs including brain and spinal cord showed no abnormalities.	[22]
34 mo male	Ipecac fluid extract administered for ingestion of baby aspirin. He failed to vomit so lavage performed. Vomited several times $2\frac{1}{2}$ - $4\frac{1}{2}$ hr later; developed clonic convulsive movements about 14 hr after Ipecac. Admitted to hospital, unconscious and convulsing. Abnormal blood studies, leukocytosis; diarrhea and vomiting began again on 4th and 5th days. Child returned to normal after several days. Sigling to 4-yr-old female above.	[22]
23 mo female	Syrup of Ipecac administered after pipamazine ingestion. Emesis not produced. Child placed on cardiac pacemaker due to cardiac irregularities, e.g., atrial irritabilities, T-wave inversion, multiple premature beats, altered PR interval.	[23]

3 yr female	Ipecac fluid extract administered for ingestion of baby aspirin. Persistant vomiting began a second time about 2 hr after Ipecac fluid administration. Eight to ten hours after drug, child had tachycardia, dehydration, hyperthemia, and convulsions. ECG changes 14-16 hr after ipecac: flat, wide T-wave, prolonged Q-T interval, some evidence of left ventricular preponderance. Apnea followed at about 20 hr, rectal bleeding no BP recorded. Laboratory studies upon admission to hospital showed leukocytosis, toxic granulation in leukocytes. Death ensued 25-27 hr after Ipecac fluid extract. Necropsy findings: Lesions confined to heart, gastrointestinal tract, kidneys, and brain. Heart: 100 gm (normal 73 gm), gross softening of endocardium, esp. over left ventricular septum; microscopic thickening and edema of endocardium; diffuse vacuolization and necrosis of cardiac muscle fibers; and generalized interstitial edema. Esophagus, stomach, and duodenum normal. Mucosa of jejenum and ileum showed diffuse superficial ulceration; thickened mesentery of small intestine with enlarged, pale lymph nodes; mucosa of ascending, transverse, and descending colon erythematous but not ulcerated. Kidneys normal on gross examination but microscopically showed loss of nuclei and granular degeneration of cells lining distal convoluted tubules. Brain weighed 1400 gm (normal 1190 gm). Dilatation and congestion of superficial cerebral vessels. Microscopic scattered hemorrhagic foci throughout. Nissl stain showed acute degenerative neuronal changes in form of chromatolysis.	[38]
2 yr female	Ipecac fluid extract administered for ingestion of baby aspirin. Persistent vomiting occurred a second time about 2 hr after Ipecac fluid extract given. Upon admission to hospital about 8-9 hr after Ipecac fluid extract, child was moderately dehydrated, no tachycardia or lower blood pressure, neurologic and mental status normal, blood count normal. About 1 hr after hospitalization, child passed red clotted blood rectally; had scattered rales in chest. Discharged after 4 days with no sequelae.	[38]

(continued)

TABLE 3. (continued)

Age/Sex	Comment	Ref.
$3\frac{1}{2}$ yr	Ipecac fluid extract administered for ingestion of baby aspirin. Vomiting occurred within minutes of Ipecac administration. No untoward effects observed.	[38]
19 mo	Ipecac fluid extract administered for ingestion of heads of book matches. Child did not vomit after 3 teaspoonfuls; vomited about 2 spoonfuls of contents after an additional 2 teaspoonfuls of ipecac fluid extract. Symptoms included: shock, lethargy, diarrhea, dehydration, convulsions, cardiorespiratory distress, pneumonia. Death ensued on 3rd day. Death was due to: shock associated with acute dysentery; emetine intoxication.	[37]
—	Syrup of Ipecac administered in two instances where patients were still conscious but overdosed on phenothiazines. Emesis not produced. Cardiac toxicity (unspecified) observed.	[32]
7 mo	Ipecac fluid extract administered for ingestion of baby lotion. General symptoms: retching; dryness of skin; erthyma of soft palate; discoloration of buccal mucosa; redness of tongue; sinus tachycardia with no arrhythmias or murmurs; slight temperature elevation after 1st day; diarrhea after 2 days; some retching occurred for several days. Child apparently returned to normal after several days.	Manno and Manno

ECG abnormalities vary; however, they may be summarized as a lowering and inversion of T waves, alterations in the QRS complex, prolongation of the PR interval, and atrial tachycardia or atrial premature beats, or both [44-50]. In fact, appearance of cardiac irregularities during emetine therapy for amebiasis has been recommended as an indication for discontinuation of emetine therapy [51]. It has been felt by some that the tachycardia or abnormal ECG which occurs precedes emetine-induced cardiac arrest. The heart is either in asystole or ventricular fibrillation at arrest [51a].

Several investigators have pursued the mechanism of cardiotoxic effects of emetine; however, the complete mechanism has not been elucidated. Dack and Moloshok [45] observed that ECG changes, when present after a course of emetine therapy, were of long duration, suggesting fixation of the drug in the myocardium. They felt that perhaps the heart is hypersensitive to emetine, especially since myocardial tissue concentrations are usually much lower than those found in skeletal muscle and other tissues [43, 45]. Histopathologic examination revealed that hearts from dogs receiving emetine were congested in appearance with generalized marked right atrial and ventricular dilation. In contrast, tissue with high emetine concentration, i.e., spleen and lung, was normal in appearance [43]. In contrast to these findings are the observations of Rinehart and Anderson [50], which include severe damage to heart muscle of rabbits after lethal or sublethal doses of emetine. A summary of studies concerning the pathologic findings and biochemical studies into the mechanism of emetine cardiotoxicity is presented in Table 4.

Negative pathologic findings have been reported in emetine myocardial toxicity; however, the data more strongly support the findings of cardiac muscle damage due to emetine administration. This is further substantiated by clinical reports of patients receiving both fatal and nonfatal doses of emetine and patients receiving fluid extract of Ipecac. Observations have also been made that emetine cardiotoxicity may occur at the time of administration of the drug but have a delayed onset of action depending on single dose size and upon multiple dose total concentration. Early investigators of emetine-induced cardiac toxicity concluded that emetine was a "muscle poison." More recent in vivo and in vitro biochemical studies have shown that emetine (a) depresses myocardial glycolysis; (b) inhibits the tricarboxylic acid or Kreb's Cycle activity in the heart; (c) affects the conversion of glycogen to contractile energy; (d) inhibits protein biosynthesis; and (e) depresses cellular respiratory enzyme activity (see Table 4). These studies support a mechanism of cardiac toxicity due to a decrease in the contractile function of the myocardium associated with depression of metabolic activity. The delay in clinical signs for a cardiotoxic response to emetine can be explained by the inhibition of leucine incorporation into soluble proteins and actinomyosin, hence an inhibition in the biosynthesis of new contractile protein components.

TABLE 4. Summary of Pathologic and Biochemical Findings in Emetine Cardiotoxicity

	Finding	Ref.
1.	Weakened, slowing heart; diastolic arrest. Conclusion: muscle poison	[26]
2.	Cardiac paralysis	[29]
3.	Ventricular fibrillation followed by abrupt fall in blood pressure with death from acute cardiac dilation	[84]
4.	Respiratory and cardiac failure after large i.v. doses of emetine. Small s.c. dose produced gastroenteric changes; heart was congested at necropsy. No detailed pathologic studies reported.	[41]
5.	Studied nitrogen metabolism in dogs. Concluded that changes observed were similar to those induced by arsenic, phosphorus, potassium cyanide, etc., due to interference with intracellular metabolism with accompanying acidosis.	[41]
6.	Fibrillary contraction of heart after lethal i.v. dose. No gross changes except pulmonary edema. After s.c. injection, observed hemorrhage of lungs, congestion of intestine, fatty changes in liver and tubulonephritis. No report on heart.	[59]
7.	Auriculoventricular dissociation and auricular fibrillation. Conclusion: cardiac poison	[60]
8.	Weakened cardiac action after therapeutic emetine use. Death may occur from auricular or ventricular fibrillation.	[61]
9.	Rabbits poisoned by emetine showed that the parenchyma of heart muscle was the earliest tissue affected. Cloudy swelling of muscle fiber; disappearance of transverse striations; muscle fiber shrinkage; atrophy of fibers with replacement by connective tissue cells.	[62]

(continued)

TABLE 4. (continued)

	Finding	Ref.
10.	Death of rabbits and guinea pigs was dose dependent in from 5-20 days; hyperemia and granular and cloudy swelling of heart muscle, skeletal muscle, kidney and liver; Wallerian degeneration in occasional fiber of sciatic nerve and chromatolysis in a few of the anterior horn cells. Conclusion: protoplasmic poison	[55]
11.	Marked degeneration of heart muscle at necropsy.	[64]
12.	Cardiac morphologic changes delayed; death in less than 48 hr due to heart failure with an interstitial edema of heart muscle; survivors of lethal and sublethal doses for 3-4 days showed necrosis of some fibers in heart muscle with degenerative swelling in remaining fibers. Given divided lethal doses, observed small cellular scars in myocardium centered about necrotic muscle fibers. Authors called attention to similarity of the Aschoff reaction of acute rheumatic fever and effects of emetine on heart.	[50]
13.	Emetine affects the conversion of glycogen to contractile energy.	[63]
14.	Interstitial myocarditis of toxic rather than inflammatory origin.	[65]
15.	Myocardial respiration inhibited in vitro.	[66]
16.	Myocardial carbohydrate metabolism depressed.	[67]
17.	Myocardial respiration inhibited in vitro.	[68]
18.	Showed that treatment of animals with low doses of emetine causes significant inhibition of myocardial cellular respiratory enzymes. This may occur at time of drug administration.	[69, 70]
19.	Showed that emetine inhibits the transfer of activated aminoacyl compounds from sRNA to ribosomes, which is similar to the effects of cycloheximide.	[71]

(continued)

TABLE 4. (continued)

	Finding	Ref.
20.	Emetine inhibits incorporation of [^{3}H]leucine into soluble proteins and actinomyosin in an in vitro system using minced rat myocardium. Incorporation of [^{3}H]leucine was also inhibited when animals were emetine pretreated for 3 days. Data suggested that emetine toxicity in the myocardium may be mediated through its effect on protein synthesis.	[72]
21.	When isolated perfused heart was used, it was shown that emetine depressed myocardial metabolism of pyruvate and glucose (uptake) but did not change palmitate uptake. Oxygen uptake and CO_2 formation significantly decreased; therefore inhibition of Krebs cycle and glycolysis occurs, resulting in decreased myocardial contractility.	[73]

Mechanism of Neuromuscular Toxicity

Emetine therapy in humans has been reported to cause a transient muscular weakness after each injection and a prolonged weakness which lasts for 1-4 weeks after drug administration has been discontinued [48]. Peripheral neuritis has also been reported [52]. Salako reported similar muscle weakness in rats after emetine treatment—patterns resembling those used in humans [53]. Weight loss has also been reported in humans [55] and in rats [53, 54]. As Salako pointed out, weight change is difficult to evaluate due to the weight loss encountered as a result of the disease state being treated by emetine, i.e., amebiasis. This is a pertinent observation applicable to weight loss in patients who suffer protracted diarrhea and vomiting as a result of administration of fluid extract of Ipecac.

Ng's [56-58] investigations indicate a blocking action of emetine on the adrenergic neurones, the ganglia, and the neuromuscular junction. He suggests that emetine blocks norepinephrine release by acetylcholine at the adrenergic nerve endings. After Ng's work demonstrated that emetine has no direct effect on muscle stimulation, Salako [53, 54] studied its effect on neuromuscular transmission. He demonstrated a reversible block of indirect muscle contraction resulting from chronic or subacute administration of emetine to rats. He, too, discounted a direct action of emetine on the muscle. Salako [53] concluded that emetine produces neuromuscular blockade by a tubocurarine-like action.

He further reasoned that neostigmine would be useful in the management of the severe muscular paralysis which is occasionally encountered with emetine therapy.

Miscellaneous Reports on Ipecac and Emetine Toxicity

A number of additional referenced [74-94] beyond the scope of a single limited review are included.

Reported Ipecac Intoxications

Case reports of persons intoxicated with fluid extract and syrup of Ipecac are summarized in Table 3. It is important to note that in syrup of Ipecac intoxication, treatment had been initiated for ingestion of drugs with potent antiemetic properties, i.e., phenothiazines. The cardiotoxic problems encountered appear to have arisen because the phenothiazines had depressed the CTZ and vomiting did not occur thereby permitting absorption of the syrup of Ipecac. It must be stressed that the use of syrup of Ipecac should be avoided in antiemetic drug overdoses, e.g., phenothiazines, as well as in the unconscious patient or after caustic, hydrocarbon, or strychnine ingestion. In instances where Ipecac preparations have been administered and vomiting does not occur within 15-30 min, especially if a second dose is given, gastric lavage should be performed. This will remove the potentially irritating and toxic compound from the gastrointestinal tract and preclude absorption of Ipecac alkaloids. Table 5 summarizes the primary signs of Ipecac toxicity.

SUMMARY

The general effectiveness and safety of Ipecac syrup, per se, has not been questioned, but rather an attempt has been made to consolidate pertinent literature dealing with the toxic manifestations of Ipecac fluid extract. Ipecac contains both emetine and cephaeline and the toxicity of Ipecac fluid extract is consistent with reports on the toxicity of both compounds. The majority of the work has involved emetine since it is in higher concentration in Ipecac fluid extract than is cephaeline. Comparison of the clinical picture presented in syrup or fluid extract of Ipecac overdose and emetine toxicity in amebiasis treatment permits us to summarize the general characteristics of Ipecac alkaloid toxicity as involving primarily gastrointestinal, cardiovascular, and neuromuscular foci.

TABLE 5. Primary Signs of Ipecac Toxicity

Gastrointestinal	Cardiovascular	Neuromuscular	Miscellaneous
Severe diarrhea	Tachycardia	Skeletal muscle	Dehydration
Nausea	ECG irregularities	weakness aching	Hyponatremia
Vomiting	Hypotension	stiffness	Fever
Abdominal cramping		Convulsion	Shock
		Mild tremor	Blood dyscrasia
		Edema	

ACKNOWLEDGMENT

We wish to thank Mrs. Hollie Owens, Mrs. Martha Elzen, and Mrs. Jo Anne Sterling for their assistance in the preparation of this review.

REFERENCES

[1] F. J. Arnold, J. B. Hodges, and R. A. Barta, in collaboration with S. Spector, I. Sunshine, and R. J. Wedgewood, Evaluation of the efficacy of lavage and induced emesis in treatment of salicylate poisoning, Pediatrics, 23, 286 (1959).
[2] R. N. Tattersall, Emetics, Practitioner, 206, 111 (1971).
[3] W. J. Decker, In quest of emesis: fact, fable, and fancy, Clin. Toxicol., 4, 383 (1971).
[4] D. G. Corby, R. C. Lisciendro, R. H. Lehman, and W. J. Decker, The efficiency of methods used to evacuate the stomach after acute ingestions, Pediatrics, 40, 871 (1967).
[5] A. H. Abadulla and A. Tye, A comparison of the efficacy of emetic drugs and stomach lavage, Am. J. Diseases Child., 113, 571 (1967).
[6] D. G. Corby, W. J. Decker, M. J. Moren, and C. E. Payne, Clinical comparison of pharmacologic emetics in children, Pediatrics, 42, 361 (1968).
[7] T. A. Hanson, Apomorphine in the management of accidental ingestion of poisons, South. Med. J., 60, 603 (1967).
[8] H. C. Shirkey, Ipecac syrup. Its use as an emetic in poison control, J. Pediat., 69, 139 (1966).
[9] M. E. Thoman, The use of emetics in poison ingestion, Clin. Toxicol., 3, 185 (1970).
[10] M. E. Thoman and H. L. Verhulst, Ipecac syrup in antiemetic ingestion, JAMA, 196, 147 (1966).
[11] G. M. Oderda, Clinical toxicology, J. Am. Pharm. Assoc., NS14, 626 (1974).
[12] H. Matthew, Acute poisoning: some myths and misconceptions, British Med. J., 10, 519 (1971).
[13] H. Matthew, Gastric aspiration and lavage, Clin. Toxicol., 3, 179 (1970).
[14] B. Karlsson and L. Norén, Ipecacuanha and copper sulphate as emetics in intoxications in children, Acta Paediat. Scand., 54, 331 (1965).
[15] T. M. Cashman and H. C. Shirkey, Emergency management of poisoning, Pediat. Clin. North Am., 17, 525 (1970).
[16] W. O. Robertson, Syrup of ipecac—a slow or fast emetic? Am. J. Diseases Child., 103, 136 (1962).

[17] L. Rogers, Further experience of the specific curative action in amoebic disease of hypodermic injections of soluble salts of emetine, Brit. Med. J., 1912-2, 405.

[18] L. Robers, The rapid cure of amoebic dysentery and hepatitis hypodermic injections of soluble salts of emetine, Brit. Med. J., 1912-1, 1424.

[19] A. L. Walters and E. W. Koch, Pharmacological studies of the ipecac alkaloids and some synthetic derivatives of cephaeline. I. Studies on toxicity, J. Pharm. Exptl. Therap., 10, 73 (1917-18).

[20] The Pharmacopeia of the United States of America (XVII), The U. S. Pharmacopeia Convention Inc., Rockville (1970).

[21] R. P. Smith and D. M. Smith, Acute ipecac poisoning: Report of a fatal case and review of the literature, N. Engl. J. Med., 265, 523 (1961).

[22] T. Bates and E. Grunwaldt, Ipecac poisoning: A report of two cases of ingestion of fluid extract of ipecac, Am. J. Diseases Child., 102, 169 (1962).

[23] J. MacLeod, Ipecac intoxication—use of a cardiac pacemaker in management, N. Engl. J. Med., 268, 146 (1963).

[24] D. Duckworth, Observations upon the action of ipecacuanha and its alkaloid emetia. (sic.), St. Bartholomew's Hospital Reports, 5, 218 (1869); 7, 91 (1871).

[25] von Podwyssotzki, Beiträge zur Kenntniss des Emetins, Arch. Exper. Path. v. Pharmakol. Leipz., xi, 231 (1879).

[26] R. B. Wild, The pharmacology of the Ipecacuanha alkaloids, Lancet, 1895-2, 1274.

[27] C. Eggleston and R. A. Hatcher, The seat of the emetic action of various drugs, J. Pharm. Exptl. Therap., 7, 225 (1915).

[28] A. L. Walters, C. R. Eckler, and E. W. Koch, Pharmacological studies of the ipecac alkaloids and some synthetic derivations of cephaeline. II. Studies on emetic effect and irritant action, J. Pharm. Exptl. Therap., 10, 185 (1917-18).

[29] C. Lowin, Beiträge zur Kenntnis der Ipecacuanha, Arch. Intern. Pharmacol. Therap., 11, 9 (1902-1903).

[30] L. Goodman and A. Gilman, The Pharmacological Basis of Therapeutics, 5th ed., Macmillan, New York, 1975, p. 1075.

[31] L. J. Thumas, Ueber das Brachcentrum und über die Wirkung einiger pharmakologischer Mittel auf dassel be, Arch. Path. Anat., etc. Berl., Cxxiii, 44, (1891).

[32] G. Bourianoff, No time for ipecac, Emergency Med., 3, 5 (1971).

[33] L. S. Goodman and A. Gilman, The Pharmacological Basis of Therapeutics, 5th ed., Macmillan, New York, 1975, p. 161.

[34] J. E. Weaver and J. F. Griffith, Induction of emesis by detergent ingredients and formulations, Toxicol. Appl. Pharm., 14, 214 (1969).

[35] R. B. Allport, Ipecac is not innocuous, Am. J. Diseases Child., 98, 786 (1959).
[36] R. T. Harrison, A case of ipecacuanha poisoning? Lancet 1908-2, 536.
[37] N. J. Rose, Report of accidental poisoning death from fluid extract of ipecac, Ill. Med. J., 137, 338 (1970).
[38] J. D. Speer, W. O. Robertson, and L. R. Schultz, Ipecacuanha poisoning: Another fatal case, Lancet, 1963-1, 475.
[39] B. N. Ghosh and P. C. Adhya, Some newer observations on the pharmacology of emetine, J. Indian Med. Assoc., 13, 37 (1943).
[40] P. Bahr-Manson, Amoebic dysentery and its effective treatment, Brit. Med. J., 1941-ii, 255.
[41] E. J. Pellini and G. B. Wallace, The pharmacology of emetine, Am. J. Med. Sci., 152, 325 (1916).
[42] R. N. Chopra, J. C. Gupta, and K. V. Pillai, Observations on the action of emetine on the gastrointestinal tract, Indian J. Med. Res., 15, 883 (1927-28).
[43] A. I. Gimble, C. Davison, and P. K. Smith, Studies on the toxicity, distribution and excretion of emetine, J. Pharm. Exptl. Therap., 94, 431 (1948).
[44] L. J. Boyd and D. Scherf, The electrocardiogram in acute emetine intoxication, J. Pharm. Exptl. Therap., 71, 362 (1941).
[45] S. Dack and R. E. Moloshok, Cardiac manifestations of toxic action of emetine hydrochloride in amebic dysentery, Arch. Intern. Med., 79, 228 (1947).
[46] M. Hardgrove and E. R. Smith, Effects of emetine on the electrocardiogram, Am. Heart J., 28, 752 (1944).
[47] L. Kent and R. C. Kingsland, Effects of emetine hydrochloride on the electrocardiogram in man, Am. Heart J., 39, 576 (1950).
[48] G. Klatskin and H. Fiedman, Emetine toxicity in man: studies on the nature of early toxic manifestations, their relation to dose level, and their significance in determining safe dosage, Ann. Intern. Med., 28, 892 (1948).
[49] W. A. Sodeman, J. S. D'Antoni, and A. A. Doerner, Emetine intoxication, Trans. Roy. Soc. Trop. Med. & Hyg., 46, 151 (1952).
[50] J. F. Rinehart and H. H. Anderson, Effect of emetine on cardiac muscle, Arch. Pathol., 11, 546 (1931).
[51] P. P. Turner, The effects of emetine on the myocardium, Brit. Heart J., 25, 81 (1963).
[51a] L. Goodman and A. Gilman, The Pharmacological Basis of Therapeutics, 2nd ed., Macmillan, New York, 1955.
[52] A. R. Kilgore, Peripheral neuritis following emetine treatment of amebic dysentery, Boston Med. Surg. J., 175, 380 (1916).
[53] L. A. Salako, Effects of emetine on neuromuscular transmission, Europ. J. Pharm., 11, 342 (1970).
[54] L. A. Salako, Inhibition of neuromuscular transmission in the intact rat by emetine, J. Pharm. Pharmacol., 22, 69 (1970).

[55] W. A. Young and G. R. Tudhope, The pathology of prolonged emetine administration, Trans. Roy. Soc. Trop. Med. & Hyg., 20, 93 (1926).
[56] K. K. F. Ng, An adrenergic neurone blocking action of emetine, J. Pharm. Pharmacol., 18, 255 (1966).
[57] K. K. F. Ng, Blockade of adrenergic and cholinergic transmission by emetine, Brit. J. Pharmacol., 28, 228 (1966).
[58] K. K. F. Ng, A new pharmacological action of emetine, Brit. Med. J., 1966-1, 1278.
[59] G. C. Lake, On the toxicity of emetine hydrochloride, with special reference to the comparative toxicity of various market preparations, Bull., Hyg. Lab., U.S. Pub. Health Serv., 2(113), 41 (1916).
[60] F. C. Arrillaga and J. Guglielmetti, Action du chlorahydrate d'emetine sur le coeur, Compt. Rend. Soc. Biol., 85, 596 (1921).
[61] R. N. Chopra and B. N. Ghosh, The therapeutics of emetine, Indian Med. Gaz., 57, 248 (1922).
[62] R. N. Chopra, B. N. Ghosh, and P. De, Some observations on the toxicity of emetine, Indian Med. Gaz., 59, 338 (1924).
[63] L. G. Parmer and C. W. Cottrill, Distribution of emetine in tissues, J. Lab. Clin. Med., 34, 818 (1949).
[64] W. J. Bais, Dood door emetine (Death from emetine poisoning), Geneesk. Tijdschr. v. Nederl.-Indie, 61, 500 (1921).
[65] T. H. Brem and B. E. Konwaller, Fatal myocarditis due to emetine hydrochloride, Am. Heart J., 50, 476 (1955).
[66] R. A. Deitrich and H. C. Heim, The effect of emetine upon rat heart respiration, J. Am. Pharm. Assoc., 45, 562 (1956).
[67] E. J. Diamont, Carbohydrate metabolism in emetine-poisoned rats, J. Pharmacol. Exptl. Therap., 122, 465 (1958).
[68] A. Mareno and S. Magliulo, The effects of emetine and embryonic heart extract upon guinea pig heart respiration, Arch. Intern. Pharmacodyn. Therap., 132, 331 (1961).
[69] G. D. Appelt and H. C. Heim, Effect of chronic poisoning by emetine on oxidative processes in rat heart. II. Effects on oxidation of citric acid cycle intermediates and nicotinamide adenine dinucleotide metabolism, J. Pharm. Sci., 54, 1621 (1965).
[70] G. D. Appelt and H. C. Heim, Effect of chronic poisoning by emetine on oxidative processes in the rat. I. Effects on lipid metabolism and oxidative phosphorylation, J. Pharm. Sci., 53, 1080 (1964).
[71] A. P. Grollman, Structural basis for the inhibition of protein synthesis by emetine and cycloheximide based on an analogy between ipecac alkaloids and glutarimide antibiotics, Proc. Natl. Acad. Sci. U.S., 56, 1867 (1966).
[72] B. M. Bellar, Observations on the mechanism of emetine poisoning of myocardial tissue, Circ. Res., 22, 501 (1968).

[73] A. J. Brink, J. C. N. Kotzé, S. P. Muller, and L. Sochner, The effect of emetine on metabolism and contractility of the isolated rat heart, J. Pharmacol. Exptl. Therap., 165, 251 (1969).
[74] H. H. Anderson and A. C. Reed, Untoward effects of anti-amebic drugs, Am. J. Trop. Med. Hyg., 14, 269 (1934).
[75] H. H. Anderson and C. D. Leake, Oral toxicity of emetine hydrochloride and certain related compounds in rabbits and cats, Am. J. Trop. Med., 10, 249 (1930).
[76] L. J. Baer, Electrocardiographic effects of emetine hydrochloride, Mil. Surgeon, 109, 120 (1951).
[77] P. W. Brown, Results and dangers in the treatment of amebiasis: a summary of fifteen years' clinical experience at the Mayo Clinic, JAMA, 105, 1319 (1935).
[78] L. J. Cera, Emetine toxicity with electrocardiographic abnormalities, Circulation, 14, 33 (1956).
[79] H. H. Dale, A preliminary note on chronic poisoning by emetine, Brit. Med. J., 1915-2, 895.
[80] W. D. Hagamen, C. M. Berry, and S. Wolf, The effect of subnauseant doses of syrup of ipecac on gastric acidity and activity, J. Pharmacol. Exptl. Therap., 105, 240 (1952).
[81] R. Heilig and S. K. Visveswar, On the cardiac effects of emetine, Indian Med. Gaz., 78, 419 (1943).
[82] H. H. Johnson and J. A. Murphy, The toxic effect of emetine hydrochloride, Mil. Surgeon, 40, 58 (1917).
[83] F. J. Leibly, Fatal emetine poisoning, due to cumulative action in amoebic dysentery, Am. J. Med. Sci., 179, 834 (1930).
[84] R. L. Levy and L. G. Rountree, On the toxicity of various commercial preparations of emetine hydrochloride, Arch. Intern. Med., 17, 420 (1916).
[85] S. Locket, Clinical toxicology. V. Evaluation of various forms of treatment administered in poisoning, Practitioner, 210, 709 (1973).
[86] E. P. Pick and R. Wasecky, Zur pharmakologischen analyse des emetins, Arch. Exptl. Pathol. Pharmakol., lxxx, 147 (1916).
[87] S. J. Powell, The cardiotoxicity of systemic amebicides: a comparative electrocardiographic study, Am. J. Trop. Med. Hyg., 16, 447 (1967).
[88] J. L. Radomski, E. C. Hagan, H. N. Fuyat, and A. A. Nelson, The pharmacology of ipecac, J. Pharmacol. Exptl. Therap., 104, 421 (1952).
[89] E. A. Rosen, R. R. Martin, and N. A. David, Cumulative toxicity of emetine hydrochloride in guinea pigs, Proc. Soc. Exptl. Biol. Med., 33, 289 (1935).
[90] D. E. Schwartz and J. Herrero, Comparative pharmacokinetic studies of dehydroemetine and emetine in guinea pigs using spectrofluorometric and radiometric methods, Am. J. Trop. Med. Hyg., 14, 78 (1965).

[91] J. M. Welchman, The cardiac toxicity of emetine, Am. J. Trop. Med. Hyg., 60, 296 (1957).
[92] N. Whittaker, The synthesis of emetine and related compounds. Part IX, The use of Wittig-type reagents in the synthesis of 2,3-dehydroemetine, J. Chem. Soc. (Org.), 1, 94 (1969).
[93] A. J. Wilmon, S. J. Powell, and E. B. Adams, The comparative value of emetine and chloroquine in amebic liver abscess, Am. J. Trop. Med. Hyg., 7, 197 (1958).
[94] The Pharmacopeia of the United States of America (XVII), The U.S. Pharmacopeia Convention, Inc., Rockville, 1965.

Some Historical Aspects of Marijuana

CHARLES L. WINEK, Ph.D.

Duquesne University School of Pharmacy
Department of Pharmacology and Toxicology
Pittsburgh, Pennsylvania

Marijuana, by whatever species of Cannabis it is called, has been known to science and medicine for almost 5000 years. It is reported to have been contained in the Chinese Emperor Nung's Herbal dated 2737 B.C. It was not given the name Cannabis sativa L. until Linnaeus named it in 1753 A.D.

In searching some of the older Materia Medica texts and journals, one finds reference to the medicinal uses of the plant and its products. In the 1868 edition (3rd) of Materia Medica for the Use of Students (Published by Lindsay & Blakiston, Philadelphia) by John B. Biddle, M.D. of the Jefferson Medical College of Philadelphia the following is given on pp. 66-67:

EXTRACTUM CANNABIS—EXTRACT OF HEMP

> An ALCOHOLIC EXTRACT of the dried tops of Cannabis sativa—variety Indica," was introduced into the Materia Medica in the edition of the U.S. Pharmacopoeia preceding the last. Cannabis sativa, or Hemp (Nat. Ord. Cannabinaceae) is a native of Persia and the northern parts of India, and is cultivated in Europe, and in the United States. Narcotic virtues appear to exist only in the Cannabis Indica or Indian variety of the plant, although there is no difference in the botanical character of the several varieties.

> The medicinal properties of the plant reside in a resinous substance, which exudes from glands upon the surface of the stalks and leaves, and the EXTRACT is made by evaporating a tincture of the dried tops. Under the name of purified extract of hemp, (extractum cannabis purificatum), the U.S. Pharmacopoeia directs a preparation made by evaporating a tincture of the crude extract, thus securing greater uniformity of strength. EXTRACT OF HEMP is of a dark, olive-green color, a fragrant narcotic odor, and a bitter, acrid taste. It is soluble in alcohol and ether, but not in water. The resin, which is probably the active principle, has received the name CANNABIN.
>
> EFFECTS AND USES—The medicinal properties of Cannabis Indica are narcotic and antispasmodic, and in India both the herb and resin are extensively used as intoxicating exhilarants, under the name of HASCHISCH. In large doses it is sedative, producing relaxation of the muscles, heavy sleep, and abatement of pain, without much affecting the secretions; but opinions are by no means settled in the United States and Great Britain as to its effects. It has been chiefly extolled as an antispasmodic in traumatic tetanus, and has been employed with success in other spasmodic diseases, chorea, hysteria, etc., and as an anodyne in rheumatism, gout, neuralgia, etc. It has also been given with advantage as an hypnotic in mania-a-potu; and its powers of exciting uterine contractions, and of checking uterine hemorrhagic discharges, are highly spoken of. Dose, from half a grain to two or more grains. The TINCTURE is made by dissolving THREE HUNDRED AND SIXTY GRAINS of the PURIFIED EXTRACT in a pint of alcohol; forty drops of this are about equal to a grain of the extract.

Please note that despite the fact that it was recognized that the narcotic virtues appear to exist only in the Indian variety, no effort was made to distinguish between marijuana, a drug plant, and marijuana, a fiber plant or nondrug plant. Marijuana was rendered an illegal substance regardless of the absence of active pharmacologic principles. Even today, the plant is controlled without regard to the concentration of active constituents. This should be changed in view of our total knowledge of marijuana.

It is noteworthy that the active principle was the resin and given the name Cannabin. Even in 1868 it appears that there was some medical controversy over the effects of marijuana preparations. As to its effects and uses there appears to be considerable agreement as to some level of antispasmodic, muscle-relaxing properties; referring to skeletal and smooth muscle with the opposite effect on uterine muscle. Further agreement existed on its analgesic, anodyne, "pain-relieving" ability. It is interesting to note the sedative-hypnotic effect and the absence of any reference to hallucinations or similar description of unusual activity associated with its use other than the "intoxicating exhilarants."

The 1866 edition of Manual of Materia Medica & Therapeutics, (published by Henry C. Lea, Philadelphia) an abridgement of the late Dr. Perpeira's Elements of Materia Medica, by F. J. Farre, M.D., contains the following on marijuana:

CANNABINACEAE, Lindl. The Hemp Order

CANNABIS SATIVA, Linn.

Common Hemp. Dioecia, Pentandria, Linn. Syst.

BOTANIC CHARACTER—Annual. STEM three to six feet high, erect, branched angular. LEAVES on long weak petioles, digitate, serrated, roughish. STIPULES subulate. FLOWERS dioecious. MALES: FLOWERS racemose. CALYX five-parted, imbricated. STAMENS five. FEMALES: FLOWERS in spikes. CALYX (bract?) one-leaved, acuminate, rolled round the ovary. OVARY roundish. STYLE short. STIGMAS tow, filiform, pubescent. FRUIT, one-celled, two-valved. The whole plant has a clammy feel.—
Rhede, Hort. Malab. plate 61, Vol. X.

HABITAT.—Cultivated in India. The plant which grows in India, and has been described by some botanists under the name of CANNABIS INDICA, or INDIAN HEMP, does not appear to possess any specific differences from the common hemp. Roxburgh and most other distinguished botanists have accordingly considered it identical with the CANNABIS SATIVA, LINN.

CANNABIS INDICA, Indian Hemp.

The flowering tops of the female plant from which the resin has not been removed, dried.
OFFICINAL CHARACTERS.—Tops consisting of one or more alternate branches, bearing the remains of the flowers and smaller leaves and a few ripe fruits, pressed together in masses which are about two inches long, harsh, of a dusky-green color and a characteristic odor.
DESCRIPTION—The dried hemp plant which has flowered, and from which the resin has not been removed, is sold, under the name of Gunjah, in the Calcutta bazaars, for smoking chiefly, in bundles of about two feet long and three inches in diameter, each containing twenty-four plants. That which

I have received from Doctor O'Shaughnessy, and also found in commerce, consists of cylindrical or fusiform masses (about the size and shape of the fingers) of a grayish or greenish-brown color, and composed of stems, leaves, and petioles pressed together. It has a faint odor and feeble, bitterish taste. The more abundant resinous secretion of the Indian plant is easily accounted for, as suggested by Dr. Royle, by its exposure to greater light and heat. The hemp cultivated in Edinburgh by Dr. Christison exhibited no resin. Plants collected in the Regen's Park contained about one-tenth as much as oriental plants. Dr. Fronmuller, of Fuerth, says that French and German hemp appear to be richer in resin, Italian still more so; while Greece and Asia Minor yield quite a powerful product; but the produce of Persia and India far exceeds them all. The resinous exudation removed from the leaves, slender stems, and flowers, is called CHURRUS. It is collected in India, Herat, and Persia, and is employed for its intoxicating effects in the East, but is not officinal in this country.

COMPOSITION—Besides the resin (cannabin), which appears to be the active ingredient, hemp contains some gum, extractive, and a little ethereal oil, about twelve drops in twenty-eight ounces (Fronmuller), but there is no evidence at present that the oil possesses any activity.

HISTORY—This plant was well known to the ancient Greeks and Romans, but they do not appear to have been acquainted with its narcotic properties. Dioscorides merely mentions that the expressed juice of the seeds of Χανναβις allays ear-ache, and the same statement is made by Galen. Herodotus mentions it, and states that the Scythians threw the seeds on red-hot stones, and used the perfumed vapor thereby obtained as a bath, which excited from them cries of exultation. This, I presume, refers to the intoxicating properties of its smoke. The hemp may have been, as Dr. Royle suggests, the "assuager of grief," or the NEPENTHES φαρμαχογγηπενθε'ς of which Homer speaks as having been given by Helen to Telemachus in the house of Menelaus. Helen is stated to have received the plant from a woman of Egyptian Thebes. It is known in India as the "increaser of pleasure," the "exciter of desire," the "cementer of friendship," the "cause of a reeling gait," and the "laughter mover."

PHYSIOLOGICAL EFFECTS—Indian hemp owes its celebrity chiefly to its exhilarating and inebriating effects on orientals. In these the inebriation or delirium produced by it is usually of an agreeable or cheerful character, exciting the individual to laugh, dance, and sing, and to commit various extravagances—acting as an aphrodisiac, and augmenting the appetite for food. In some it occasions a kind of reverie. It renders others excitable and quarrelsome, and disposes to acts of violence. It may also produce a cataleptic condition, in which the muscles are moderately contracted, but flexible and pliant, and the limbs retain any position or attitude in which they may be placed. The following illustrative cases are taken from Dr. O'Shaughnessy's paper on Indian hemp: "At two P.M. a grain of the resin of hemp was given to a rheumatic patient. At four P.M. he was very talkative, sang, called loudly for an extra supply of food, and declared himself in perfect health. At six P.M. he was asleep. At eight P.M. he was found insensible, but breathing with perfect regularity, his pulse and skin natural, and the pupils freely contractile on the approach of light. Happening by chance to lift up the patient's arm, I found that it remained in the posture in which I placed it. It required but a very brief examination of the limbs to find that the patient had, by the influence of this narcotic, been thrown into the state of CATALEPSY. We raised him to a sitting posture, and placed his arms and limbs in every imaginable attitude. A waxen figure could not be more pliant or more stationary in each position, no matter how contrary to the natural influence of gravity on the part. To all impressions he was meanwhile almost insensible. He continued in this state till one A.M., when consciousness and voluntary motion quickly returned. Another who had taken the same dose, fell asleep, but was aroused by the noise in the ward. He seemed vastly amused at the strange aspects of the statue-like attitudes in which the first patient had been placed. On a sudden he uttered a loud peal of laughter, and exclaimed that four spirits were springing with his bed into the air. In vain we attempted to pacify him; his laughter became momentarily more and more uncontrollable. We now observed that his limbs were rather rigid, and in a few minutes more his arms and legs could be bent and would remain in any desired position. His limbs in less than an hour gained their natural condition, and in two hours he expressed himself perfectly well and excessively hungry." In Europeans I have never heard of a cataleptic state being produced by this drug. In a case of tetanus under my care in the Longon Hospital, and which was carefully watched by Dr. O'Shaughnessy and myself, the resinous extract of Indian hemp was given in increasing doses up to twenty grains. It caused stupor and cessation of spasms, but no perfectly cataleptic state. The only tendency to this condition which was observed was when the arm of the patient was lifted and then cautiously let go: it fell slowly and gradually, not quickly as it would have done under ordinary conditions; the patient was at this time quite insensible. (The exhilarating effects so constantly experienced by Asiatics, appears to be almost equally unknown in this country. The cause of this may be in great part due to the difference in the European and Asiatic temperaments; but probably the hemp loses some of its properties during its transmission; for in the author's large work are described by Drs. Taylor and Rees the inebriating and phantasmic effects on Mr. B. Taylor while at Damascus, which are not surpassed by any of the extravagances to which it gives rise in Asiatics. —Ed.) Dr. Fronmuller thinks it probable that the Indian hemp contains some ethereal ingredient which is dissipated on the passage. (See Composition.) Dr. O'Shaughnessy, when in England, satisfied himself of the difference of the effect of Indian hemp in this country and in Bengal; and he observed, that while in India he had seen marked effects from half a grain of the extract, or even less, and had been accustomed to consider one grain and a half a large dose; in England he had given ten or twelve or more grains to produce the desired effect. Dr. Fronmuller, who has used it in 1,000 cases, considers eight grains of the extract the smallest dose. By internal use it acts as a MYDRIATIC, causing preternatural dilation of the pupil. But Dr. Lawrie states that when applied around the eye it does not cause dilatation of the pupil. Indian hemp does not appear much to affect the secretions. It neither excites nausea nor lessens the appetite. It neither causes dryness of the tongue nor constipation of the bowels. It does not appear to check or otherwise affect the bronchial secretions.

THERAPEUTICS.—Indian hemp is chiefly employed as a medicine for its hypnotic, anodyne, and antispasmodic properties; occasionally, also, as a phrenic. As a HYPNOTIC, I have used it with advantage in spirit drinkers, and have succeeded in one or two cases in producing sleep with it where large doses of morphia had failed. Dr. Fronmuller ranks it next to opium. As an anodyne it is, I think, in general, decidedly inferior to opium; but in acute and subacute rheumatism, in gout, and in neuralgia, it frequently alleviates the pain.

As an ANAESTHETIC, Mr. Donovan found that under its influence his sense of touch and feeling gradually became obtuse, until at length he lost all feeling unless he pinched himself severely. As an ANTISPASMODIC, it has been employed in tetanus, hydrophobia, and chorea. In the cases of tetanus (both traumatic and idiopathic) and of hydrophobia which I have seen treated with it, it completely failed to give permanent relief. Mr. O'Brien treated seven cases of tetanus in the native hospital, Calcutta, with ten grain doses of the extract. Four of these recovered. Professor Miller, of Edinburgh, records three successful cases of traumatic tetanus in children about seven years of age, who took thirty drops of the tincture every half hour, and all of whom recovered; but most of the cases recorded are examples of its failure. In chorea I have found it serviceable, sometimes as an antispasmodic, at others as a hypnotic; and the same may be said of its use in hysteria. As a PHRENIC, or medicinal agent affecting the mental functions, Indian hemp has also been employed. Dr. Clendinning speaks favorably of its use as a nervine stimulant, in removing languor and anxiety, and raising the pulse and spirits; and Dr. Conolly thinks that it may be useful in some chronic forms of mania. Dr. Sutherland has not obtained any good effect from it.

(EXTRACTUM CANNABIS PURIFICATUM, U.S., Purified Extract of Hemp.—"Take of extract of hemp, two troyounces; alcohol, a sufficient quantity. Rub the extract with two fluidounces of alcohol until they are thoroughly mixed; and, having added twelve fluidounces of alcohol, allow the mixture to macerate for twenty-four hours. Then filter the tincture through paper, passing sufficient alcohol, through the filter, to exhaust the dregs completely. Lastly, by means of a water bath, at a temperature not exceeding 160°, evaporate to dryness." U.S.)

The dose of the alcoholic extract of Indian hemp is generally from one grain to five. I have usually found one grain of the extract kept in the London shops to act as a narcotic. The Messrs. Smith state that two-thirds of a grain of the pure resin produced on themselves and others powerful narcotic effects. In a case of tetanus under my care in the London Hospital, the dose of the extract (supplied by Dr. O'Shaughnessy, who watched the case with me) was gradually increased to gr. xx. (I have already stated that Dr. O'Shaughnessy considered that ten or twelve grains are required in England to produce the effects which follow one grain in India, and that Dr. Fronmuller considers eight grains of the extract THE SMALLEST DOSE.—Ed.) (There is no other officinal drug which is at once so powerful and so utterly uncertain. I have known one-eighth of a grain, repeated every three or four hours, after three or four doses, to cause great mental disturbance, amounting almost to delirium. On the other hand, ten or even fifteen grains

frequently fail to produce any symptoms. One great cause of these differences is no doubt the bad quality and worthlessness of much of the extract kept in the shops—but it has seemed to me that there is a very remarkable difference in the susceptibility of patients to the influence of the same preparation. Any one who habitually used five or even two grains of the purified extract as a COMMENCING dose, would certainly sooner or later meet with a case in which it would produce serious and alarming, if not fatal, symptoms. The practitioner should be assured that his preparation is good and then carefully feel his way with the small fractional doses.—W.)
(It may be administered in the form of pill; or better, by diffusion through an emulsion (prepared by rubbing and extract with olive oil, in a warm mortar, and gradually adding mucilage, and afterwards water.)

TINCTURA CANNABIS INDICAE, Tincture of Indian Hemp. (TINCTURA CANNABIS, U.S.)—Take of extract of Indian hemp, one ounce; rectified spirit, one pint. Dissolve the extract of hemp in the spirit. ("Take of purified extract of hemp, three hundred and sixty grains; alcohol, a pint. Dissolve the extract in the alcohol, and filter through paper." U.S.).
The tincture is prepared from the alcoholic extract instead of from the herb, to secure greater uniformity of strength, as the latter varies much in the quantity of resinous secretion. The proportions are those directed to be used by Dr. O'Shaughnessy; but, probably by a typographical error, he has ordered PROOF spirit instead of rectified spirit. The tincture may be administered in an emulsion or mucilaginous mixture, or in water sweetened with sugar. It should be swallowed soon after it has been added to the aqueous liquid, as the resin is precipitated, and is apt to adhere to the side of the vessel.
Dose from mix to fl. drm. j. Dr. O'Shaughnessy gives in tetanus a fluidrachm every half hour until the paroxysms cease or catalepsy is induced; in cholera, ten drops every half hour. (If, however, we adopt the doses of the extract recommended for Europeans by Dr. O'Shaughnessy and Dr. Fronmuller, we shall probably find it necessary to give somewhat larger doses of the tincture, as one fluidrachm is only equivalent to two and a half grains of the extract. I have found one-drachm doses well borne in chorea by children twelve or fourteen years of age.—Ed.)

Here we find descriptions of the effects of marijuana on the sensorium and note that the physicians were aware of the variance of potency among the marijuana products of other countries. It seems apparent that the differences in effects described are due to the dose received on a weight basis, the potency of the drug used, the disease state or health of the patient (including mental health), and possibly the setting, i.e., time of day, surroundings. Reference is made to the "hungry patient" upon returning to normalcy. Internal use produced a mydriatic effect as described by Dr. Fronmuller which is in opposition to the slight miotic effect described by Dr. Edward F. Domino (National Institute of Mental Health). Again there is reference to its chief uses as an hypnotic, anodyne, and antispasmodic.

The Journal of Materia Medica devoted to Materia Medica, Pharmacy, Chemistry, and edited by Joseph Bates, M.D. and H. A. Tilden and published by Tilden & Co., Publishers, New Lebanon, N. Y. contained references to marijuana. In Volume 13, 1874, p. 350, the following "letter to the editor" type communication is found:

CANNABIS INDICA

> Your Cannabis Indica I find useful in many cases. I had a singular instance of the value of this agent where I little expected to find any medical treatment of service. It was a case of senile trembling, where the patient had not been able to dress herself for three years. During that period she had not been able to fasten her clothes. She was nearly eighty years of age. For the six months preceeding the time she came under my care, her mental and bodily power had slowly and surely failed. Her friends desired me to see her, and if possible, give her some aid. I noticed considerable mental excitement and hallucinations, and saw that, indeed, her mental and bodily strength was failing. Her advanced age, indeed, made such a course of events, nothing to be surprised at. With the hope of alleviating her condition—and a very faint hope—but with little thought of any decided improvement—I prescribed.
>
> ℞ Fl. Ext. Cannabis Indica . . . . gutt. cxcij.
> Spts. Lav. Comp . . . .
> Spts. Ether, Comp . . . . aa q. s. to
> make Sig. Teaspoonful three times a day in a
> little sugar and water. M.
>
> In two weeks my patient surprised her daughter by coming out of her room all dressed, in the morning, much pleased

that she could once more "dress herself." The mental excitement seemed allayed, bodily strength improved, and a return to the use of her mental faculties accomplished.

With my regards, respectfully yours,
Albert N. Gould, M.D., Great Falls, N. H.

This, of course, sounds like a "miracle" or a testimonial for "Hadacol." One wonders what role in her apparent mental reversal was played by alcohol, ether, lavender, etc., as well as the marijuana. The polypharmacy of the time makes cause-effect relationships difficult.

In an earlier issue of the journal (vol. 2, 1860) on p. 474 the following is found:

CANNABIS INDICA AS A HYPNOTIC—Dr. Fronmuller, after a large number of experiments, draws the following resume of the value of this drug.
Of all anaesthetics ever proposed, Indian hemp is the one which produces a narcotism most closely resembling the natural sleep without causing any extraordinary excitement of the vessels, or any particular suspension of secretions, or without fear of a dangerous reaction, and consecutive paralysis. It acts neither as violently nor as surely as opium. It can be given in all acute inflammatory diseases as well as typhoid affections. It is well adapted as an alternate with opium in case this ceases to act. Its best mode of administration consists in pills of the alcoholic extract and powdered seed. The smallest dose susceptible of producing sleep is eight grains in pills of one grain. This dose, however, must be rapidly augmented. The action on the skin, the kidneys and sexual organs, attributed to Indian hemp is without any practical importance.—

Prager Vierteljahrschrift, 1860

One wonders about how large the number of experiments was? Could someone use this type of language in today's journals? I note that a negative notice is given for the action of marijuana on the sexual organs. Of course they had no erotic films to use when observing the effects of marijuana as is done in one of the $300,000.00 studies in the U.S. The claim of producing sleep most closely resembling natural sleep reminds us of some of our former TV commercials for sleeping aids.

In Vol. 3, 1861, the journal contained the following prescription for consumption (I assume tuberculosis or some other wasting disease) was found:

PRESCRIPTION FOR CONSUMPTION

> Dr. C. T. Horton (Baltimore Journal of Medicine), uses the following prescription in the treatment of consumption, bronchitis, etc.:
>
> ℞ Etherial tincture of Indian Hemp. . 1/2 pint
> Extract of liquorice. . . . . 1/2 pound (Troy?)
> Carbonate of potassa . . . . 1/2 "
> Warm water . . . . 1 gallon
>
> The dose of this is a tablespoonful three times a day, gradually increased to two. The ethereal tincture is obtained by dissolving two ounces of the alcoholic extract of hemp in a pint of sulphuric ether.

This prescription was apparently ignored by Dr. Fronmuller who states some years later (see above) that there is no suspension of secretions. The polypharmacy effect is seen again. He also indicated no suspension of secretion in his 1860 report on the anesthetic effect of cannabis.

FREE COMMUNICATION

Acute and Subacute Toxicology and Safety Evaluation of SMA 1440-H Resin

C. L. WINEK and JAMES J. BURGUN

Duquesne University School of Pharmacy
Department of Pharmacology and Toxicology
Pittsburgh, Pennsylvania

INTRODUCTION

SMA resins [1] are low molecular weight copolymers of styrene and maleic anhydride. They were developed to fill the need for resins having low solution viscosity, high functionality, and light color. They are used widely in floor polishes as leveling resins, in emulsion polymerization as protective colloids and stabilizers, in paint as pigment dispersants, in thermostat coatings as vehicles, and numerous other applications [2].

The majority of SMA resins are partial esters whereby the copolymer has been esterfied with a select alcohol to afford specific properties. SMA 1440-A is highly esterfied with a water-soluble alcohol, thus giving it very low anhydride functionality. SMA 1440-H is the 35% (w/v) ammoniacal solution of SMA 1440-A. Because or its negatively charged chemical structure and complementary design of hydrophobic-hydrophilic properties, SMA 1440-H can effectively disperse and stabilize many different types of pigments in latex paint formulations. The copolymer becomes water insoluble as the paint film cures and therefore contributes to film reinforcement [3].

In the present study SMA 1440-H was evaluated to determine possible toxic reactions resulting from exposure in the industrial setting. Subacute oral toxicity, teratogenic and feticidal activity, and an acute oral LD_{50} were determined in rats. Acute and subacute dermal toxicity tests and eye irritation studies were performed in rabbits. Finally, skin sensitization reactions were studied in guinea pigs.

METHODS

Acute Oral LD_{50} Determination

Twenty-four albino Sprague-Dawley rats of each sex were divided into four groups of six animals each. The animals were dosed at levels of 10.0, 13.0, 17.0, and 22.0 ml/kg. The rats were observed for 14 days and mortality data recorded. Autopsies were performed as soon as possible after death and the tissues examined for pathologic changes.

Subacute Oral Toxicity

Sixty male and sixty female albino weanling rats, weighing 60 to 90 gm, were divided into six groups of ten rats per group. The compound was fed to the rats at dietary levels of 0, 1, 10, 100, 1000, and 10,000 ppm for a period of 90 days. The following studies were performed on days 45 to 90 on one animal from each group: hematocrit, serum glutamic oxalacetic transaminase (SGOT), organ to body weight ratios of the heart, lungs, kidneys, liver, and spleen, and examination of these organs at autopsy. The animals were weighed weekly and a weight-growth curve plotted for each dose level.

Acute Dermal Toxicity

Seven male and seven female New Zealand strain rabbits were used in this study. The animals were prepared by clipping the skin of the back free of hair followed by application of a commercial depilatory agent, after which they were allowed to recover for 24 hr prior to dosing. The rabbits were divided into three dose levels with four animals (2 males and 2 females) per dose level. The dose levels employed were 3.9, 6.0, and 9.4 ml/kg. One male and one female of each group were further prepared by making epidermal abrasions with a scalpel every few centimeters over the area of exposure. The single male and female control rabbits underwent similar preparation with the exception that each had 50% of its back abraded. The material was poured on the animals' backs and a rubber sleeve then wrapped completely around the animals' bodies and the edges secured with adhesive tape. The rabbits were then immobilized for 24 hr. At the end of this 24-hr exposure period the sleeves were removed and the backs examined for gross pathology. The animals were observed for 14 days during which time any animals that died were autopsied and the heart, lungs, kidneys, liver, and spleen examined for pathologic changes. After this period of time the surviving animals were sacrificed and the organs examined.

Subacute Dermal Toxicity

Sixteen male and 16 female rabbits were used in this study. The animals were prepared by clipping the skin of the trunk free of hair. Eight animals of each sex were nonabraded and eight were abraded as previously described. The eight abraded and eight nonabraded of each sex were divided into four groups of two animals each. Two animals were not dosed and served as controls, two were dosed at a level of 2 ml/kg, two at 4 ml/kg, and two at 8 ml/kg. The material was applied to the backs of the animals by gentle rubbing with a glass rod; applications were made daily for 14 consecutive days. After the final application the rabbits were observed for 2 weeks for signs of toxicity. After this period the animals were sacrificed and autopsies performed.

Teratogenic Study

Twenty-four rats, obtained as timed pregnancies, were used in this study. The rats were divided into three groups of eight animals each. In each group six animals were dosed at a level of 4 ml/kg and two, serving as controls, were dosed at a level of 4 ml/kg with distilled water. Group 1 was dosed on day 1 through day 7 of pregnancy, group 2 on day 8 through day 14, and the third group on day 14 through 20. All animals were sacrificed on day 20 and the uterus removed. The pups were examined for terata, average pup weight, crown-rump distance, number of pups per litter, and the uterus examined for any resorption sites.

Eye Irritation Studies

Nine albino rabbits were used in this study. One-tenth of a milliliter of SMA 1440-H was instilled into the conjunctival sac of one eye while the other eye remained untreated and served as the control. In the case of the first three rabbits the treated eye remained unwashed. In three other rabbits the eye was washed with approximately 20 ml of lukewarm water 2 sec after instillation of the substance. In the last three rabbits the eyes were washed 4 sec after instillation. The eyes were observed at 24, 48, and 72 hr and at 4 and 7 days after treatment and scored according to the method of Draize [4].

Skin Sensitization

Twelve male albino guinea pigs were prepared by shaving the hair from the back and flanks followed by application of a depilatory. The animals were allowed to recover for 24 hr prior to dosing. One-tenth of a milliliter of a 0.1% solution of SMA 1440-H in normal saline was injected every other day until a total of 10 injections had been made. The injections were made at random in the area of the back and upper flanks. Following the tenth injection the animals were housed under normal conditions for two weeks, after which they were challenged by a final injection of 0.05 ml.

RESULTS

The rats dosed at a level of 10 ml/kg showed no signs of toxicity at any time. The rats dosed at 13 ml/kg appeared lethargic shortly after dosing. One male rat died three days later. At 17 ml/kg all rats had a mild, bloody diarrhea. One female rat died three days later. At 22 ml/kg all of the male rats had mild bloody diarrhea. One rat died on the day of dosing. The female rats at 22 ml/kg dose level had severe bloody diarrhea. All six rats were dead the following day. The rats were autopsied shortly after death and all had greatly distended stomachs due to the volume of the compound. All organs, including the lungs, appeared normal. The LD_{50} value is greater than 20 ml/kg in female rats and 22 ml/kg in male rats.

All animals on all of the dose levels appeared normal throughout the 90-day course of the study. All rats showed weight gain comparable with the controls. Hematocrit and SGOT determinations were within normal range. All organs appeared normal at autopsy.

None of the rabbits in the acute dermal study exhibited edema or erythema, nor were pathologic signs noted in the animals that were autopsied.

The rabbits in the 14-day dermal toxicity study showed no signs of toxicity during or after the application of SMA 1440-H. The skin showed no sign of irritation and hair regrowth occurred on all of the animals. No pathologic signs were noted in the animals that were autopsied.

The control rats and the rats dosed with 4 ml/kg SMA 1440-H produced litters which were comparable in all parameters studied: number of pups per litter, average pup weight, and crown-rump distance.

In no cases were resorption sites noted nor terata observed.

The group of rabbits whose eyes were topically dosed with SMA 1440-H but not followed by eye irrigation showed, at 24 hr after application, a slight redness and swelling of the conjunctivae and a small amount of discharge. The cornea exhibited scattered areas of opacity as shown by fluorescein stain and in every case the details of the iris were clearly visible. At 48 hr after application these reactions were almost entirely cleared, and by 72 hr no evidence of injury remained. The rabbits who received a 2- or 4-sec wash showed no signs of irritation or injury at any time.

SMA 1440-H did not produce skin sensitization under the conditions of the experiment. No local or systemic reactions occurred either during the course of the initial 10 injections nor after the challenge dose.

DISCUSSION

The acute oral toxicity studies indicate that SMA 1440-H would not be classified as a toxic substance as defined in the regulations in the Federal Hazardous Substances Labeling Act [5].

The 90-day feeding study revealed that rats receiving up to 1% of SMA 1440-H in their daily diet exhibited no toxic effects.

The 24-hr acute and the 14-day subacute dermal toxicity tests show that the compound is not a corrosive or toxic substance when applied to the skin nor does it appear to have significant potential for percutaneous absorption.

The evaluation of SMA 1440-H in timed-pregnancy rats yielded negative results regarding teratogenic and feticidal activity.

The rabbit eye irritation studies showed that SMA 1440-H would be classified as an eye irritant, but since the lesions cleared within three days, it would not be classified as a severe eye irritant.

The guinea pig experiment revealed that the compound is not a skin sensitizer under the conditions of this experiment.

REFERENCES

[1] B. G. Gower, "SMA Resins: Properties and Applications," Polymer Synthesis, Petrochemicals Division, Sinclair Research Inc., Harvey, Illinois

[2] "SMA 1440-H for Aqueous Pigment Dispersion," Application Bulletin No. 202-A. Sinclair Petrochemicals Inc., New York, N. Y.

[3] M. N. Gleason, R. E. Gosselein, H. C. Hodge, and R. P. Smith, Clinical Toxicology of Commercial Products, 3rd ed., Williams and Wilkins, Baltimore, Maryland, 1969.
[4] "Toxicity of SMA resins," Sinclair Petrochemicals Inc., 600 Fifth Avenue, New York, N. Y.
[5] C. Weil, Biometrics, VIII, iii, 249 (1952).
[6] "Appraisal of the Safety of Chemicals in Foods, Drugs, and Cosmetics," The Association of Food and Drug Officials of the United States, Topeka, Kansas (2nd printing 1965).
[7] "Prinicples and Procedure for Evaluating the Toxicity of Household Substances," National Academy of Sciences-National Research Council Publication No. 1138. Washington, D.C., 1964.
[8] SMA Product Data Bulletin No. 101. Sinclair Petrochemicals Inc., New York, N. Y.

Appendix

ORGANIZATIONS IN TOXICOLOGY

American Academy of Forensic Sciences
Toxicology Section
Executive Director
1140 Rockville Pike, Suite 515
Rockville, Maryland 20852
(301) 881-0537

American Academy of Clinical Toxicology
Secretary-Treasurer, Franklin D. Aldrich, Ph.D., M.D.
M.I.T. Room
77 Massachusetts Avenue
Cambridge, Massachusetts 02139

American Industrial Hygiene Association
Managing Director, William E. McCormick
66 South Miller Road
Akron, Ohio 44313
(216) 836-9537

American Board of Forensic Toxicology
Secretary, Dr. Leo A. DalCortiva
Division of Medical Legal Investigation & Forensic Sciences
Suffolk County Office Building
Hauppauge, New York 11787

American Board of Veterinary Toxicology
President, Dr. H. E. Smalley
P. O. Drawer GE
College Station, Texas 77840

American Association of Poison Control Centers
Secretary-Treasurer, Dr. Wm. O. Robertson
Children's Orthopedic Hospital
Seattle, Washington 98105

American Society for Clinical Pharmacology and Therapeutics
Clinical Pathology & Human Toxicology Section
Chairman, Dr. Robert B. Forney
Indiana University, Medical School
1040 West Michigan Street
Indianapolis, Indiana 46207

American College of Veterinary Toxicologists
Office of Secretary-Treasurer
Comparative Toxicology Laboratory
Kansas State University
Manhattan, Kansas 66506

Academy of Pharmaceutical Sciences
Pharmacology-Toxicology Section
2215 Constitution Avenue, N.W.
Washington, D.C. 20037

The Association of Drug Detection Laboratories
Ms. Celia Bobette Zettel
P. O. Box 2565
Houston, Texas 77001

Addiction Research Foundation
33 Russell Street
Toronto, Ontario M5S 2S1

The Association of Official Analytical Chemists
Box 540 Benjamin Franklin Station
Washington, D.C. 20044

Canadian Association for Research in Toxicology
Secretary, Dr. R. G. Bunford
G. D. Searle & Co. of Canada, LTD.
400 Iroquois Shore Road
Oakville, Ontario, Canada

The Canadian Society of Forensic Science
63 Kilbarry Crescent
Ottawa, Ontario K1K OH2

Chemical Industry Institute of Toxicology
Dr. Leon Golberg
P. O. Box 12137
Research Triangle Park, N. Carolina 27709

European Society of Toxicology
Secretariat
B. P. No. 37
34430 Saint Jean De Vedas, France

Forum for the Advancement of Toxicology
Dr. John Autian
College of Pharmacy and Dentistry
University of Tennessee, Center for the Health Sciences
Memphis, Tennessee 38163

The Forensic Science Society
P. O. Box 41
Harrogate, Yorkshire, England HG1 2LF

International Society on Toxinology
Instituto Clodomiro Picado
Universidad De Costa Rica
Ciudad Universitaria, Costa Rica
Att: Dr. Roger Bolanos

International Association of Forensic Toxicologists
Dr. N. Dunnett
Home Counties Forensic Science Laboratory
Aldermaston, Berkshire, RG7 4PH, U.K.

National Center for Toxicological Research
Jefferson, Arkansas 72079
(501) 536-6200

Pharmaceutical Manufacturers Association
Toxicology Section
1155 Fifteenth Street, N.W.
Washington, D.C. 20005

The Society of Forensic Toxicologists
Dr. J. H. Bidanset
P. O. Box 160
East Meadow, New York 11554

The Society of Toxicology
Office of the Secretary, Gale C. Boxill
Wyeth Laboratories
Box 861
Paoli, Pennsylvania 19301
(215) 644-8000

INDEX